Carotenoids: Importance in Human Nutrition and Health

Carotenoids: Importance in Human Nutrition and Health

Edited by Julia Murphy

hayle medical

New York

Hayle Medical,
750 Third Avenue, 9th Floor,
New York, NY 10017, USA

Visit us on the World Wide Web at:
www.haylemedical.com

ISBN: 978-1-64647-535-3

Cataloging-in-Publication Data

Carotenoids : importance in human nutrition and health / edited by Julia Murphy.
p. cm.
Includes bibliographical references and index.
ISBN 978-1-64647-535-3
1. Carotenoids. 2. Carotenoids--Nutritional aspects. 3. Carotenoids--Health aspects.
4. Nutrition. I. Murphy, Julia.
QP671.C35 C37 2023
612.015 28--dc23

Table of Contents

Preface

Carotenoids are a class of phytonutrients synthesized by plants, algae and photosynthetic bacteria. These richly colored molecules are responsible for the yellow, orange and red colors of many fruits and vegetables. Carotenoids can be broadly classified as carotenes and xanthophylls based on the chemical contained in them. There are several types of dietary carotenoids such as α-carotene, β-carotene, β-cryptoxanthin, lutein, zeaxanthin, and lycopene. Mangoes, papayas, carrots, sweet potatoes, spinach, and pumpkins are some good sources of β-carotene. Carotenoids play diverse roles in promoting human health. They act as antioxidants in the human body and have strong cancer-fighting properties. The body converts some carotenoids into vitamin A, which is essential for vision, normal growth and development. The anti-inflammatory and immune system benefits of carotenoids can help in preventing cardiovascular diseases. The book outlines the importance of carotenoids in human health in detail. With its detailed analyses and data, it will prove immensely beneficial to nutritionists, registered dieticians, and medical students involved in the field of clinical nutrition and dietetics at various levels.

All of the data presented henceforth, was collaborated in the wake of recent advancements in the field. The aim of this book is to present the diversified developments from across the globe in a comprehensible manner. The opinions expressed in each chapter belong solely to the contributing authors. Their interpretations of the topics are the integral part of this book, which I have carefully compiled for a better understanding of the readers.

At the end, I would like to thank all those who dedicated their time and efforts for the successful completion of this book. I also wish to convey my gratitude towards my friends and family who supported me at every step.

Editor

1

The Benefits and Risks of Certain Dietary Carotenoids that Exhibit both Anti- and Pro-Oxidative Mechanisms

Homer S. Black [1,*], Fritz Boehm [2], Ruth Edge [3,*] and T. George Truscott [4]

1 Department of Dermatology, Baylor College of Medicine, Houston, TX 77030, USA
2 Photobiology Research, Internationales Handelszentrum (IHZ), Friedrichstraße 95, 10117 Berlin, Germany; fritz.boehm@gmx.de
3 Dalton Cumbrian Facility, Westlakes Science Park, The University of Manchester, Cumbria CA24 3HA, UK
4 School of Chemical and Physical Sciences, Keele University, Keele, Staffordshire ST5 5BG, UK; t.g.truscott@keele.ac.uk
* Correspondence: hblack@bcm.edu (H.S.B.); ruth.edge@manchester.ac.uk (R.E.)

Abstract: Carotenoid pigments, particularly β-carotene and lycopene, are consumed in human foodstuffs and play a vital role in maintaining health. β-carotene is known to quench singlet oxygen and can have strong antioxidant activity. As such, it was proposed that β-carotene might reduce the risk of cancer. Epidemiological studies found inverse relationships between cancer risk and β-carotene intake or blood levels. However, clinical trials failed to support those findings and β-carotene supplementation actually increased lung cancer incidence in male smokers. Early experimental animal studies found dietary β-carotene inhibited UV-induced skin cancers. Later studies found that β-carotene supplementation exacerbated UV-carcinogenic expression. The discrepancies of these results were related to the type of diet the animals consumed. Lycopene has been associated with reduced risk of lethal stage prostate cancer. Other carotenoids, e.g., lutein and zeaxanthin, play a vital role in visual health. Numerous studies of molecular mechanisms to explain the carotenoids' mode of action have centered on singlet oxygen, as well as radical reactions. In cellular systems, singlet oxygen quenching by carotenoids has been reported but is more complex than in organic solvents. In dietary β-carotene supplement studies, damaging pro-oxidant reactivity can also arise. Reasons for this switch are likely due to the properties of the carotenoid radicals themselves. Understanding singlet oxygen reactions and the anti-/pro-oxidant roles of carotenoids are of importance to photosynthesis, vision and cancer.

Keywords: carotenes; cancer; porphyria; macular degeneration; singlet oxygen; radical reactions; β-carotene; lycopene

1. Introduction

Carotenoids are profuse throughout both plant and animal kingdoms although, in plants, their presence is often masked by chlorophyll. These pigments are widely distributed as naturally occurring constituents of fruits and vegetables, as well as causing the coloration of a wide variety of flowers, birds and marine animals. Over 600, now estimated by some to be around 750, carotenoids have been identified with about 100 finding their way into foodstuffs consumed by humans [1]. As well as fruit and vegetable intake, they are often added to human foodstuffs in order to achieve acceptable food coloration as they strongly absorb light in the region of 400–500 nm and are colored red, orange, and yellow. Chemically these pigments are tetraterpenoid, C40 compounds, consisting of eight isoprenoid residues (Figure 1).

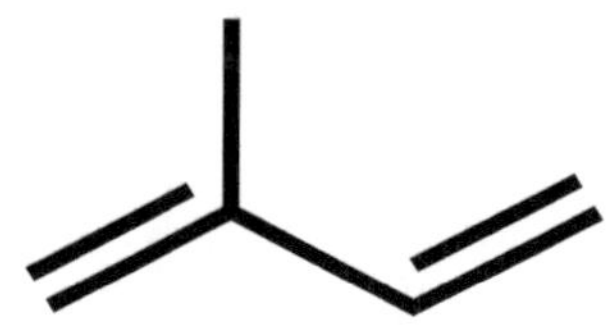

Figure 1. Isoprene unit.

The central unit normally contains 22 carbon atoms, with nine double bonds and four side-chain methyl groups, but rearrangements of this are still classified as carotenoids if the two central methyl groups are retained. The end groups are often cyclized, and do not have to be identical. They are each affixed a Greek letter name (Figure 2) and, when the end groups are not identical, the Greek letter prefixes are given in alphabetical order, with the first end group having the unprimed numbers in the numbering system of the hydrocarbon chain (Figure 2). Although the numbering system provides a means of naming a carotenoid so that its structure can be identified, the most common carotenoids are typically given commonplace names.

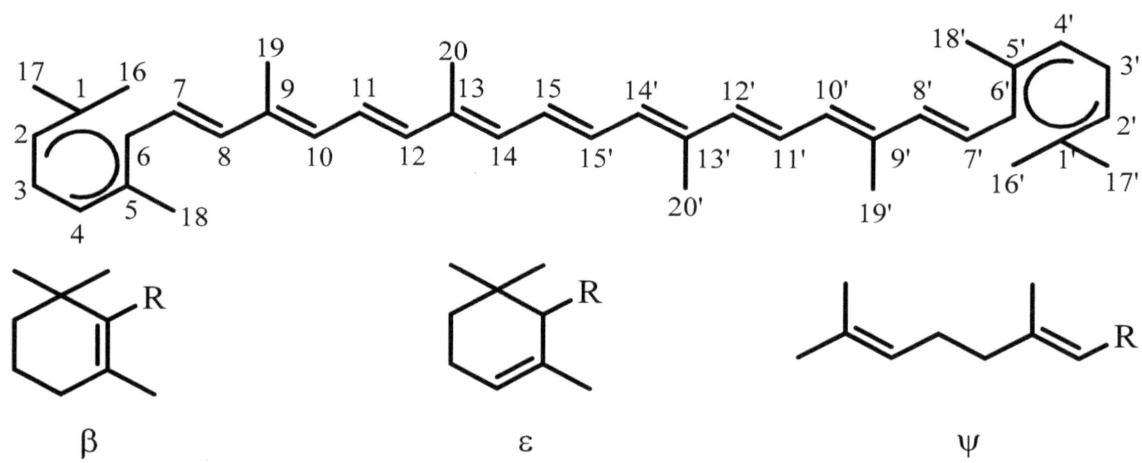

Figure 2. The numbering system of the stem name 'carotene' and three of the seven prefixes which designate the end groups found in natural carotenoids.

β-Carotene is the orange pigment in carrots, from where this class of pigments gets its name; it is the carotenoid which is the most well-known and considered to be the 'parent' carotenoid. All carotenoids which contain oxygen moieties are collectively termed xanthophylls. These may contain, for example, hydroxyl, methoxyl, aldehyde or carboxylic acids, most commonly in the 1–6 or 1′–6′ ring positions.

Carotenoids which have over 40 carbon atoms are known as homo-carotenoids, while those with fewer than 40 are termed apo-carotenoids when carbon atoms have been removed from the end of the molecule, or nor-carotenoids when they have been lost from within the chain. The general name of retro-carotenoid is given to those where the single and double bonds within the conjugated chain have been shifted by one position.

The majority of carotenoids found in nature are in their all-trans (all-E) forms, with only a few exceptions, such as those in photosynthetic reaction centers. Chirality can also be observed within carotenoids, with the C-3 of the 3-hydroxy-β-ring being the most common chiral center, as seen for the stereoisomers zeaxanthin and meso-zeaxanthin. Their structures, and those of the various carotenoids discussed in this review, are given in Figure 3.

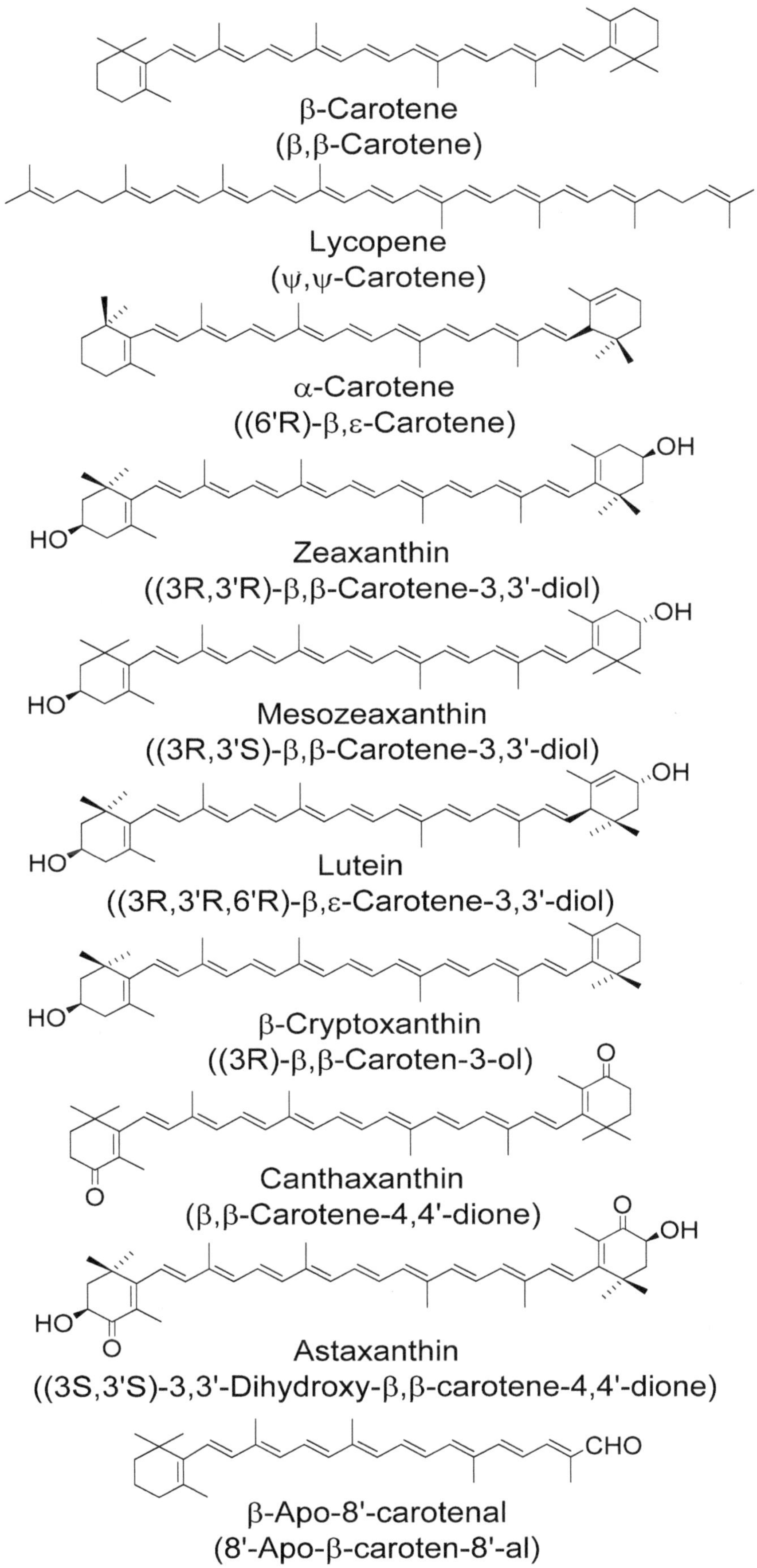

Figure 3. Structures of all-trans carotenoids and analogues.

Most carotenoids are insoluble in water but dissolve readily in hydrocarbon solvents, such as benzene and hexane. The xanthophylls also dissolve in alcohols, but hydrocarbon carotenoids only dissolve to a small extent in such solvents. Of course, the shape and size of a carotenoid will affect its ability to fit into cellular membrane structures. All-trans isomers, which are rigid linear molecules, aggregate more readily than cis isomers [2]. The nature of the end groups is also of importance; for example, carotenoids containing polar groups can interact with molecules at the water–membrane interface, e.g., lutein and zeaxanthin. In some cases, they can also span the membrane, thus, increasing membrane rigidity and mechanical strength, e.g., zeaxanthin [3].

While carotenoids are eaten in significant quantities in foodstuffs present in a normal diet, more recently, they are also consumed via food supplementation. A major reason for this may well be due to claims that they offer significant health benefits; however, there are also counter claims that they can be damaging to human health. This 'switch' may well be linked to anti- and pro-oxidation processes involving carotenoids and, in this review, we discuss in vitro, ex vivo, animal and human studies. Carotenoids are considered to be antioxidants due to their ability to quench many reactions that lead to lipid peroxidation.

The beneficial and deleterious roles on human health of the dietary carotenoids may be due to several factors, but antioxidant and pro-oxidant processes seem to be particularly important. Other factors not discussed in this review include the effects of carotenoids on gap junction potentials [4] and insulin-like growth factors [5]. The antioxidant behavior concerns two distinct oxidizing species (i) singlet oxygen—sometimes called 'active' oxygen and (ii) free radicals of which there are several different types (discussed below). The pro-oxidative, deleterious effects are also believed to involve free radicals—often where the carotenoid itself behaves as an oxidizing radical. In some processes, high oxygen tension (above 150 Torr, the O_2 pressure in normal air) has been shown to lead to a switch to such pro-oxidative damage.

Carotenoids serve in a protective role against photosensitization, generating singlet oxygen via endogenous photosensitizers such as porphyrins. For example, β-carotene is an important micronutrient that effectively prevents lethal hematoporphyrin photosensitization in mice and is employed in the treatment of protoporphyrin-induced photosensitivity in the human genetic disease erythropoietic protoporphyria (EPP) [6,7]. However, its role (and that of other dietary carotenoids) in affecting a reduction in other serious diseases, for example, cancer and heart disease, are in question [8,9].

In this review we attempt to link the clinical, in vivo and ex vivo results with the underlying molecular mechanisms obtained from in vitro studies, with an emphasis on antioxidative processes and the possible switch to damaging pro-oxidation.

2. Epidemiological Studies and Clinical Trials

2.1. Porphyria

The intermediates in the formation of haem are porphyrins (natural tetra pyrrole metabolites). Haem is composed of an iron atom in the ferrous state, chelated to a specific tetrapyrrole called protoporphyin IX. Enzymic dysfunction can lead to a group of diseases called porphyria. These diseases can be acquired or inherited. When protoporphyrin IX (PPIX) builds up, the consequence is severe skin photosensitivity [10]. Other porphyrins are associated with different porphyria. Thus, when uroporphyrin I (UPI) builds up, in the urine and plasma [10], the result is the disease *porphyria cutanea tarda* (PCT) causing both photosensitivity and actinic elastosis. On exposure to light, the porphyrins are converted to their triplet excited states and these, in turn, transfer their excess energy to molecular oxygen, resulting in the formation of singlet oxygen ($^1O_2$) which causes the photosensitivity. As well as $^1O_2$, other reactive oxygen species (ROS) can be formed and these include peroxyl radicals, hydroxy radicals, the superoxide radical anion and hydrogen peroxide, and these can also lead to cell membrane damage [10–12], which is discussed further below. β-carotene is widely used to treat the skin photosensitivity which arises in EPP [13–15] but it is much less useful in ameliorating the photosensitivity associated with PCT [7]. However, it is possible that other carotenoids may be more effective and that combinations of antioxidants may enhance the protective effects.

β-Carotene has been used for over 30 years to ameliorate the skin photosensitivity arising from excess protoporphyrin. In the early studies of Mathews-Roth and co-workers [7], about 84% of those with EPP benefited from large daily doses of β-carotene. Currently the normal dose used is 75–150 mg/day. The molecular mechanisms associated with such photosensitivity are discussed below.

PCT has also been considered for treatment with β-carotene. Unlike PPIX, uroporphyrin is soluble in water. (Interestingly, it is this disease which is associated with the myths concerning vampires!). β-carotene does not appear to protect against the photosensitivity in PCT; however, it may be that combinations of antioxidants, with or without β-carotene, may enhance skin protection [16]. These investigators used various cell lines and human cell cultures and compared PPIX and UPI as photosensitizers. While both β-carotene and lycopene gave significant protection for PPIX photosensitization, neither protected against UPI photosensitization. However, a triple combination of β-carotene plus vitamin C and E (α-tocopherol) did give significant protection against UPI photosensitization, approximately the same protection as a triple combination with PPIX. The vitamin C and E alone gave no protection and while no molecular mechanism has been published for this finding, a possible role of vitamin C with UPI is discussed below.

β-carotene is also used to treat other diseases associated with UV, such as solar urticaria, polymorphic light eruptions (PLE), and photoallergic drug reactions, although in some cases the outcome seems variable. Mathews-Roth [7] found only 33% benefited from β-carotene against PLE and only 20% for other forms of UVB-induced photosensitivity. However, other researchers [17] claim significant benefits for β-carotene, with over 50 of the 66 patients studied reporting significantly increased tolerance to sunlight. The detailed molecular mechanisms of PLE/β-carotene are not understood—the UV absorbing chromophores are not established, as there is no excess porphyrin for these diseases. Of course, several possibilities exist for UVB absorbers, including the amino acid moieties tryptophan, tyrosine and cysteine, as well as flavins, etc. A range of ROS may then be formed and at least some of these could be ameliorated by carotenoids, such as β-carotene.

2.2. Cancer

A seminal study, in 1981, reported that individuals that consumed a greater amount of green leafy and yellow vegetables exhibited a lower risk for cancer [18]. Aware that these types of vegetables were rich in carotenoids, particularly β-carotene, and aware of the latter's singlet oxygen quenching and antioxidant capacity, the authors suggested that β-carotene might be responsible for the anti-cancer effect observed. Later, that same year, a report of a 19-year longitudinal case-control study concluded that smokers had a much greater incidence of lung cancer than non-smokers and that the greatest incidence occurred in the quartile that reflected the lowest β-carotene intake [19]. Almost all of a large number of prospective and retrospective epidemiological studies of either the intake of foods rich in β-carotene or high blood levels of β-carotene reported a strong association with reduced risks of various kinds of cancers including lung, skin, colon, breast, and prostate [1,20]. For example, almost all of nine major case-controlled studies of lung cancer found a lower risk for persons with a higher intake of carotenoids [1]. Furthermore, significant inverse associations of lung cancer with blood (plasma or serum) β-carotene concentrations were found in seven nested case-controlled studies [1]. The incidence of non-melanoma skin cancer (NMSC) was also found to be inversely associated with serum β-carotene levels in a case-control study [21]. It is with skin and lung cancer that these associations have been the strongest, whereas associations of dietary intake of β-carotene and other cancers have largely been inconclusive. One reason for this is that in epidemiological studies, such as in case-control design, data for intake of fruits and vegetables may suffer from patient dietary recall and selection bias.

The effects of carotenoids, mainly β-carotene and lycopene, on a range of cancer biomarkers have been reported. These include those for lung cancer [22,23], colon cancer [24] and breast cancer [25,26].

The outcome frequently depends on a range of factors, such as cell type. A particularly important biomarker for prostate cancer is the Protein Specific Antigen (PSA), and this is discussed in some detail below. For many of the cancers, the results of the biomarker studies suggest beneficial effects of carotenoids—but not in some specific cases (as discussed below for lung cancer, β-carotene increases lung cancer in heavy smokers).

2.2.1. Breast Cancer

A pooled analysis of cohort studies found non-significant associations for total fruit, total vegetables, and total fruit and vegetable intake and breast cancer [27]. In this regard, a systematic review and meta-analysis of prospective studies of dietary intake and blood concentrations of six dietary carotenoids found that blood concentrations of carotenoids are more strongly associated with reduced breast cancer risk than carotenoids assessed by dietary questionnaires [28]. A longitudinal study, in which serum concentrations of β-carotene, α-carotene, β-cryptoxanthin, lycopene, and lutein plus zeaxanthin were measured at baseline, and repeated across time, indicated that α- and β-carotene were inversely associated with breast cancer in postmenopausal women [29]. A positive association was observed for lycopene, although the sample size was small. Contrarily, an epidemiologic cohort study based on blood carotenoid intake as a biomarker for consumption of fruits and vegetables found no significant associations between breast cancer risk and serum carotenoids in postmenopausal women [30]. More recently, a nested case control study of plasma carotenoids and breast cancer risk, over 20 years of follow-up in the Nurses' Health Study, found that higher concentrations of α-carotene, β-carotene, lycopene and total carotenoids were associated with an 18–28% statistically significant lower risk of breast cancer [31]. This was particularly the case for more aggressive and fatal disease. It is difficult to draw clear conclusions about the role of carotenoids in breast cancer incidence from the many conflicting studies. Nevertheless, studies of subgroups of pre- and postmenopausal women may provide further insight into the role of specific carotenoids in this disease.

2.2.2. Prostate Cancer

As noted previously, dietary factors have been implicated as risk factors for prostate cancer [32]. Studies into the role of carotenoids in reducing prostate cancer risk have been as contradictory and inconclusive as with other cancers. The first epidemiological study (case-control) to demonstrate a reduced risk of prostate cancer with increased intake of β-carotene was initiated in 1981 [33]. A number of studies followed that supported an association of β-carotene with reduced prostate cancer risk, whereas others did not [34]. As individual carotenoid concentrations began to be investigated with regard to cancer risk, lycopene became the carotenoid of interest. A study involving 47,365 persons, the so-called Health Professionals Follow-Up Study, examined the role of lycopene upon prostate cancer risk through the evaluation of tomato products. Participants with high tomato sauce (a strong predictor of plasma lycopene) and lycopene intake were at reduced risk of prostate cancer [35]. A pooled analysis of 15 studies involving 11,239 cases of prostate cancer and 18,541 controls examined associations of the concentrations of seven carotenoids and risk of prostate cancer and associations by stage or grade of disease [36]. None of the carotenoids tested, including lycopene, were associated with an overall risk of prostate cancer. However, lycopene exhibited a statistically significant heterogeneity related to the stage of the disease, i.e., the risk of aggressive disease was inversely associated with lycopene. A phase II randomized and controlled clinical trial was conducted to evaluate the safety and effect of several doses of lycopene to men with clinically localized prostate cancer and to assess the impact on intermediate endpoints [37]. Serum-free testosterone decreased and total estradiol increased significantly in those patients receiving 30 mg lycopene daily, while no significant increases in serum prostate specific antigen (PSA) occurred, although these changes were not significant compared to the control arm of the study. Nevertheless, the authors suggested that mechanisms other than antioxidant activity, perhaps mediated by steroid hormones, might also be responsible for lycopene's beneficial effect. A meta-analysis of 34 observational studies (10 cohort, 11 nested case-control and 13 case-control studies) reported that both α-carotene and lycopene were inversely associated with the risk of prostate cancer, although neither could lower the risk of advanced prostate cancer [38], while β-carotene intake or its blood levels were not associated with a lower prostate cancer risk. A randomized double-blind placebo-controlled phase I-II study examined the effects of dietary supplements, including lycopene, in men with multifocal high grade prostatic intraepithelial neoplasia and/or atypical small acinar proliferations (precancerous prostatic lesions) [39]. The investigators found that the administration of high doses (35 mg) of lycopene was associated with a higher incidence of prostatic cancer at re-biopsy and recommended that this supplement should be avoided. However, in updated results, Giovannucci et al. [35] have shown that lycopene is associated with a reduced risk of lethal prostate cancer rather than indolent prostate cancer. Indeed, this may explain the variation in outcomes discussed above. Presumably, lethal prostate cancer is the preferred endpoint, rather than total prostate cancer, for epidemiological studies into the value of lycopene against prostate cancer [36].

Indeed, several small clinical trials have shown benefits against prostate cancer for lycopene, employing typical doses around 15 mg/day. One such trial [40] was based on PSA measurement over one year in a group of patients, all of whom had established prostate cancer, and suggested that over 60% benefited from the reduced rate of acceleration of PSA or, in about 20% of the cases, an actual reduction in PSA. In another trial, patients who were scheduled to undergo radical prostatectomy received supplementation with lycopene or did not [41]. It was found that the plasma PSA level decreased by 18% in the intervention group, while it increased by 14% in the control group. They also reported that, following the prostatectomy, about twice as many men in the lycopene group had tumors of 4cc or less, compared to the control group. These researchers point out that carotenoids (such as lycopene and β-carotene) may modulate processes related to mutagenesis, carcinogenesis, cell differentiation and proliferation independently of their role as antioxidants, one such role being to increase gap junction intercellular communication.

Of course, as noted above, intake of dietary antioxidants other than lycopene may also contribute to benefits against prostate cancer [33]. More recently, Vance and co-workers [42] have demonstrated that the intake of antioxidants was associated with less oxidative stress among men with incident prostate cancer. Their results indicate additional research on the relationship between dietary antioxidants and prostate tissue redox status and carcinogenesis is needed to confirm if such a relationship may influence disease severity, progression and recurrence.

2.2.3. Colon Cancer

Fruit, vegetables and, by association, carotenoid intake have also been implicated in the prevention of colon cancer [43]. Only half of the six studies reviewed reported that the combined consumption of vegetables and fruit reduced colorectal cancer risk. Because of these inconsistencies, a Canadian study (case-control) was undertaken to examine the association between dietary carotenoids and colon cancer risk [44]. Overall, no association was found between dietary intake of carotenoids and colon cancer risk. However, among never-smokers, a significant reduced risk was associated with intake of β-carotene. An inverse association was found between lycopene intake and colon cancer risk among smokers. In a multi-ethnic cohort study, using a quantitative food frequency questionnaire and carotenoid densities, the researchers reported no significant associations between intake of individual and total carotenoids and colorectal cancer risk in either men or women, depending upon the model employed in analysis (basic or multivariate [45]). β-cryptoxanthin showed a small protective effect in men. Lycopene intake was related to an increased risk of rectal cancer in men. Total β-carotene decreased the risk of colorectal cancer in male smokers (this is an interesting observation considering what has been reported in lung cancer). A Chinese case-control study measured serum levels of α-carotene, β-carotene, β-cryptoxanthin, lycopene and lutein/zeaxanthin and found that colorectal cancer incidence was associated with lower levels of α-carotene, β-cryptoxanthin and lycopene among the specific Chinese population [46]. Thus, the role of carotenoids in the risk of colorectal cancer is as inconclusive as with other cancers.

2.2.4. Skin Cancer

It was assumed that Non-Melanoma Skin Cancer (NMSC) risk could be ameliorated by β-carotene based upon its known strong singlet oxygen quenching and antioxidant properties. A case-control study found that the incidence of NMSC was inversely related to the level of serum β-carotene [21]. However, in a controlled clinical trial in which 50 mg of oral β-carotene was administered daily, there were no significant differences in any of the primary endpoints after five years [8]. The amount of β-carotene administered in this study increased the plasma carotenoid levels nearly 10-fold above that of controls. A second randomized trial in Australia examined the influence of 30 mg/day supplementation of β-carotene on the incidence of basal and squamous cell carcinomas over a four-year period [47]. A small, but statistically insignificant, increase (1508 vs 1146/100,000; 1.315 (0.84–2.19) in the incidence of squamous cell carcinoma was observed with β-carotene supplementation. The investigators concluded that there were no beneficial or detrimental effects on skin cancer rates as a result of β-carotene supplementation. Further evaluations from nested case-control studies showed that β-carotene supplementation had no effect on any of the controlled patient subgroups, i.e., numbers of previous skin cancers, age, gender, smoking, skin type or baseline plasma β-carotene levels [48,49]. Interestingly, those persons who were in the highest quartile of the initial plasma β-carotene level had the lowest risk of death from all causes, but β-carotene supplementation did not affect mortality.

Few studies have examined the influence of β-carotene on the occurrence of melanoma skin cancer. Nevertheless, in three case-control studies, no association was found between blood carotenoid levels and the risk of melanoma [50–52]. In one of these studies the risk of melanoma among men and women in the three highest quartiles of β-carotene intake actually increased by 40–50%, albeit neither the risk for the fourth quartile nor the test for trend was statistically significant [52]. A side note of interest is that β-carotene supplementation (50 mg/day for 36 months) has been reported to have beneficial effects in dysplastic nevus syndrome, producing a statistically significant retardation in the size of dysplastic nevi on some body sites. β-Carotene did not have a significant effect on the average number of newly developed nevi [53]. A meta-analysis of randomized controlled trials found that β-carotene supplementation had no effect on the incidence of melanoma (RR, 098; 95% CI, 0.65–1.46) nor upon NMSC risk (RR, 0.99; 95% CI, 0.93–1.05) [54].

2.2.5. Lung Cancer

As noted above, a 1981 19-year longitudinal case-control study found that smokers had a markedly greater incidence of lung cancer, compared to non-smokers, and that the greatest incidence occurred in the quartile that exhibited the lowest carotene intake [19]. Furthermore, of nine major case-control studies of lung cancer and carotene intake, all showed a lower risk of lung cancer among persons with a higher intake of carotenoids [1]. In addition, seven nested case-control studies of lung cancer and blood (plasma or serum) β-carotene levels found significant inverse associations when controlled for tobacco use and other confounding factors. It is interesting to note that the majority of these studies found stronger inverse trends with fruit and vegetable intake than that with carotenoid intake, providing a hint that the combination of β-carotene with other micronutrients may have had a greater effect than the carotenoid alone. Thus, almost all of the large number of prospective and retrospective epidemiological studies of either the intake of foods rich in β-carotene, or high levels of blood β-carotene, reported a strong association with reduced risks of lung cancer [55]. With overwhelming epidemiological evidence for the cancer-preventive effect of β-carotene, it was both surprising and disturbing when results from the eight-year intervention trial of the Alpha-Tocopherol, Beta-Carotene Cancer Prevention Study (known as the ATBC trial) reported an 18% increase in the incidence of lung cancer in male smokers who were administered 20 mg/day of a β-carotene supplement, compared to non-supplemented controls [56]. Previously, five intervention trials had been undertaken. Except for a trial in which β-carotene had been co-administered with selenium and α-tocopherol, none of these provided evidence of a protective effect of β-carotene [1]. A second lung cancer chemoprevention trial, the β-carotene and retinol efficacy trial (known as CARET), sought to determine whether the combination of β-carotene, with its presumed antioxidant effects, and the tumor-suppressing molecular actions of vitamin A could reduce the incidence of lung cancer in high risk populations [57]. Participants in the intervention arm of the study received 30 mg/day of β-carotene plus 25,000 IU daily of retinol. β-carotene plus retinol was associated with an increased incidence of lung cancer among the entire cohort of 18,314 smokers, former smokers and asbestos-exposed participants (RR, 1.28; 95% CI, 1.04–1.57; $p = 0.02$). In view of the ATBC trial results and in consideration of the safety of participants in the CARET trial, the intervention was halted about 21 months early. This pretty much signaled the end of β-carotene clinical trials. However, as discussed above, very high doses (75–150 mg/day) of β-carotene continue to be used to treat skin photosensitivity. This is discussed by Bayerl [58] who points out both the criticisms of the ATBC and CARET trials and also suggests that the use of β-carotene should be discussed with patients only after weighing the risk/benefit ratio.

2.3. *Age-Related Macular Degeneration (AMD)*

AMD is the leading cause of blindness in the Western world. The carotenoid (xanthophyll) pigments lutein and zeaxanthin accumulate in the macula (zeaxanthin is in two stereo isomeric forms, one of which is called meso-zeaxanthin—the structures are given in Figure 3). AMD may be associated with low levels of lutein and zeaxanthin in the diet, serum or retina, and exposure to blue light. The area on the retina that can perceive the finest details is known as the "yellow spot" or "macula". It surrounds the fovea, which contains the highest density of visual cells. These molecules in the macula lutea are concentrated up to a combined concentration of about 1 mM, (ratio 1:1:1) the highest concentration of carotenoids found anywhere in the primate body [59]. Epidemiological findings over many years show how lutein, zeaxanthin and mesozeaxanthin could contribute to a risk reduction of drusen formation, neovascularisation and, especially, Age-Related Macular Degeneration based on both a 'simple' light filter effect and also reduced damage by quenching various forms of Reactive Oxygen Species, including both singlet oxygen and various free radicals [60].

At least two roles for the macular pigments are likely—a simple light-filter effect, and an antioxidant effect to minimize the damage due to $^1O_2$ and other ROS (the macula has a high metabolic rate and, as a consequence, a high oxygen requirement). While several roles may be important, in this review, we concentrate on the anti/pro-oxidation processes involving the macular carotenoids. Some proposed mechanisms concerning such processes are given below, suggesting distinct roles for lutein, zeaxanthin and also for lycopene (even though lycopene does not accumulate in the macula).

3. Animal Studies

As noted earlier, β-carotene was shown to prevent lethal hematoporphyrin photosensitization in mice and is employed in the treatment of protoporphyrin-induced photosensitivity in the human genetic disease erythropoietic protoporphyria (EPP) [6,7]. In addition to their original investigations of EPP, Mathews-Roth et al. [13,14,61] showed that β-carotene exerted a small, but statistically significant, increase in the minimal erythema dose (MED) of sunburn in man. These studies were extended to show a similar protective effect with phytoene in guinea pigs [62]. Phytoene is the triene precursor to β-carotene and absorbs strongly in the UVB range of the electromagnetic spectrum.

Based upon these observations, Epstein examined the potential influence of intraperitoneally injected β-carotene on UV-induced tumor formation in the hairless mouse [63]. The carotenoid was found to exert a limited, but protective, effect with regard to time of tumor appearance and tumor growth. In mixed chemical/UV carcinogenic protocols, oral administration of β-carotene or canthaxanthin was found to delay the appearance of skin tumors [64]. Employing a UV-carcinogenic protocol and the Skh-Hr-1 hairless mouse model, it was determined that canthaxanthin, but not β-carotene or phytoene, could slow the development of subsequent tumors if administered immediately after development of the primary tumor, indicating a promotion stage effect [65]. Nevertheless, phytoene, when administered (injected intraperitoneally) for ten weeks prior to exposure to a single, large, tumor-initiating fluence of UV was photoprotective. Additional studies confirmed that oral (dietary) administration of 0.1% (w/w) of either β-carotene or canthaxanthin, for six weeks prior to exposure to a single, tumor-initiating UV dose, and then continuing carotenoid administration during the progression stage of carcinogenesis, could significantly prevent the development of skin tumors [66]. β-carotene, when administered only before UV exposure, provided no significant protection. Thus, in this study, it was inferred that photoprotection resulted only when the carotenoid was administered during the progression phase of tumor development [67]. Subsequently, in a somewhat complicated protocol (complicated from the standpoint that animals received the varying levels of carotenoids in different "run-in" feeding periods ranging from 4 days to one month and that animal ages at the time of irradiation ranged from 8 to 20 weeks), the investigators found that both canthaxanthin and β-carotene provided significant photoprotection to carcinogenesis when the pigment was administered throughout the course of the study and at a level of 0.07% (w/w) in the diet [68]. Lower levels did not provide significant protection. Employing the C3H/HeN mouse model in an UV-carcinogenic protocol, a diet supplemented with 1% (w/w) canthaxanthin significantly reduced the average skin tumor burden, although the tumor latent period was unaffected [69,70].

At this point, there seemed to be overwhelming experimental evidence to substantiate the anti-UV-carcinogenic potential of β-carotene. However, in 1998, a laboratory study employing a semi-defined diet, compared to the earlier studies employing commercial closed-formula diets in which photoprotection was observed, not only failed to provide protection against UV-carcinogenesis, but resulted in significant exacerbation by β-carotene and astaxanthin, but not by lycopene [71].

Matrix analyses of experimental variables in those studies showing photo-protection or exacerbation of carcinogenesis indicated that animal age, carotenoid dose, or type of diet were the most probable causes of the divergent responses to β-carotene. No significant differences in the tumor latent period occurred in young animals (2.5 months of age) fed the semi-defined diet, regardless of β-carotene dose (either 0.07% or 0.3% (w/w) of diet)) Nevertheless, tumor multiplicity was significantly increased at each higher dose of the carotenoid. Both young and older animals were equally responsive to exacerbation of UV-carcinogenesis with respect to this tumor parameter [72]. Thus, animal age was not an adequate determinant of carcinogenic response to β-carotene.

It seemed logical that the presence and interactions with other dietary factors in the closed-formula diet, and the lack thereof in the semi-defined diet, might be responsible for the disparate influence of β-carotene on UV-carcinogenesis [73]. An explanation of the two types of rations employed in the β-carotene studies is warranted. Commercial rodent rations are examples of closed-formula diets. They are composed of feedstuffs such as milled grains, alfalfa, and so forth. The composition of these diets will vary with season, regional locale of source, and market prices. Thus, the specific composition of each lot will vary, making it impossible to quantitatively duplicate. It was this type of ration that was employed in the earlier studies in which photo- protection was observed. Semi-defined diets are those formulated from refined foodstuffs, e.g., corn starch, refined oils, casein, and defined vitamin and mineral supplements. It is this type of diet that was employed where exacerbation of UV-carcinogenesis was observed. Indeed, the influence of β-carotene-supplemented diets is reflected in Table 1 [74]. Care was taken in this study to ensure that comparable levels of the carotenoid were consumed in both diets and none of the effects, or lack thereof, on carcinogenic expression could be attributed to differential carotenoid intake [74]. Here, it is worth pointing out that the 0.07% β-carotene supplementation in the mouse is equivalent to consumption, on a body weight basis, to ~160-fold higher levels than that employed in many clinical trials (50 mg/day per ~75 kg body weight). The practical relevance of employing a higher dose of the carotenoid, even if effective as a photo-protectant, would be questionable. Nevertheless, it is apparent from these studies that dietary components, such as other carotenoids, their isomers, or some unidentified phytochemicals, are present in the closed-formula ration that are absent in the semi-defined diet and which potentiate the carcinogenic response to β-carotene. Moreover, β-carotene has been shown to exhibit either limited antioxidant protection or to behave as a pro-oxidant under oxidative stress conditions [75]. The possible molecular mechanisms and the role of oxygen concentration are discussed below. Some of these mechanisms suggest a role for the interaction of vitamin C with carotenoid radicals. There was no listed vitamin C content in the commercial closed-formula ration in those studies in which β-carotene had provided photo-protection or in those in which no effects of the carotenoid were observed [76]. Studies in which β-carotene induced exacerbation of carcinogenic expression employed the semi-defined diet to which vitamin C had been added. The same exacerbation occurred, however, when the semi-defined diet was devoid of vitamin C. In previous studies, it was proposed that either a lack of adequate levels of vitamin C in smokers or an excess of vitamin C could stoichiometrically drive the proposed repair mechanism (see reaction Equations (7)–(10) in Molecular Mechanisms, Section 4.12) to a pro-oxidant state that, in turn, would lead to an increased level of β-carotene radical cation and block the effective antioxidant activity of vitamin E. This might explain the divergent results obtained from the two diets [77].

Table 1. Influence of diet on β-carotene-mediated UV-carcinogenic expression *.

Diet	Median Tumor Time, Weeks	Tumors/Animal
Closed formula		
Control	20.6	0.52
0.07% β-Carotene	20.0	0.60
Semi-defined		
Control	19.5	0.60
0.07% β-Carotene	17.2	1.63

* There was no significant influence of β-carotene on tumor latent period (median time to tumor) or tumor multiplicity (mean number of tumors/animal) in animals fed the closed-formula diet. Nor were there differences in either tumor parameter between closed-formula and semi-defined control diets. However, β-carotene supplementation of the semi-defined ration significantly shortened the tumor latent period ($p < 0.002$) and increased tumors ($p < 0.03$) [74].

Hairless mice were fed β-carotene-supplemented semi-defined diets containing varying levels of vitamins C and E (either increasing their concentrations or reducing them to reflect levels found in closed-formula rations) and subjected to a UV-carcinogenic protocol). The addition of high levels of vitamin E (10-fold) or vitamin C (six-fold) did not ameliorate the exacerbated effects of β-carotene on carcinogenesis, nor did the complete removal of vitamin C from the diet have an effect. However, by reducing the level of vitamin E in the semi-defined diet to that present in the closed-formula ration, there was a significant (nearly two-fold) increase of exacerbation of UV-carcinogenesis [78]. These effects are depicted in Table 2 [79].

Table 2. Influence of varying levels of vitamins C and E on β-carotene-modulated tumor multiplicity (average number of tumors per animal at median tumor time).

Control (−βCar) [a]	(+βCar) [b]	(+βCar, −Vit C) [c]	(+βCar, −Vit C, low Vit E) [d]
1.05	3.20	3.45	5.90

[a] Control, semi-defined diet containing 110 mg vitamin E and 990 mg vitamin C/kg of diet; [b] (+βCar): semi-defined diet containing 0.79g/kg diet of β-carotene with equivalent levels of vitamins C and E as Control; [c] (+ βcar, −Vit C): same composition as + βCar but with no vitamin C; [d] (+βCar, −Vit C, low Vit E): same composition as +βCar, −Vit C but with only 49 mg/kg diet of vitamin E, the same as in closed-formula ration [79]. (Reprinted by permission of the publisher Taylor and Francis, Ltd., http://tandfonline.com).

When compared to the control, it can be seen that β-carotene supplementation of the semi-defined diet, at the lower level of vitamin E, significantly ($p = 0.0065$) increased tumor multiplicity nearly six-fold. These data suggest that β-carotene and vitamin E interact to partially meliorate the pro-carcinogenic influence of the former. The data with vitamins C and E supplementation also suggest that antioxidant supplementation has a limited range of upregulation in healthy, well-nourished individuals.

While proposed/speculated mechanisms are discussed below, it is clear that dietary factors can have a profound influence on β-carotene's capacity to influence carcinogenic expression [74]. It has been suggested that β-carotene, so prevalent in the green and yellow vegetables and fruits (which led to the proposal that the carotenoid could reduce cancer risk), merely cloaks the potential anti-cancer agent [80]. The results from the ATBC and CARET clinical trials of β-carotene and lung cancer, along with the experimental results with the carotenoid and UV-carcinogenesis, have raised concern regarding the safety of β-carotene supplementation and the warning that it should not be used in cancer prevention in the general population [1,81].

Meanwhile, efforts continue (discussed below, in Molecular Mechanisms) to explain how β-carotene, a molecule with excellent antioxidant capacity under specific conditions and a singlet oxygen quencher, can act as a pro-carcinogen in UV-carcinogenesis and in lung cancer patients.

4. Molecular Mechanisms

4.1. *Singlet Oxygen—General*

Singlet oxygen is a significantly damaging species, both because it is energetic enough to react with most biological substrates and because it has an inherent long lifetime. It arises in nature mainly from substrates which absorb light, converting to their lowest triplet state (e.g., porphyrins and chlorophylls). These triplet states react with normal, ground state oxygen to generate $^1O_2$. Other generation routes are possible, such as enzymatic processes and processes related to stress response [82,83]. Many $^1O_2$ quenchers, such as all dietary carotenoids, also directly quench photosensitizer triplets, including porphyrins and chlorophylls, (to produce the carotenoid triplet, followed by loss of the energy as heat). Therefore, they can protect by reducing the $^1O_2$ yield without actually quenching $^1O_2$. However, in homogeneous solvents, such as hexane, benzene and xanthophylls that are soluble in alcohols, it is possible to adjust the concentrations to minimize this direct energy transfer and, hence, study only the quenching of the $^1O_2$ by the so-called quencher (the carotenoid). However, in a real-life situation, this may not be so simple and could make studies of $^1O_2$ in such model ex vivo systems less easy to understand—this is discussed further below with respect to HeLa cells.

4.2. *Singlet Oxygen—Simple Solvents, Micelles and Liposomes*

In homogeneous solvents, it is well established that most non-aggregated carotenoids are extremely efficient quenchers of $^1O_2$. This efficiency is reduced by several factors—aggregation, isomerization and the number (n) of conjugated double bonds in the carotenoid. A good example of the effects of aggregation is shown by zeaxanthin in deuterated methanol/water mixtures [84].

As can be seen in Figure 4, at 20% D_2O, the quenching rate constant falls and at 37.3% D_2O, there is effectively no quenching of $^1O_2$; this corresponds to the water concentration, causing carotenoid aggregation. Such aggregation is also shown by Oliveros et al. [85] at the reduced rate, by an order of magnitude of $^1O_2$ quenching by β-carotene in alcohol compared to benzene.

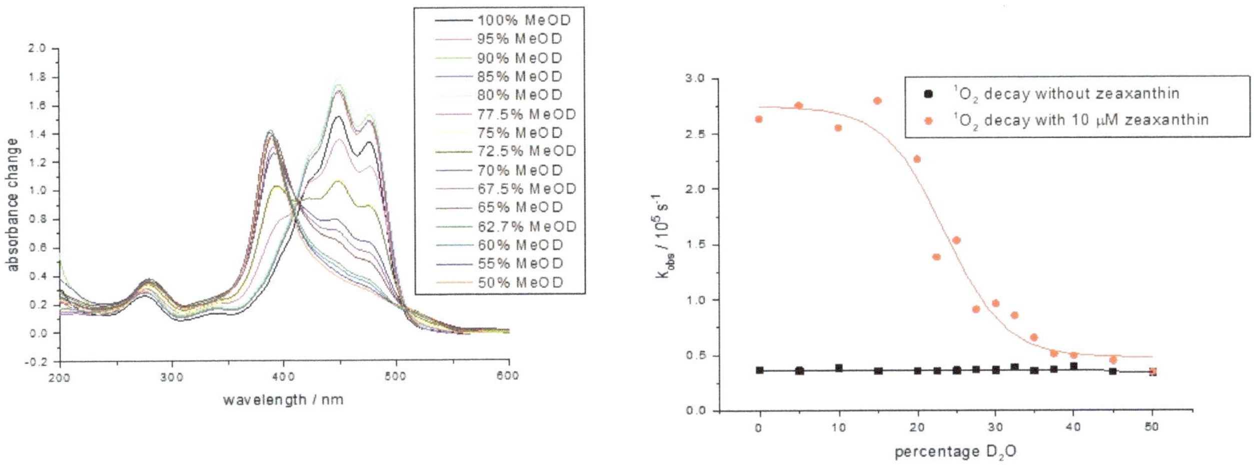

Figure 4. Left: ground state absorption spectra of 1×10^{-5} M zeaxanthin in various MeOD/D_2O mixtures. Right: the effect of increasing D_2O (inducing zeaxanthin aggregation) on $^1O_2$ deactivation efficiency of zeaxanthin.

Studies, using benzene, have also shown cis carotenoids are less efficient at quenching $^1O_2$ than all-trans isomers. For example, the rate constant decreases for β-carotene as the cis bond moves towards the end of the molecule from 13.5×10^9 dm^3 mol^{-1} s^{-1} for the all-trans β-carotene to 8.99×10^9 dm^3 mol^{-1} s^{-1} for the 9-cis β-carotene [86]. A time-resolved resonance Raman has an additional band—the so-called cis peak—which could affect the results from steady-state studies.

An important example of the effect of the conjugated double bond length on the $^1O_2$ quenching, for dietary carotenoids is for lutein (n = 10) compared to zeaxanthin (n = 11). However, for α-carotene (n = 10), this effect is less marked. A further reduction of n (to nine, for example, as in septapreno-β-carotene) leads to a dramatic reduction in the quenching rate constant—see Table 3, below [86].

Table 3. Second-order rate constants (k_q) for the carotenoid quenching of $^1O_2$ in benzene.

Carotenoid	n	$k_q/10^9$ dm^{3}mol^{-1}s^{-1}
lycopene	11	17.0
β-carotene	11	13.0
zeaxanthin	11	12.6
Meso-zeaxanthin	11	12.2
α-carotene	10	12.0
lutein	10	6.64
septapreno-β-carotene	9	1.38

It has also been established that all β-carotene isomers share a common triplet state, twisted about the middle carbon–carbon double bond, compared to the ground state [87]. Additionally, when using hexane as a solvent, it has been demonstrated that cis isomers are formed after the reaction of the all-trans isomers with $^1O_2$ for both β-carotene and lycopene and, furthermore, that lycopene prevents β-carotene isomerization [88]. Since the absorption spectra of the cis isomers has an additional band—the so-called cis peak—this could affect the results from steady-state studies.

Studies have also been undertaken using micelles [86,89] and liposomes [90–92] as cell models. The $^1O_2$ quenching rate constants are still rather high (>10^8 dm^3 mol^{-1} s^{-1}). In the liposome, the quenching of $^1O_2$ did not depend on the site of the $^1O_2$ generation (the $^1O_2$ was generated by a water or lipid soluble photosensitizer). However, there was a significant difference in quenching by xanthophylls in liposomes compared to micelles—rate constants fell by up to 30 times in liposomes, while the quenching rate constant for β-carotene in liposomes was similar to that in neutral micellar solutions (Triton-X100). However, this seems to depend on the detergent micelle and the carotene studied. In early work β-carotene was shown not to quench $^1O_2$ in charged sodium dodecyl sulfate (SDS) and cetyltrimethylammonium bromide (CTAB) micelles [93]. However, there was efficient quenching by xanthophylls in the charged micelles [94], while, for alpha-carotene, little quenching was observed in SDS [95].

A significant concentration effect on $^1O_2$ quenching was also observed for xanthophylls in liposomes (especially for zeaxanthin), suggesting, as in alcohol–water mixtures, aggregation lowers quenching efficiency. Furthermore, in contrast to organic solvents, the quenching abilities of lycopene and β-carotene toward $^1O_2$ are virtually identical in mixed micelles of Triton-X100 and Triton-X405, and also in dipalmitoylphosphatidylcholine (DPPC) liposomes. Indeed, in multi-lamellar environments, lycopene is seen to be a poorer quencher of $^1O_2$ than β-carotene—8×10^9 compared to 19×10^9 $dm^3\ mol^{-1}\ s^{-1}$ (unpublished—Cantrell and Truscott, 2002). A related liposome study using dimyristoylphosphatidylcholine (DMPC), reported the inhibition of $^1O_2$-induced lipid peroxidation and showed that inhibition by β-carotene, canthaxanthin and astaxanthin was similar but that such inhibition by lycopene was significantly less (10-fold) [92]. A more recent study has also demonstrated inhibition of $^1O_2$-induced plasma lipid oxidation by both β-carotene and fucoxanthin [95], with fucoxanthin being the better inhibitor, even though the rate constant of $^1O_2$ quenching by fucoxanthin is lower than that of β-carotene [96].

4.3. Singlet Oxygen—Ex Vivo Cell Studies

Boehm and co-workers [97] used lymphocytes from human blood and water-soluble β-carotene beadlets to study the possible ex vivo quenching of $^1O_2$. These researchers reported a significant quenching of $^1O_2$ near to that observed in homogeneous organic solvents [98] and they suggest that this implies that these preparations lead to the β-carotene being bound at or near the cell surface, rather than embedded in the cell membrane, although, as noted above for liposomes, the $^1O_2$ quenching by carotenoids was independent of the site of generation of $^1O_2$ (in the region 10^8–10^9 $dm^3\ mol^{-1}\ s^{-1}$). In a more detailed study, using similar cell models [99], four carotenoids were studied using water soluble beadlets (β-carotene, lycopene, astaxanthin and canthaxanthin). All except canthaxanthin showed a marked quenching of $^1O_2$. These researchers also measured a cell protection factor for membrane damage by each preparation and showed the carotenoids reduced the cell damage by about a factor of two. Finally, this work also studied the effect of β-carotene taken orally rather than via incubation as beadlets. Once again, $^1O_2$ quenching was observed at β-carotene concentrations which may be used in everyday supplementation. However, the effect was somewhat less marked than with the water soluble beadlets. Boehm and co-workers [100] also reported a protection factor for lycopene taken from the diet (from boiled tomato juice) of over six.

The ability of β-carotene to quench $^1O_2$ in cellular environments has been questioned by Ogilby and co-workers [101]. Using individual HeLa mammalian cells and microscope-based time resolved 1275 nm luminescence, these researchers could observe no quenching of the $^1O_2$ by β-carotene (these researchers gave careful consideration to concentrations and rates of reaction in viscous intracellular environments). However, as they comment, such whole-cell systems are complex. Indeed, in a totally different cellular system, related to photosynthesis studies, Telfer and co-workers [102] used time-resolved direct detection of $^1O_2$ at 1270 nm and steady state methods to demonstrate the formation of $^1O_2$ in isolated Photosystem II (PSII) reaction centers and other researchers [103] have suggested quenching of such $^1O_2$ by β-carotene. These, and related studies, have been reviewed more recently by Telfer [104]. This review addresses the roles of β-carotene bound to the PSII reaction centers where it is well known that $^1O_2$ arises. By using chemical techniques to vary the concentration of the carotenoids, Telfer and co-workers [105] show that carotenoids quench some of the $^1O_2$ but not all, due to the distance of the carotenoids from the source of the $^1O_2$. This work in PSII systems suggest that, in a specific biological environment, quenching will only be efficient when the carotenoid is sufficiently close to the source of the $^1O_2$. Clearly, there is more to learn about the interaction of β-carotene with $^1O_2$ in an ex vivo situation. See Figure 5 for an overview of carotenoid-$^1O_2$ reactions.

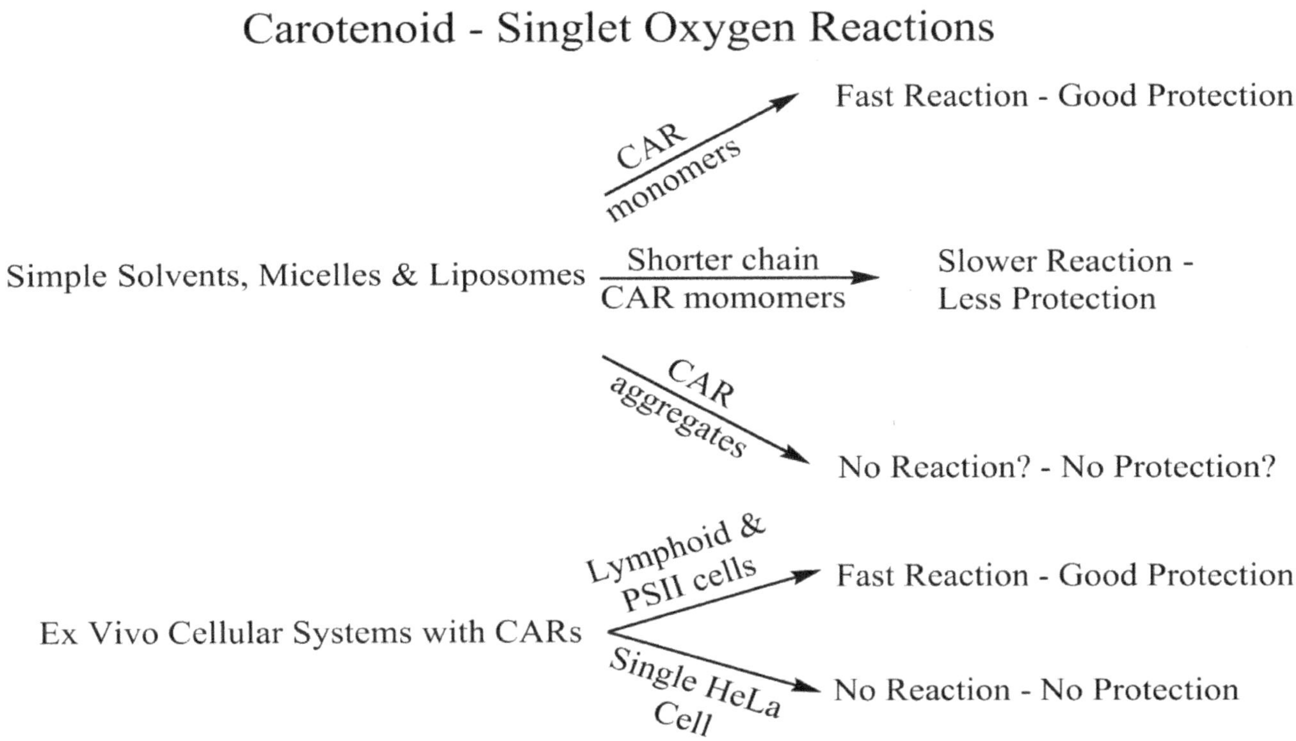

Figure 5. Summary scheme of carotenoid reactions with singlet oxygen.

4.4. Singlet Oxygen—Porphyria

Two processes are believed to be associated with the observed protection against porphyria by β-carotene. One is just 'simple' light absorption by the β-carotene—i.e., an 'inner filter' effect—and the second is that the $^1O_2$ and/or porphyrin triplet state, formed upon light absorption, is efficiently quenched by the β-carotene. Within this second process, whichever quenching mechanism predominates will depend on the site-specific concentrations of oxygen and β-carotene. Clearly, the nearer the skin surface, the higher the oxygen concentration, thus, $^1O_2$ quenching will likely predominate with direct triplet quenching being less important. PPIX has been detected in both the dermis and epidermis [106] and during both the quenching processes discussed here. All-trans β-carotene is converted to a cis–trans mixture, as has been observed previously and discussed above [87,88]. Since it is well established that cis isomers absorb light around 330 nm, some inner filter effects may arise from such cis isomers, which may somewhat increase the importance of this mechanism of protection and cis carotenoids quench $^1O_2$ less efficiently than all-trans isomers [86], so the $^1O_2$ quenching mechanism will be decreased.

4.5. Singlet Oxygen—Cancers

While $^1O_2$ can be generated non-photochemically [82,83], its generation via light in the skin and the eyes is of most importance. The possibility that dietary carotenoids, especially β-carotene, might reduce human cancers, including those in the skin due to UV/visible radiation and ROS, including singlet oxygen, has been discussed for many years, (see, for example, [107]) with contradictory claims both with respect to its effectiveness and its safety. As noted above, the results from the ATBC and CARET clinical trials of β-carotene and lung cancer, along with experimental results from carotenoids and UV-carcinogenesis, have raised concerns regarding the safety of β-carotene supplementation and the warning that it should not be used in cancer prevention in the general population [1,81]. However, as summarized by Bayerl [58] and Góralczyk [108], the methodology of these studies has been questioned. There seems no doubt that the use of β-carotene to treat EPP and other photosensitive diseases is worthwhile, but clearly smoking should be strongly discouraged for such people. Furthermore, this review suggests short term use (e.g., for vacations in regions with high UV exposure), particularly for non-smokers, would be worth considering.

There are also differences in the claims for β-carotene benefits against squamous cell carcinoma, ranging from inhibition of the proliferation of these cells [109] to no evidence being found that carotenoids play an important protective role against incident squamous cell carcinoma of the skin [110]. However, there is some degree of agreement that a combination of carotenoids with other antioxidants, including vitamin E and C, are likely to offer some skin protection [16,111,112].

Several other carotenoids have been discussed as possible beneficial antioxidants in the skin, including lycopene, astaxanthin, lutein and, to some extent, such benefits for the skin seem likely [113,114]. Perhaps the most exciting claims concern zeaxanthin and skin melanomas [115] and earlier studies with fucoxanthin. However, these findings do not involve $^1O_2$ and are out of the scope of this review.

The overall situation is summarized in a recent review [113]. As these researchers point out, although UV radiation is a main factor in the development of non-melanoma skin cancer and melanoma, studies do not, for certain, confirm the protective role of carotenoids in skin photocarcinogenesis.

In the eye, there is little or no involvement of carotenoids and $^1O_2$ with regard to the development of cancer. However, there are claims, as noted above, that zeaxanthin (which can significantly help against AMD, see below) may also have anti-carcinogenic properties which have been studied for the treatment of various cancers. These do not appear to include melanoma of the eye [116]. However, one speculation [117] does concern $^1O_2$ and both eu- and phaeomelanin. Both these melanins bind transition metals and, hence, can lead to radicals via Fenton reactions. The melanins associate with the minor grooves in DNA which allow them to both damage DNA and reduce access to DNA repair enzymes. However, melanin can react with $^1O_2$ [118], possibly leading to structural modifications in the melanin itself and, hence, affecting the role of the transition metals redox reactions. This work suggests a dual role for melanins as pro- and antioxidants and may offer improved strategies for using PDT to treat melanoma. In a somewhat related study [119], models of both melanins have been shown to react with both oxidizing and reducing radicals.

4.6. Singlet Oxygen—Age-Related Macular Degeneration (AMD)

AMD is a major cause of loss of sight in the Western world. Of the over 25 or so carotenoids in human serum only lutein and zeaxanthin accumulate in the macula (zeaxanthin is in two stereo isomeric forms, one of which is called meso-zeaxanthin—the structures are given in Figure 3). AMD may well be related to reduced levels of lutein and zeaxanthin (macular pigment) in the diet, serum or retina, and blue light exposure. However, several groups claim that lycopene also has a role in reducing AMD even though there is no lycopene in the macula [120–122]; a possible molecular mechanism, based on radical reactions, is discussed below.

Somewhat related to the mechanisms associated with porphyria, at least two roles for the macular pigments are now accepted [123]—a simple filter effect and an antioxidant effect to minimize the damage due to $^1O_2$ and other ROS. As shown in Table 3 above, the efficiency of quenching $^1O_2$ is about double for zeaxanthin and meso-zeaxanthin than lutein in benzene. Furthermore, in liposomes, the quenching rate constants for zeaxanthin and lutein show a similar ratio—2.3 and 1.1×10^8 dm^3 mol^{-1} s^{-1}, respectively. These results possibly suggest that a major role of zeaxanthin in the macula is $^1O_2$ quenching, but that such quenching may be a less important function of lutein [90]. However, as the concentration of the carotenoid increases (in the liposomes) there are significant differences between lutein and zeaxanthin. The lutein quenches the $^1O_2$ in a linear manner at all concentrations used (up to 70 μM), while the quenching by zeaxanthin starts to become less efficient above about 30 μM. Indeed, at 70 μM zeaxanthin shows no $^1O_2$ quenching at all under these conditions when the $^1O_2$ is generated in the aqueous phase (using rose bengal, a water-soluble sensitizer to generate the $^1O_2$). When the $^1O_2$ is generated within the liposome, the loss of quenching efficiency is less marked, but is still evident above about 40 μM. Since the macular pigment concentrations are relatively high, this may suggest $^1O_2$ quenching is important for lutein and that the results in simple organic solvents such as benzene do not account for this aggregation effect.

It is noteworthy that the efficiency of $^1O_2$ quenching by other dietary carotenoids in liposomes are much higher [90] (e.g., β-carotene = 24×10^8 dm^3 mol^{-1} s^{-1}) and, of course, there is much more β-carotene in our diet than any of the macular pigments. Thus, the reasons for the specific carotenoid pigments accumulated in the macula are far from just that of efficient $^1O_2$ quenchers. Overall, the possible role of the different carotenoids with respect to the efficiency of $^1O_2$ in the macula is still not totally understood.

4.7. Radicals—General (In Vitro)

As noted above, epidemiological studies have linked the intake of carotenoids with the reduced risk of degenerative diseases. However, trials using dietary carotenoid supplements have led to the possibility that damaging pro-oxidant reactivity can also arise. Likely reasons for such a switch in behavior include the properties of the carotenoid radicals themselves.

Carotenoid interaction with oxidizing radicals (and, to a lesser extent, with reducing radicals) is far more complex than with $^1O_2$. This is because several quite different radicals are important and several types of reaction, with oxidizing radicals, can occur. For example, the hydroxyl radical (OH•) and some sulfur-based radicals add to carotenoids to give a neutral adduct radical, while nitrogen dioxide (NO_2•) and thionyl (RSO_2•) radicals can oxidize a carotenoid to its corresponding radical cation and the superoxide radical anion ($O_2\bullet^-$) is generally regarded as unreactive. The corresponding conjugate acid, HO_2•, is much more reactive than $O_2\bullet^-$ ($O_2\bullet^-$/HO_2• pKa is 4.7) and reactivity for $O_2\bullet^-$ at pH values near neutrality could be due to the small amounts of HO_2•, present even at such pH values. Theoretical studies, not reviewed here, claim carotenoids may undergo an electron transfer with $O_2\bullet^-$ to yield the corresponding carotenoid radical anion—this is quite different from the oxidation of carotenoids by a number of other oxidizing free radicals [124].

Neutral carotenoid radicals, including adducts, are not easy to study, both because their spectra often overlap with the intense ground state absorption and because there are several possible neutral radicals—see below. A further complexity arises because, once formed, neutral radicals can add molecular oxygen, forming peroxyl radicals, and this can lead to a switch from the antioxidant to pro-oxidant behavior of carotenoids. This has been observed for β-carotene in a non-biological environment [76] and, more recently, for lycopene in human cells [125]. Such anti-/pro-oxidant roles of carotenoids and xanthophylls are of particular interest to photosynthesis, vision and cancer.

4.8. Radicals—Simple Solvents, Micelles and Liposomes

Early work, using pulse radiolysis [126], subsequently [127,128] established the spectra of the carotenoid radical cations ($CAR\bullet^+$). These radicals can also be generated in other ways, such as by flash photolysis [129–131], electrochemically [132,133] and chemically [134]. Pulse radiolysis was also used to generate and characterize the radical anions of the carotenoids [126,135].

These techniques have led to the measurement of the one-electron oxidation potentials of a number of carotenoids to be measured for aqueous micellar solutions—they are all near 1000 mV, which means carotenoid radical cations are quite strong oxidizing agents themselves [127,128,136,137]. Thus, carotenoid radical cations may oxidize important biomolecules, such as tyrosine, tryptophan and cysteine. Moreover, electron transfer between many pairs of carotenoids have been observed. This allowed the relative one-electron oxidation potentials of several carotenoids to be obtained. Such studies demonstrated that lycopene has the lowest potential, i.e., it is the most easily oxidized of the carotenoids. A consequence of this could be that lycopene is the "sacrificial" carotenoid in vivo, when there is a mixture of carotenoids present, and this may be related to health benefits often reported for dietary lycopene—see, for example, [122,138].

The high-energy fast reaction technique of pulse radiolysis has also demonstrated that water-soluble antioxidants, such as vitamin C, can convert (water-insoluble) carotenoid radical cations back to the parent carotenoid [137]. Thus, a potentially deleterious pro-oxidant effect due to the oxidizing potential of carotenoid radical cations may be reduced by ascorbic acid. It is also established that the free radicals in cigarette smoke will reach the lungs. For heavy smokers, it has been shown that a high concentration of dietary β-carotene can have a damaging effect, and a possibility is that this may be related, in part, to smoke-based free radicals (e.g., $NO_2\bullet$) reacting with β-carotene to produce the β-carotene radical cation, which can then damage bio-substrates. A related and interesting observation, with respect to the mechanisms of photosynthesis, has come from work reported by Skibsted et al. [130,131]. These studies used pH conditions where the standard reduction potentials were the same for tyrosine and tryptophan. They found that tyrosine reacted with the carotenoid radical cation an order of magnitude faster than tryptophan and suggest that this may be related to tyrosine, rather than tryptophan, being the protein moiety reacting with β-carotene in the protective mechanism, which operates in the photosynthetic reaction center. These researchers also point out that the driving force in such processes depends on the "local" pH, so the reverse reaction between a tyrosine radical and β-carotene may also be important in proteins.

Finally, more than one neutral radical can arise from various routes:

$$HCAR\bullet^{+} \rightarrow CAR\bullet + H^{+} \quad (1)$$

(note: here, we have abbreviated the radical cation as $HCAR\bullet^{+}$ rather than $CAR\bullet^{+}$ to illustrate the deprotonation),

$$HCAR = O\bullet^{-} + H_2O \rightarrow HCAR\text{-}OH\bullet + OH^{-} \quad (2)$$

where the radical anion of a carbonyl containing carotenoid reacts with water to give a neutral adduct, and:

$$CAR + RS\bullet \rightarrow CAR\text{-}RS\bullet \text{ and } CAR + OH\bullet \rightarrow CAR\text{-}OH\bullet \quad (3)$$

Carotenoid radicals have also been generated and studied in micelles and liposomal cell models. These reactions and subsequent processes have been reviewed recently [139].

Carbon tetrachloride is known to cause various types of tissue injury and, using trichloromethylperoxyl radical ($CCl_3O_2\bullet$) as a model of alkylperoxyl radicals, and Triton X micelles as a cell membrane model, Hill and co-workers [140] reported that pulse radiolysis gave two distinct species, a rapidly formed carotenoid radical cation and a species assigned to an addition product, the addition product decaying to give a more radical cation, i.e., the $CAR\bullet^{+}$ is formed via the fast:

$$CCl_3O_2\bullet \rightarrow CAR\bullet^{+} + CCl_3O_2\bullet^{-}, \quad (4)$$

and slower:

$$CAR\text{-}CCl_3O_2\bullet \rightarrow CAR\bullet^{+} + CCl_3O_2\bullet^{-} \quad (5)$$

(with astaxanthin, only the slow process was observed).

Results from comparing the detergent and totally non-polar environments (benzene) suggest there is more than one distinct environment for β-carotene in these micellar cell membrane models. Indeed, if the TX 100 is a useful cell model, this suggests such a range of 'sites' may well have biological consequences.

4.9. Radicals—Ex Vivo Cell Studies

Boehm and co-workers [125] have reported the significant effect of the concentration of oxygen on the protection of human lymphoid cells against high-energy γ-radiation by lycopene. In this study, volunteers either took a large lycopene diet or near-zero lycopene and their lymphoid cells were irradiated with γ-radiation from a ^{60}Co source. This radiation leads mainly to the production of two reactive radical species:

$$H_2O \rightarrow OH\bullet + e_{aq}^{-} \quad (6)$$

(plus a small amount of H• and non-radical species).

In the presence of nitrous oxide (N_2O), the solvated electrons are converted to more OH• and, with oxygen-flushed formate solutions, virtually only $O_2\bullet^-$ is generated [141].

These researchers used standard cell-staining techniques with eosin and measured membrane destruction and cell death. Using γ-radiation doses up to 5000 Gy (and normal atmospheric conditions), the dietary lycopene was found to protect the cells four to five times more efficiently compared to a virtually zero lycopene diet. Interestingly, a really substantial effect of oxygen concentration was also reported. Thus, at near zero concentrations of oxygen the cells were totally protected by the lycopene, while at 100% oxygen there was no protection at all by the lycopene [125]. A similar effect was seen for β-carotene with more or less the same protection from zero to 20% oxygen as for lycopene (to be published). At very high oxygen concentrations (above 60%), the β-carotene was a more efficient protector than lycopene. Moreover, in preliminary studies, the macular pigments, zeaxanthin and lutein, were shown to offer more protection as the oxygen concentration increases—far better than for either lycopene or β-carotene (to be published). These researchers compared this 'oxygen' effect to the earlier observations of Burton and Ingold [75] who used non–biological conditions. A proposed mechanism involved cell protection via quenching of the reactive OH• by lycopene (either by hydrogen abstraction or addition) then the formation of a reactive peroxyl neutral radical via oxygen addition. This peroxyl radical was proposed as the major species leading to the cell membrane destruction. Whatever the mechanism (e.g., involving neutral lycopene radicals and oxygen addition) this, substantial difference, in cell protection, due to oxygen concentration, may (with appropriate methods) be useful clinically by leading to a mitigation of damage caused by radiation treatment of tumors. From a simplistic point of view (after a high lycopene diet), saturating the tumor with oxygen should cause no effect on the radiation therapy benefit, while flushing the non-necrotic areas with, say, nitrogen could protect against the unwanted radiation damage. This oxygen addition mechanism may also offer another explanation for the (lung) damaging effect of high doses of β-carotene in heavy smokers discussed above. If radicals, such as $NO_2\bullet$, present in cigarette smoke can also add to β-carotene (as well as oxidize it as described above), then the high oxygen concentration in the lungs could increase the possibility of oxygen addition to the initial neutral radical adducts, leading to a damaging carotenoid peroxyl radical. For $NO_2\bullet$ itself, the adduct (if formed) is short-lived, so this may not be an important process, but, of course, it could be important for other radicals present in cigarette smoke. We have previously noted vitamin C can convert damaging carotenoid radical cations (which can result from oxidation by, for example, $NO_2\bullet$) back to the parent carotenoid, but there is no information on a corresponding process with carotenoid peroxyl radicals.

The radiation protection study described above [125] allowed a comparison of the effects of the radicals generated on cell kill. Under typical conditions, a cell death of 5.60%, 8,75% and $\leq$ 2.18% was detected for OH•, $O_2\bullet^-$ and e_{aq}^-, respectively, which indicated that solvated electrons are inefficient at inducing cell kill, whilst superoxide radical is the most effective radical at causing cell death.

Furthermore, as noted above, other dietary antioxidants may interact with free radicals and this can lead to enhanced protection. However, in this study, no such enhancement was observed for the cell protection by lycopene, with the addition of vitamins C and E. This implies that lycopene radical cation is not produced during the process of lycopene protection against γ-radiation.

As noted in [125], metal ions may also be involved in cell damage via Fenton reactions [142], but these are not involved in the above study.

A wide range of other ex vivo studies on skin models, atherosclerosis, AMD and cancers have been reported previously [84,139].

4.10. Radicals—The Skin and EPP

It is generally accepted that EPP involves light absorption by PPIX, leading to the PPIX triplet state followed by energy transfer to oxygen to generate $^1O_2$, which then damages the skin. The protective mechanism of β-carotene is believed to be based on the efficient quenching of the $^1O_2$ by the β-carotene.

However, as discussed above, Ogilby and co-workers [101] have been unable to detect singlet oxygen in a single cell, laser-based system. Thus, other protective processes involving β-carotene should be considered. One such non-radical process is direct quenching of the PPIX triplet state by β-carotene. This leads to the triplet of the quencher (β-carotene) which then dissipates the energy as heat. This seems somewhat unlikely due to the mobility of the oxygen. However, it must be remembered that the quenching of the PPIX triplet by normal (ground state triplet oxygen) is nearly an order of magnitude less than the diffusion-controlled rate constant (i.e., only about one ninth of the collisions between the oxygen and the triplet PPIX will result in $^1O_2$).

Perhaps more likely is the formation of a range of free radicals due to UVA/UVB incident on the skin, which leads to porphyrin radicals which, in turn, can be quenched by the β-carotene. However, the generally accepted mechanism of $^1O_2$ generation from the PPIX triplet seems more likely at this time.

4.11. Radicals—Eye Cancers and AMD

UVA and long wavelength UVB radiation is virtually completely filtered out before it reaches the macula. However, there are a variety of endogenous photosensitizers within the retina which can be excited by the light that does reach it. The outer retina (containing the photoreceptors and retinal pigment epithelium (RPE)), is immediately adjacent to the choroidal blood supply and, as such, is highly oxygenated. Therefore, favorable conditions for photodynamic damage arise. The fact that there is a strong dependence of oxygen concentration on the susceptibility of the retina to photodamage suggests that light-induced damage to the retina is indeed due to the photodynamic processes leading to singlet oxygen production, and is related to AMD and not cancers. However, other parts of the eye have much less light/UV filtering and this can lead to ocular melanoma. Eye melanoma most often affects the middle layer of the eye (uvea), the colored portion of the eye (iris), the muscle fibers around the eye's lens (ciliary body), and the layer of blood vessels that line the back of the eye (choroid). The iris is exposed to both visible and UV radiation, even though some of the UV is removed by the cornea, with the precise amount depending, of course, on the specific wavelength. This light exposure can lead to iris melanoma. The iris contains various pigments including melanins and haemoglobin. The melanin is reduced upon aging, typically by about half at 65 years of age. It is well established that the melanin has a major protective role via sequestering metal ions, and light absorption. There are two major classes of melanin, black–brown eumelanin and yellow–red sulfur-containing phaeomelanin. Both types of melanin can be free radical quenchers for both oxidizing and reducing radicals [143].

While the biological relevance of this ability to quench free radicals is not fully established, these results do show that melanins may act as a protector against free radical damage, including cancers, by this additional protective role. However, interactions with dietary carotenoids are less well established. The iris, ciliary body, and RPE/choroid (the uveal structures) contain about 30% of the eye's lutein and zeaxanthin, plus other carotenoids. As noted above, when carotenoids react with some oxidizing radicals, such as $NO_2\bullet$, the carotenoid radical cation is formed as a consequence of the removal of the damaging $NO_2\bullet$. Since, as shown above, such radical cations are rather strongly oxidizing themselves, this can lead to a switch to pro-oxidative damage rather than anti-oxidative protection. However, Edge and co-workers [141] have shown that both types of melanin can react with carotenoid radical cations (including lutein and zeaxanthin) and reduce them back to the parent carotenoid. The melanins act as a free radical 'sink', but the reactivity of melanins with carotenoid radical cations may be an additional role for melanins in protecting the in vivo system from oxidative damage by carotenoid radical cations. Moreover, where the concentration of carotenoids are low but pivotal to the protective processes, this behavior of the melanins may help to maintain the concentration of the key carotenoids, such as lutein and zeaxanthin.

A surprising observation concerns a role for lycopene in protecting against AMD [120,122]. We suggest the most likely mechanism for such a protection is based in the relative redox properties of lycopene compared to lutein and zeaxanthin.

Using pulse radiolysis, we have shown the order of such potentials, as shown in Figure 6 [136]. Thus, it seems possible, that lycopene, even though it is not found in the macula, can help to preserve the lutein and zeaxanthin en route to the macular. If this is true it would suggest that protection against AMD should not just be linked to lutein and zeaxanthin supplementation, but also to a diet rich in tomato lycopene.

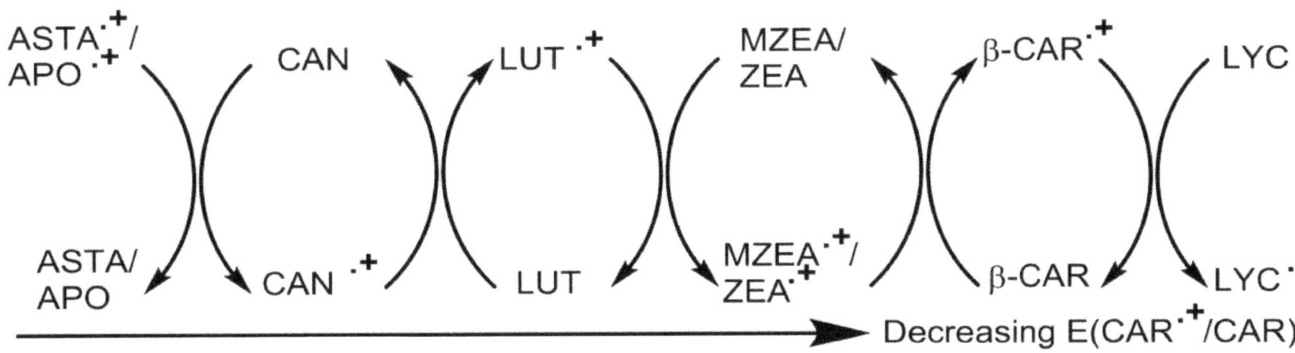

Figure 6. Scheme showing the relative ordering of the one-electron reduction potentials of several carotenoid radical cations in benzene.

4.12. Radicals—Cancer

The benefits and problems associated with carotenoids and cancer are summarized above. Despite many in vitro and ex vitro studies indicating the antioxidant benefits of carotenoids against many cancers via free radical quenching, there is little or no certainty that carotenoids reduce the incidence of cancer by such a simple mechanism. As well as such possible antioxidant benefits, carotenoids may also influence several aspects of carcinogenesis. A wide range of cancers and the possible benefits of carotenoids have been reviewed by Rock [144].

As described above, animal studies have compared closed-formula and semi-defined diets with β-carotene, with some work reported on lycopene and astaxanthin. Understanding the molecular mechanisms associated with β-carotene-fed animal studies and UV radiation is problematical for several reasons. Firstly, there is a significant difference between the so-called closed-formula diet and the semi-defined diets (see above). The 'closed formula' diet can vary from experiment to experiment and show the photoprotective effect of the carotenoid. However, the semi-defined diet (where, amongst other factors, the vitamin supplements are defined) show not only no protection of β-carotene against UV-induced tumors, but also a significant exacerbation. This effect, for the semi-defined diet, was also observed with β-carotene replaced by astaxanthin, but not by lycopene. Another factor not always discussed in such work (and other studies using UV radiation) is that the UV will produce not just a single oxidizing radical, but several radicals so that the damage can result from more than one mechanism.

Moreover, important in explaining the different responses caused by β-carotene is the finding that β-carotene shows efficient radical trapping antioxidant behavior at normal oxygen concentrations (i.e., normal partial pressure), while at higher oxygen concentrations, the carotenoid changes from being an antioxidant and exhibits pro-oxidant properties [75,145]. Thus, β-carotene has been shown to have either limited antioxidant protection or to be a pro-oxidant under oxidative stress conditions [146]. The carotenoid reacts efficiently with peroxyl radicals ($RO_2\bullet$) where the reaction (electron transfer) produces the carotenoid radical cation ($CAR\bullet^+$), as shown in Equation (7) [147].

$$RO_2\bullet + \beta\text{-CAR} \rightarrow RO_2^- + \beta\text{-CAR}\bullet^+ \quad (7)$$

Whether the physiological environment, e.g., oxidative stress, can modulate the likelihood of this reaction is uncertain. However, as described above, carotenoid radical cations are quite strong oxidizing species, with a reduction potential of about 1000 mV [127,128,147]. Such radicals, if formed, could contribute both directly to membrane damage, and indirectly to the pro-oxidant capacity of the 'parent' carotenoid. This may well be related to whether the carotenoid radical cation could be repaired. Based on electron transfer rate constants between various carotenoids and their interactions with vitamin E (α-tocopherol, (TOH) and vitamin C ($AscH^-$), both components of animal rations, a mechanism was suggested for the interaction of β-carotene that would lead the repair of the β-carotene radical cation (Equations (8)–(10)) [136,137].

$$RO_2\bullet + TOH \rightarrow TOH\bullet^+ + ROOH \quad (8)$$

$$TOH\bullet^+ + \beta\text{-CAR} \rightarrow TOH + \beta\text{-CAR}\bullet^+ \quad (9)$$

$$\beta\text{-CAR}\bullet^+ + AscH^- \rightarrow \beta\text{-CAR} + Asc\bullet- + H^+ \quad (10)$$

Such a mechanism suggests vitamin E reacting with an oxy-radical to form the vitamin E radical cation and β-carotene repairing this radical cation to form the β-carotene radical cation (β- $CAR\bullet^+$), as in (9). This, in turn, could be repaired by vitamin C as in (10). That is, β-carotene would not only protect by directly quenching the reactive oxy-radical, as shown in Equation (7), but also enhance the radical protective properties of both vitamins E and C, shown in Equations (8)–(10). Of course, UV can produce many other radicals and oxidizing radicals, e.g., ($RO_2\bullet$), and these may also react with β-carotene to produce the carotenoid radical cation directly.

Overall, these animal dietary studies do not support a proposed scheme, as suggested by Equation (10), of the β-carotene radical cation being repaired by ascorbic acid. If the mechanism does not apply, then the reduced intermediates, in the case of the β-carotene radical cation, behave as pro-oxidants. While the mechanism may remain uncertain, it is obvious that dietary factors can have a significant effect on the capacity of β-carotene to influence carcinogenic expression [74]. These factors may, of course, be other carotenoids, their isomers, or some yet unidentified phytochemical (Equation (11)).

$$\beta\text{-CAR}\bullet^+ + ? \rightarrow \beta\text{-CAR} + H^+ + ? \quad (11)$$

The ex vivo results, discussed above (Section 4.9) for β-carotene and other carotenoids, may suggest that an important factor is molecular oxygen. Once a neutral radical such as OH• has formed a neutral adduct with β-carotene (to give HO-Carotene•), an oxygen molecule can be added to give a damaging peroxyl radical (HO-Carotene-OO•), leading to enhanced cell membrane damage and, hence, possibly to increased cancer risk.

It has been suggested that β-carotene, (which is so prevalent in the green and yellow vegetables and fruits, and which led to the proposal that the carotenoid could reduce cancer risk), merely cloaks the real anti-cancer agent [80] The results from the ATBC and CARET clinical trials of β-carotene and lung cancer, along with the experimental results with the carotenoid and UV-carcinogenesis, have raised concerns regarding the safety of β-carotene supplementation and the warning that it should not be used in cancer prevention in the general population [1,81].

The various molecular mechanisms for radicals and carotenoids can be summarized in the following scheme (Figure 7):

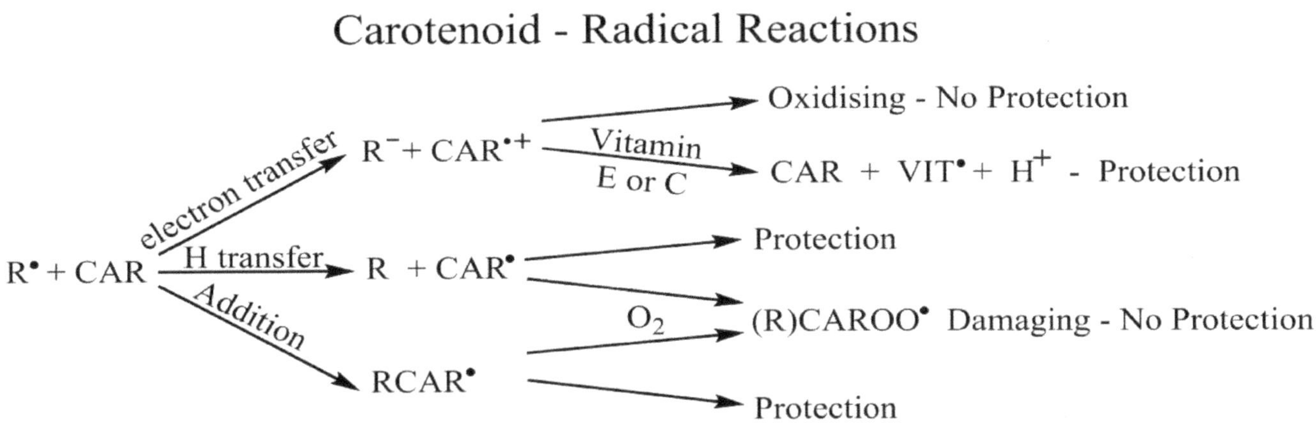

Figure 7. Summary scheme of carotenoid reactions with free radicals.

5. Summary

Carotenoids are widespread in nature and in commercial use. From photosynthesis to porphyria and from cancer to commercial food dyes, they play varied and pivotal roles. Indeed, in photosynthesis, they both protect the system from too much light and act as auxiliary pigments when the light is insufficient for efficient photosynthesis. Apart from photosynthesis, the carotenoids' major roles in human health are as protective pigments and, for β-carotene, precursors for essential vitamins and metabolites that are requisites for good health. In the commercial world, their main use is as "natural" colorants - both directly, as additives to our foods, and indirectly via feeding materials for, for example, chickens and salmon.

However, the protective function of certain carotenoids, particularly β-carotene and lycopene, has been challenged as a result of clinical trials where β-carotene supplementation in male smokers resulted in significantly increased incidence of lung cancer, and from animal studies in which β-carotene supplementation resulted in the exacerbation of UV-carcinogenic expression. Indeed, dietary studies have shown diet influences the carcinogenic response to β-carotene and that β-carotene, per se, is pro-carcinogenic in UV-carcinogenesis. These findings challenge the use of β-carotene as an anti-cancer agent for the general population.

If we are to understand the contradictory reports of beneficial associations and detrimental effects in clinical trials and experimental animal studies, we must first understand the molecular mechanisms involving singlet oxygen and antioxidant reactions in which carotenoids are involved. Furthermore, we must understand the individual properties of the carotenoid in participating in such reactions and recognize that some carotenoids, e.g., β-carotene, may act as a pro-oxidant under specific conditions. Thus, the introduction of an antioxidant carotenoid into the complex milieu of a cell can result in unexpected consequences.

Among the molecular mechanisms, singlet oxygen is a highly damaging species and dietary carotenoids directly quench the source of singlet oxygen-photosensitizer triplets, such as those of porphyrins and chlorophylls. A significant quenching of singlet oxygen itself, of a magnitude observed in organic solvents, was also reported from human lymphocytes and water-soluble β-carotene. Although slightly lower, similar quenching was observed with oral intake of β-carotene at concentrations used in everyday supplementation. Lycopene, from the diet, also provided a significant protection factor for singlet oxygen quenching. Nevertheless, the ability of β-carotene to quench this oxygen species has been questioned after studies where individual cells reported no such quenching. On the other hand, it has been demonstrated that β-carotene does quench some singlet oxygen in isolated PSII II. Singlet oxygen quenching by β-carotene is a major process in the protection mechanism in porphyria. Related mechanisms associated with porphyria are now accepted for AMD. One mechanism is that the carotenoids exhibit antioxidant effects that minimize singlet oxygen quenching and other ROS. The generation of singlet oxygen by UV/visible light in the skin is of importance and is a primary reason for the speculation that β-carotene might reduce cancer risk. However, the role of β-carotene quenching of singlet oxygen in the etiology of skin cancer has been controversial. One major observation from all of these studies, particularly those of PSII, is that the proximity of the carotenoid to the singlet oxygen source is a major consideration for quenching to occur.

Pulse radiolysis was used to establish the spectra of carotenoid radical cations and radical anions. This technique also allowed the one-electron oxidation potentials of several carotenoids to be measured in aqueous micellar solution. The radical cations typically exhibited an oxidation potential of near 1000 mV, indicating that they are strong oxidizing agents. It has been suggested that the β-carotene radical cation could be involved in the damaging effects to lungs of heavy smokers, particularly those with low levels of ascorbic acid that have the potential of reducing the carotenoid radical cation. Such a mechanism has been proposed for the pro-carcinogenic activity of β-carotene in UV-carcinogenesis, although, in the latter, dietary studies have shown that vitamin C level has no potentiating effect on β-carotene exacerbation on UV-carcinogenesis. It must be remembered that mice are able to synthesize their own vitamin C requirement and the proposed mechanism for lung damage in humans should still be considered as a serious proposal; however, it would be much stronger if the carotenoid radical cation could be identified in the target tissue.

Aware of the unique property of β-carotene and lycopene to "switch" from antioxidant to pro-oxidant under varying oxygen concentrations, investigators have reported a substantial effect of oxygen concentration on the protection of human cells against Y-radiation by lycopene. At very high oxygen concentrations, β-carotene was a more efficient protector than lycopene. Y-radiation leads, mainly, to two reactive radical species—hydroxyl radical and superoxide anion. At zero-oxygen concentration, cells containing lycopene exhibited virtually no damage due to the high-energy radiation, whereas lycopene gave no protection at all at 100% oxygen concentration. Furthermore, no enhancement with supplemental antioxidants, vitamins C and E, occurred, indicating that the lycopene radical cation was not involved in the γ-radiation protection mechanism and it is likely to involve addition processes with both a (neutral) radical and oxygen, giving damaging peroxyl radicals. These observations may have important clinical potential for protecting normal tissue when exposed to high radiation levels during the treatment of affected target cells.

There was formidable epidemiological evidence, before the β-carotene intervention trials were conducted, that the carotenoid would exhibit anti-cancer properties. Indeed, β-carotene was known to be a strong singlet oxygen quencher and antioxidant, and this formed the basis for the enthusiasm that the carotenoid would act as an anti-cancer agent. However, the study of the molecular mechanism(s) of β-carotene has revealed knowledge of the carotenoid and its chemical properties under various microenvironments that clearly demonstrate that the carotenoid's interactions are complex and must be taken into account to explain the volumes of research and clinical results observed. The fact that it can act as antioxidant or pro-oxidant, the fact that the carotenoid can form radical ions that themselves may participate in cellular damage, the conditions under which β-carotene acts as an efficient singlet oxygen quencher and knowledge of the conditions in which the carotenoid is introduced are all conditions to be considered before declaring its biological response. It is only through continued study of the "antioxidant" itself that we will be able to assess the potential beneficial and/or harmful effects of the respective carotenoids. Whereas a diet rich in carotenoid-containing fruits and vegetables may be beneficial in the fight against some diseases, one must remain cognizant of the potential risks that carotenoid supplementation may pose.

Author Contributions: All authors (H.S.B., F.B., R.E., T.G.T.) contributed actively to the preparation of this review manuscript; writing—original draft preparation, H.S.B., F.B., R.E., and T.G.T.; writing—review and editing, H.S.B., F.B., R.E., and T.G.T. All authors have read and agreed to the published version of the manuscript.

References

1. IARC Working Group on the Evaluation of Cancer-Preventive Agents. *IARC Handbooks of Cancer Prevention: Carotenoids*; IARC: Lyon, France, 1998.
2. Britton, G. Structure and properties of carotenoids in relation to function. *FASEB J.* **1995**, *9*, 1551–1558. [CrossRef]
3. Lazrak, T.; Milon, A.; Wolff, G.; Albrecht, A.-M.; Miehe, M.; Ourisson, G.; Natatani, Y. Comparison of the effects of inserted C_{40}- and C_{50}-terminally dihydroxylated carotenoids on the mechanical properties of various phospholipid vesicles. *Biochim. Biophys. Acta* **1987**, *903*, 132–141. [CrossRef]
4. Bertram, J.S.; Vine, A.L. Cancer prevention by retinoids and carotenoids: Independent action on a common target. *Biochim. Biophys. Acta* **2005**, *1740*, 170–178. [CrossRef] [PubMed]
5. Chan, J.M.; Stampfer, M.J.; Giovannucci, E.; Gann, P.H.; Ma, J.; Wilkinson, P. Plasma insulin-like growth factor-I and prostate cancer risk: A prospective study. *Science* **1998**, *279*, 563–566. [CrossRef]
6. Mathews, M.M. Protective effect of β-carotene against lethal photosensitization by haematoporphyrin. *Nature* **1964**, *203*, 1092. [CrossRef]
7. Mathews-Roth, M.M.; Pathak, M.A.; Fitzpatrick, T.B.; Haber, L.H.; Kass, E.H. Beta-carotene therapy for erythropoietic protoporphyria and other photosensitivity diseases. *Arch. Dermatol.* **1977**, *113*, 1229–1232. [CrossRef]
8. Greenberg, E.R.; Baron, J.A.; Stukel, T.A.; Stevens, M.M.; Mandel, J.S.; Spencer, S.K.; Elias, P.M.; Lowe, N.; Nierenberg, D.W.; Bayrd, G.; et al. A clinical trial of β-carotene to prevent basal-cell and squamous-cell cancer of the skin. *N. Engl. J. Med.* **1990**, *323*, 789–795. [CrossRef]
9. Rissanen, T.; Voutilainen, S.; Nyyssönen, K.; Lakka, T.A.; Salonen, R.; Kaplan, G.A.; Salonen, J.T. Low serum lycopene is associated with excess risk of acute coronary events and stroke: The Kuopio Ischaemic Risk Factor Study. *Br. J. Nutr.* **2001**, *85*, 749–754. [CrossRef]
10. Menon, I.A.; Persad, S.D.; Hasany, S.M.; Basu, P.K.; Becker, M.A.C.; Haberman, H.F. Reactive species involved in phototoxicity of photoporphyrin and uroporphyrin on bovine corneal endothelium. In *Oxidative Damage and Repair, Proceedings of the 5th International Society for Free Radical Research, Bienial Meeting, Pasadena, CA, USA, 14–20 November 1990*; Davies, K.J.A., Ed.; Pergamon Press: Oxford, UK, 1991; pp. 321–325.
11. Menon, I.A.; Becker, M.A.; Persad, S.D.; Haberman, H.F. Quantitation of hydrogen peroxide formed during UV–visible irradiation of protoporphyrin, coproporphyrin and uroporphyrin. *Clin. Chim. Acta* **1990**, *186*, 375–381. [CrossRef]
12. Pathak, M.A. Reactive oxygen species in inflammatory cutaneous photosensitivity reactions—A new insight. *Clin. Exp. Dermatol.* **1986**, *11*, 204.
13. Mathews-Roth, M.M.; Pathak, M.A.; Fitzpatrick, T.B.; Harber, L.C.; Kass, E.H. Beta-carotene as a photoprotective agent in erythropoietic protoporphyria. *N. Engl. J. Med.* **1970**, *282*, 1231–1234. [CrossRef] [PubMed]
14. Mathews-Roth, M.M. Carotenoids in erythropoietic protoporphyria and other photosensitivity diseases. *Ann. N. Y. Acad. Sci.* **1964**, *691*, 127–138. [CrossRef] [PubMed]
15. Lehmann, P.; Scharffetter, K.; Kind, P.; Goerz, G. Erythropoetische protoporphyrie: Synopsis von 20 patienten. *Hautarzt* **1991**, *42*, 570–574. [PubMed]
16. Bohm, F.; Edge, R.; Foley, S.; Lange, L.; Truscott, T.G. Antioxidant inhibition of porphyrin-induced cellular phototoxicity. *J. Photochem. Photobiol. B Biol.* **2001**, *65*, 177–183. [CrossRef]
17. Jansen, C.T. β-Carotene treatment of polymorphous light eruptions. *Dermatologica* **1974**, *149*, 363–373. [CrossRef] [PubMed]
18. Peto, R.; Doll, R.; Buckley, J.D.; Sporn, M.B. Can dietary β-carotene materially reduce human cancer rates? *Nature* **1981**, *290*, 201–208. [CrossRef]
19. Shekelle, R.B.; Liu, S.; Raynor, W.J.; Leeper, M.; Maliza, C.; Rossof, A.H.; Pau, O.; Shryock, A.M.; Stamler, J. Dietary vitamin A and risk of cancer in the Western Electric study. *Lancet* **1981**, *318*, 1185–1190. [CrossRef]
20. Fairfield, K.M.; Fletcher, R.H. Vitamins for chronic disease prevention in adults. *JAMA* **2002**, *287*, 3116–3126. [CrossRef]
21. Kune, G.A.; Bannerman, S.; Field, B.; Watson, L.F.; Cleland, H.; Merenstein, D.; Vitetta, L. Diet, alcohol, smoking, serum β-carotene, and vitamin A in male nonmelanocytic skin cancer patients and controls. *Nutr. Cancer* **1992**, *18*, 237–244. [CrossRef]

22. Liu, C.; Wang, X.-D.; Mucci, L.; Gaziano, J.M.; Zhang, S.M. Modulation of lung molecular biomarkers by β-carotene in the physicians' health study. *Cancer* **2009**, *115*, 1049–1058. [CrossRef]
23. Kim, J.; Kim, Y. Animal models in carotenoids research and lung cancer prevention. *Transl. Oncol.* **2011**, *4*, 271–281. [CrossRef] [PubMed]
24. Costea, T.; Hudita, A.; Ciolac, O.-A.; Galateanu, B.; Ginghina, O.; Costache, M.; Ganea, C.; Mocanu, M.-M. Chemoprevention of colorectal cancer by dietary compounds. *Int. J. Mol. Sci.* **2018**, *19*, 3787. [CrossRef] [PubMed]
25. Chalabi, N.; Le Corre, L.; Maurizis, J.-C.; Bignon, Y.-J.; Bernard-Gallon, D.J. The effects of lycopene on the proliferation of human breast cells and BRCA1 and BRCA2 gene expression. *Eur. J. Cancer* **2004**, *40*, 1768–1775. [CrossRef]
26. Gloria, N.F.; Soares, N.; Brand, C.; Olivera, F.L.; Borojevic, R.; Teodoro, A.J. Lycopene and beta-carotene induce cell-cycle arrest and apoptosis in human breast cancer cell lines. *Anticancer Res.* **2014**, *34*, 1377–1386.
27. Smith-Warner, S.A.; Spiegelman, D.; Yaun, S.S.; Adami, H.O.; Beeson, W.L.; van den Brandt, P.A.; Folsom, A.R.; Fraser, G.E.; Freudenheim, J.L.; Goldbohm, R.A.; et al. Intake of fruits and vegetables and risk of breast cancer: A pooled analysis of cohort studies. *JAMA* **2001**, *285*, 769–776. [CrossRef]
28. Aune, D.; Chan, D.S.; Vieira, A.R.; Navarro-Rosenblatt, D.A.; Vieira, R.; Greenwood, D.C.; Norat, T. Dietary compared with blood concentrations of carotenoids and breast cancer risk: A systemic review and meta-analysis of prospective studies. *Am. J. Clin. Nutr.* **2012**, *96*, 356–373. [CrossRef]
29. Kabat, G.C.; Kim, M.; Adams-Campbell, L.L.; Caan, B.J.; Chlebowski, R.T.; Neuhouser, M.L.; Shikany, J.M.; Rohan, T.E.; WHI Investigators. Longitudinal study of serum carotenoid, retinal, and tocopherol concentrations in relation to breast cancer risk among postmenopausal women. *Am. J. Clin. Nutr.* **2009**, *90*, 162–169. [CrossRef]
30. Maillard, V.; Kuriki, K.; Lefebvre, B.; Boutron-Ruault, M.C.; Lenoir, G.M.; Joulin, V.; Clavel-Chapelon, F.; Chales, V. Serum carotenoid, tocopherol and retinol concentrations and breast cancer risk in the E3N-EPIC study. *Int. J. Cancer* **2010**, *127*, 1188–1196. [CrossRef]
31. Eliassen, A.H.; Liao, X.; Rosner, B.; Tamimi, R.M.; Tworoger, S.S.; Hankinson, S.E. Plasma carotenoids and risk of breast cancer over 20 y of follow-up. *Am. J. Clin. Nutr.* **2015**, *101*, 197–205. [CrossRef]
32. Glade, M.J. Food, nutrition, and the prevention of cancer: A general global perspective. *Nutrition* **1999**, *15*, 523–526. [PubMed]
33. Ohno, Y.; Yoshida, O.; Oishi, K.; Okada, K.; Yamabe, H.; Schroeder, F.H. Dietary β-carotene and cancer of the prostate: A case-control study. *Cancer Res.* **1988**, *48*, 1331–1336. [PubMed]
34. Wu, K.; Erdman, J.W.; Schwartz, S.J.; Platz, E.A.; Leitzmann, M.; Clintom, S.K.; DeGroff, V.; Willett, W.C.; Giovannucci, E. Plasma and dietary carotenoids and the risk of prostate cancer. *Cancer Epidemiol. Biomark. Prev.* **2004**, *13*, 260–269. [CrossRef] [PubMed]
35. Giovannucci, E.; Rimm, E.B.; Liu, Y.; Stampfer, M.J.; Willett, W.C. A prospective study of tomato products, Lycopene, and prostate cancer risk. *J. Natl. Cancer Inst.* **2002**, *94*, 391–398. [CrossRef] [PubMed]
36. Key, T.J.; Appleby, P.N.; Travis, R.C.; Albanes, D.; Alberg, A.J.; Barricarte, A.; Black, A.; Boeing, H.; Bueno-de-Mesquita, H.B.; Chan, J.M.; et al. Carotenoids, retinol, tocopherols, and prostate cancer risk: Pooled analysis of 15 studies. *Am. J. Clin. Nutr.* **2015**, *102*, 1142–1157. [CrossRef] [PubMed]
37. Kumar, N.B.; Besterman-Dahan, K.; Kang, L.; Pow-Sang, J.; Xu, P.; Allen, K.; Riccardi, D.; Krischer, J.P. Results of a randomized clinical trial of the action of several doses of lycopene in localized prostate cancer: Administration prior to radical prostatectomy. *Clin. Med. Urol.* **2008**, *1*, 1–14. [CrossRef] [PubMed]
38. Wang, Y.; Cui, R.; Xiao, Y.; Fang, J.; Xu, Q. Effect of carotene and lycopene on the risk of prostate cancer: A systematic review and dose-Response meta-analysis of observational studies. *PLoS ONE* **2015**, *10*, e0137427. [CrossRef]
39. Gontero, P.; Marra, G.; Soria, F.; Oderda, M.; Zitella, A.; Baratta, F.; Chiorino, G.; Gregnanin, I.; Daniele, L.; Cattel, L.; et al. A randomized double-blind placebo controlled phase I-II study of clinical and molecular effects of dietary supplements in men with precancerous prostatic lesions. Chemoprevention or "Chemopromotion"? *Prostate* **2015**, *75*, 1177–1186. [CrossRef]
40. Barber, N.J.; Zhang, X.; Zhu, G.; Pramanik, R.; Barber, J.A.; Martin, F.L.; Morris, J.D.; Muir, G.H. Lycopene inhibits DNA synthesis in a primary prostate epithelial cells in vitro and its administration is associated with a reduced prostate-specific antigen velocity in a phase II clinical study. *Prostate Cancer Prostatic Dis.* **2006**, *9*, 407–413. [CrossRef]

41. Kucuk, O.; Sarkar, F.H.; Sakr, W.; Djuric, Z.; Pollak, M.N.; Khachik, F.; Li, Y.W.; Banerjee, M.; Grignon, D.; Bertram, J.S.; et al. Phase II randomized clinical trial of lycopene supplementation before radical prostatectomy. *Cancer Epidemiol. Biomark. Prev.* **2001**, *10*, 861–868.
42. Vance, T.A.; Azabdaftari, G.; Pop, E.A.; Lee, S.G.; Su, L.J.; Fontham, E.T.H.; Bensen, J.T.; Steck, S.E.; Arab, L.; Mohler, J.L.; et al. Intake of dietary antioxidants is inversely associated with biomarkers of oxidative stress among men with prostate cancer. *Br. J. Nutr.* **2016**, *115*, 68–74. [CrossRef]
43. Marques-Vidal, P.; Ravasco, P.; Ermelinda Camilo, M. Foodstuffs and colorectal cancer risk: A review. *Clin. Nutr.* **2006**, *25*, 14–36. [CrossRef] [PubMed]
44. Nkondjock, A.; Ghadirian, P. Dietary carotenoids and risk of colon cancer: Case-control study. *Int. J. Cancer* **2004**, *110*, 110–116. [CrossRef] [PubMed]
45. Park, S.-Y.; Nomura, A.M.Y.; Murphy, S.P.; Wilkens, L.R.; Henderson, B.E.; Kolonel, L.N. Carotenoid intake and colorectal cancer risk: The multi-ethnic cohort study. *J. Epidemiol.* **2009**, *19*, 63–71. [CrossRef]
46. Huang, J.; Lu, M.-S.; Fang, Y.-J.; Xu, M.; Huang, W.Q.; Pan, Z.-Z.; Chen, Y.M.; Zhang, C.X. Serum carotenoids and colorectal cancer risk: A case-control study in Guandong, China. *Mol. Nutr. Food Res.* **2017**, *61*. [CrossRef]
47. Green, A.; Williams, G.; Neale, R.; Hart, V.; Leslie, D.; Parsons, P.; Marks, G.C.; Gaffney, P.; Battistuta, D.; Frost, C.; et al. A daily sunscreen application and beta carotene supplementation in prevention of basal-cell and squamous-cell carcinomas of the skin: A randomized trial. *Lancet* **1999**, *354*, 723–729. [CrossRef]
48. Greenberg, E.R.; Baron, J.A.; Karagas, M.R.; Stukel, T.A.; Nierenberg, D.W.; Stevens, M.M.; Mandel, J.S.; Haile, R.W. Mortality associated with low plasma concentration of beta carotene and the effect of oral supplementation. *JAMA* **1996**, *275*, 699–703. [CrossRef]
49. Karagas, M.R.; Greenberg, E.R.; Nierenberg, D.; Stukel, T.A.; Morris, J.S.; Stevens, M.M.; Baron, J.A. Risk of squamous cell carcinoma of the skin in relation to plasma selenium, α-tocopherol, β-carotene, and retinol: A nested case-control study. *Cancer Epidemiol. Biomark. Prev.* **1997**, *6*, 25–29.
50. Stryker, W.S.; Stampfer, M.J.; Stein, E.A.; Kaplan, L.; Louis, T.A.; Sober, A.; Willett, W.C. Diet, plasma levels of β-carotene and alpha-tocopherol, and risk of malignant melanoma. *Am. J. Epidemiol.* **1990**, *131*, 597–611. [CrossRef]
51. Kiripatrick, C.S.; White, E.; Lee, J.A.H. Case-control study of malignant melanoma in Washington State. *Am. J. Epidemiol.* **1994**, *139*, 869–880. [CrossRef]
52. Breslow, R.A.; Alberg, A.J.; Helzlsouer, K.J.; Bush, T.L.; Norkus, E.P.; Morris, J.S.; Spate, V.E.; Comstock, G.W. Serological precursors of cancer: Malignant melanoma, basal and squamous cell skin cancer, and prediagnostic levels of retinol, β-carotene, lycopene, α-tocopherol, and selenium. *Cancer Epidemiol. Biomark. Prev.* **1995**, *4*, 837–842.
53. Bayerl, C.; Schwarz, B.; Jung, E.G. Beneficial effect of β-carotene in dysplastic nevus syndrome—A randomized trial (abstract 068). In Proceedings of the 8th Congress of the European Society for Photobiology, Granada, Spain, 3–8 September 1999; p. 89.
54. Druesne-Pecollo, N.; Latino-Martel, P.; Norat, T.; Barradon, E.; Bertrais, S.; Galan, P.; Hercberg, S. Beta-carotene supplementation and cancer risk: A systematic review and metaanalysis of randomized controlled trials. *Int. J. Cancer* **2010**, *127*, 172–184. [CrossRef] [PubMed]
55. Black, H.S.; Lambert, C.R. Radical reactions of carotenoids and potential influence of UV carcinogenesis. In *Oxidants and Antioxidants in Cutaneous Biology*; Thiele, J., Elsner, P., Eds.; Karger: Basel, Switzerland, 2001; Volume 29, pp. 140–156.
56. The α-Tocopherol, β-Carotene Cancer Prevention Study Group. The effect of vitamin E and β-carotene on the incidence of lung cancer and other cancers in male smokers. *N. Engl. J. Med.* **1996**, *330*, 1029–1035.
57. Omenn, G.S. Chemoprevention of lung cancer: The rise and demise of beta-carotene. *Ann. Rev. Public Health* **1998**, *19*, 73–99. [CrossRef] [PubMed]
58. Bayerl, C. Beta-carotene in dermatology: Does it help? *Acta Dermatoven APA* **2008**, *17*, 160–166.
59. Landrum, J.T.; Bone, R.A.; Moore, L.L.; Gomez, C.M. Analysis of zeaxanthin distribution within individual human retinas. *Methods Enzymol.* **1999**, *299*, 457–467. [PubMed]
60. Holz, F.G.; Pauleikhoff, D.; Spaide, R.F.; Bird, A.C. (Eds.) *Age-Related Macular Degeneration*; Springer: Berlin/Heidelberg, Germany, 2013.

61. Mathews-Roth, M.M.; Pathak, M.A.; Parrish, J.; Fitzpatrick, T.B.; Kass, E.H.; Toda, K.; Clemens, W. A clinical trial of the effects of beta-carotene on the responses of human skin to solar radiation. *J. Investig. Dermatol.* **1972**, *59*, 349–353. [CrossRef] [PubMed]
62. Mathews-Roth, M.M.; Pathak, M.A. Phytoene as a protective agent against sunburn (>280 nm) radiation in guinea pigs. *Photochem. Photobiol.* **1975**, *21*, 261–263. [CrossRef]
63. Epstein, J.H. Effects of β-carotene on UV-induced skin cancer formation in the hairless mouse skin. *Photochem. Photobiol.* **1977**, *25*, 211–213. [CrossRef]
64. Santamaria, L.; Bianchi, A.; Arnaboldi, A.; Andreoni, L. Prevention of benzo(α)-pyrene photocarcinogenic effect by β-carotene and canthaxanthin. *Med. Biol. Environ.* **1981**, *9*, 113–120.
65. Mathews-Roth, M.M. Antitumor activity of β-carotene, canthaxanthin, and phytoene. *Oncology* **1982**, *38*, 33–37. [CrossRef]
66. Mathews-Roth, M.M. Carotenoid pigment administration and delay in development of UV-B-induced tumors. *Photochem. Photobiol.* **1983**, *37*, 509–511. [CrossRef] [PubMed]
67. Mathews, M.M.; Krinsky, N.I. Carotenoids affect development of UV-B induced skin cancer. *Photochem. Photobiol.* **1987**, *46*, 507–509. [CrossRef] [PubMed]
68. Mathews-Roth, M.M.; Krinsky, N.I. Carotenoid dose level and protection against UV-B- induced skin tumors. *Photochem. Photobiol.* **1985**, *42*, 35–38. [CrossRef] [PubMed]
69. Gensler, H.L.; Aickin, M.; Peng, Y.M. Cumulative reduction of primary skin tumor growth in UV-irradiated mice by the combination of retinyl palmitate and canthaxanthin. *Cancer Lett.* **1990**, *53*, 27–31. [CrossRef]
70. Rybski, J.A.; Grogan, T.M.; Gensler, H.L. Reduction of murine cutaneous UVB-induced tumor-inflitrating T lymphocytes by dietary canthaxanthin. *J. Investig. Dermatol.* **1991**, *97*, 892–897. [CrossRef]
71. Black, H.S. Radical interception by carotenoids and effects on UV carcinogenesis. *Nutr. Cancer* **1998**, *31*, 212–217. [CrossRef]
72. Black, H.S.; Okotie-Eboh, G.; Gerguis, J. Aspects of β-carotene-potentiated photocarcinogenesis. *Photochem. Photobiol.* **1999**, *69*, 32S.
73. Black, H.S. Reassessment of a free radical theory of cancer with emphasis on ultraviolet carcinogenesis. *Integr. Cancer Ther.* **2004**, *3*, 279–293. [CrossRef]
74. Black, H.S.; Okotie-Eboh, G.; Gerguis, J. Diet potentiates the UV-carcinogenic response to β-carotene. *Nutr. Cancer* **2000**, *37*, 173–178. [CrossRef]
75. Burton, G.W.; Ingold, K.U. β-carotene: An unusual type of lipid antioxidant. *Science* **1984**, *224*, 569–573. [CrossRef]
76. *Nutrient Requirements of Laboratory Animals*, 3rd ed.; Research Council/National Academy of Science: Washington, DC, USA, 1978; pp. 38–53.
77. Black, H.S. Pro-carcinogenic activity of β-carotene, a putative systemic photoprotectant. *Photochem. Photobiol. Sci.* **2004**, *3*, 753–758. [CrossRef] [PubMed]
78. Black, H.S.; Gerguis, J. Modulation of dietary vitamins E and C fails to ameliorate β-carotene exacerbation of UV Carcinogenesis in mice. *Nutr. Cancer* **2003**, *45*, 36–45. [CrossRef] [PubMed]
79. Black, H.S. Interaction of ascorbic acid and tocopherol on β-carotene modulated carcinogenesis. *Hemoglobin* **2010**, *34*, 284–290. [CrossRef] [PubMed]
80. Black, H.S.; Edge, R.; Truscott, T.G. β-carotene: Radical reactions and cancer associations – leading down a rabbit hole? *J. Integr. Oncol.* **2018**, *7*, 3. [CrossRef]
81. *Food, Nutrition, Physical Activity, and the Prevention of Cancer: A Global Perspective*; A Project of the World Cancer Research Fund/American Institute for Cancer Research (AICR): Washington, DC, USA, 2007.
82. Kanofsky, J.R. Singlet oxygen production by biological systems. *Chem. Biol. Interact.* **1989**, *70*, 1–28. [CrossRef]
83. Klotz, L.-O.; Kröncke, K.-D.; Sies, H. Singlet oxygen-induced signalling effects in mammalian cells. *Photochem. Photobiol. Sci.* **2003**, *2*, 88–94. [CrossRef]
84. Böhm, F.; Edge, R.; Truscott, T.G. Interactions of dietary carotenoids with activated (singlet) oxygen and free radicals: Potential effects for human health. *Mol. Nutr. Food Res.* **2012**, *56*, 205–216. [CrossRef]
85. Oliveros, E.; Braun, A.M.; Aminian-Saghafi, T.; Sliwka, H.-R. Quenching of singlet oxygen ($^1\Delta_g$) by carotenoid derivatives: Kinetic analysis by near-infrared luminescence. *New J. Chem.* **1994**, *18*, 535–539.
86. Edge, R.; McGarvey, D.J.; Truscott, T.G. The carotenoids as antioxidants—A review. *J. Photochem. Photobiol. B Biol.* **1997**, *41*, 189–200. [CrossRef]

87. Teraoka, J.; Hashimoto, H.; Matsudaira, S.; Koyama, Y. Resonance Raman spectra of excited triplet states of β-carotene isomers. *Chem. Lett.* **1985**, *14*, 311–314. [CrossRef]
88. Heymann, T.; Heinz, P.; Glomb, M.A. Lycopene inhibits the isomerization of β-carotene during quenching of singlet oxygen and free radicals. *J. Agric. Food. Chem.* **2015**, *63*, 3279–3287. [CrossRef] [PubMed]
89. Mukai, K.; Ouchi, A.; Azuma, N.; Takahashi, S.; Aizawa, K.; Nagaoka, S. Development of a singlet oxygen absorption capacity (SOAC) assay method. Measurements of the SOAC values for carotenoids and α-tocopherol in an aqueous Triton X-100 micellar solution. *J. Agric. Food Chem.* **2017**, *65*, 784–792. [CrossRef] [PubMed]
90. Cantrell, A.; McGarvey, D.J.; Truscott, T.G. Singlet oxygen quenching by dietary carotenoids in a model membrance environment. *Arch. Biochem. Biophys.* **2003**, *412*, 47–54. [CrossRef]
91. Fukuzawa, K. Singlet oxygen scavenging in phospholipid membranes. *Methods Enzymol.* **2000**, *319*, 101–110. [PubMed]
92. Fukuzawa, K.; Inokami, Y.; Tokumura, A.; Terao, J.; Suzuki, A. Rate constants for quenching singlet oxygen and activities for inhibiting lipid peroxidation of carotenoids and α-tocopherol in liposomes. *Lipids* **1998**, *33*, 751–756. [CrossRef]
93. Lindig, B.A.; Rodgers, M.A.J. Rate parameters for the quenching of singlet oxygen by water-soluble and lipid-soluble substrates in aqueous and micellar systems. *Photochem. Photobiol.* **1981**, *33*, 627–634. [CrossRef]
94. Edge, R. Spectroscopic and Kinetic Investigations of Carotenoid Radical Ions and Excited States. Ph.D. Thesis, Keele University, Keele, UK, 1998.
95. Morita, M.; Naito, Y.; Yoshikawa, T.; Niki, E. Rapid assessment of singlet oxygen-induced plasma lipid oxidation and its inhibition by antioxidants with diphenyl-1-pyrenylphosphine (DPPP). *Anal. Bioanal. Chem.* **2016**, *408*, 265–270. [CrossRef]
96. Sachindra, N.M.; Sato, E.; Maeda, H.; Hosokawa, M.; Niwano, Y.; Kohno, M.; Miyashita, K. Radical scavenging and singlet oxygen quenching activity of marine carotenoid fucoxanthin and its metabolites. *J. Agric. Food Chem.* **2007**, *55*, 8516–8522. [CrossRef]
97. Böehm, F.; Haley, J.; Truscott, T.G.; Schalch, W. Cellular bound β-carotene quenches singlet oxygen in man. *J. Photochem. Photobiol. B Biol.* **1993**, *21*, 219–221. [CrossRef]
98. Conn, P.F.; Schalch, W.; Truscott, T.G. The singlet oxygen and carotenoid interaction. *J. Photochem. Photobiol. B Biol.* **1991**, *11*, 41–47. [CrossRef]
99. Tinkler, J.H.; Böhm, F.; Schalch, W.; Truscott, T.G. Dietary carotenoids protect human cells from damage. *J. Photochem. Photobiol. B Biol.* **1994**, *26*, 283–285. [CrossRef]
100. Boehm, F.; Edge, R.; Burke, M.; Truscott, T.G. Dietary uptake of lycopene protects human cells from singlet oxygen and nitrogen dioxide - ROS components from cigarette smoke. *J. Photochem. Photobiol. B Biol.* **2001**, *64*, 176–178. [CrossRef]
101. Bosio, G.N.; Breitenbach, T.; Parisi, J.; Reigosa, M.; Blaikie, F.H.; Pedersen, B.W.; Silva, E.F.F.; Martire, D.O.; Ogilby, P.R. Antioxidant β-carotene does not quench singlet oxygen in mammalian cells. *J. Am. Chem. Soc.* **2013**, *135*, 272–279. [CrossRef] [PubMed]
102. Macpherson, A.N.; Telfer, A.; Truscott, T.G.; Barber, J. Direct detection of singlet oxygen from isolated photosystem two reaction centres. *Biochim. Biophys. Acta* **1993**, *1143*, 301–309. [CrossRef]
103. Harayama, O.; Nakamura, K.; Hamada, S.; Kobayasi, Y. Singlet oxygen quenching ability of naturally occurring carotenoids. *Lipids* **1994**, *29*, 149–150. [CrossRef] [PubMed]
104. Telfer, A. Singlet oxygen production by PSII under light stress: Mechanism, detection and the protective role of β-carotene. *Plant Cell Physiol.* **2014**, *55*, 1216–1223. [CrossRef] [PubMed]
105. Telfer, A.; Dhami, S.; Bishop, S.M.; Phillips, D.; Barber, J. β-carotene quenches singlet oxygen formed by isolated photosystem II reaction centres. *Biochemistry* **1994**, *33*, 14469–14474. [CrossRef]
106. Rossetti, F.C.; Depieri, L.V.; Tedesco, A.C.; Bentley, M.V.L.B. Fluorometric quantification of protoporphyrin IX in biological skin samples from in vitro penetration/permeation studies. *Braz. J. Pharm. Sci.* **2010**, *46*, 753–760. [CrossRef]
107. Palozza, P.; Krinsky, N.I. Antioxidant effects of carotenoids in vivo and in vitro: An overview. *Methods Enzymol.* **1992**, *23*, 403–422.
108. Góralczyk, R. β-Carotene and lung cancer in smokers: Review of hypotheses and status of research. *Nutr. Cancer* **2009**, *61*, 767–774. [CrossRef]

109. Schwarz, J.I.; Singh, R.P.; Teicher, B.; Wright, J.E.; Trites, D.H.; Shklar, G. Induction of a 70 kD protein associated with the selective cytotoxicity of beta-carotene in human epidermal carcinoma. *Biochem. Biophys. Res. Commun.* **1990**, *29*, 941–946. [CrossRef]
110. Fung, T.T.; Spiegelman, D.; Egan, K.M.; Giovannucci, E.; Hunter, D.J.; Willett, W.C. Vitamin and carotenoid intake and risk of squamous cell carcinoma of the skin. *Int. J. Cancer* **2003**, *103*, 110–115. [CrossRef] [PubMed]
111. Cesarini, J.P.; Michel, L.; Maurette, M.; Adhoute, H.; Bejot, M. Immediate effects of UV radiation on the skin: Modification by an antioxidant complex containing carotenoids. *Photoderm. Photoimmunol. Photomed.* **2003**, *19*, 182–189. [CrossRef] [PubMed]
112. Yeum, K.-J.; Beretta, G.; Krinsky, I.N.; Russell, R.M.; Aldini, G. Synergistic Interactions of Antioxidant Nutrients in a Biological Model system. *Nutrition* **2009**, *25*, 839–846. [CrossRef]
113. Balić, A.; Mokos, M. Do we utilize our knowledge of the skin protective effects of carotenoids enough? *Antioxidants* **2019**, *8*, 259. [CrossRef] [PubMed]
114. Davinelli, S.; Nielsen, M.E.; Giovanni Scapagnini, G. Astaxanthin in skin health, repair, and disease: A comprehensive review. *Nutrients* **2018**, *10*, 522. [CrossRef]
115. Juin, C.; de Olivera Junior, R.G.; Fleury, A.; Oudinet, C.; Pytowski, L.; Bérard, J.-B.; Nicolau, E.; Thiéry, V.; Lanneluc, I.; Beaugeard, L.; et al. Zeaxanthin from *Porphtridium purpureum* induces apoptosis in human melanoma cells expressing the oncogegnic BRAF V600E mutation and sensitizes them to the BRAF inhibitor vemurafenib. *Rev. Bras. Farmacogn.* **2018**, *28*, 457–467. [CrossRef]
116. Wu, N.-L.; Chiang, Y.-C.; Huang, C.-C.; Fang, J.-Y.; Chen, D.-F.; Hung, C.-F. Zeaxanthin inhibits PDGF-BB-induced migration in human dermal fibroblasts. *Exp. Dermatol.* **2010**, *19*, e173–e181. [CrossRef]
117. Suzukawaa, A.A.; Vieiraa, A.; Winnischofer, S.M.B.; Scalfob, A.C.; Di Mascio, P.; da Costa Ferreira, A.M.; Ravanat, J.-L.; de Luna Martinse, D.; Rocha, M.E.M.; Martinez, G.R. Novel properties of melanin include promotion of DNA strand breaks, impairment of repair, and reduced ability to damage DNA after quenching of singlet oxygen. *Free Radic. Biol. Med.* **2012**, *52*, 1945–1953. [CrossRef]
118. Sarna, T.; Menon, I.A.; Sealy, R.C. Photosensitization of melanin: A comparative study. *Photochem. Photobiol.* **1985**, *42*, 529–532. [CrossRef]
119. Rozanowska, M.; Sarna, T.; Land, E.J.; Truscott, T.G. Free radical scavenging properties of melanin: Interaction of eu- and pheo-melanin models with reducing and oxidizing radicals. *Free Radic. Biol. Med.* **1999**, *26*, 518–525. [CrossRef]
120. Mares-Perlman, J.A.; Brady, W.; Klein, R.; Klein, B.; Bowen, P.; Stacewiczsapuntzakis, M.; Palta, M. Serum antioxidants and age-related macular degeneration in a population-based case-control study. *Arch. Ophthalmol.* **1995**, *113*, 1518–1523. [CrossRef] [PubMed]
121. Simonelli, F.; Zarrilli, F.; Mazzeo, S.; Verde, V.; Romano, N.; Savoia, M.; Testa, F.; Vitale, D.F.; Rinaldi, M.; Sacchetti, L. Serum oxidative and antioxidant parameters in a group of Italian patients with age-related maculopathy. *Clin. Chim. Acta* **2002**, *320*, 111–115. [CrossRef]
122. Cardinault, N.; Abalain, J.-H.; Sairafi, B.; Coudray, C.; Grolier, P.; Rambeau, M.; Carré, J.-C. Lycopene but not lutein nor zeaxanthin decreases in serum and lipoproteins in age-related macular degeneration patients. *Clin. Chim. Acta* **2005**, *357*, 34–42. [CrossRef]
123. Li, B.; Bernstein, P.S. Macular pigment carotenoids and their role in human eye health and diseases. In *Studies on Retinal and Choridal Disorders, Oxidative Stress in Applied Basic Research and Clinical Practice*; Stratton, R.D., Hauswirth, W.W., Gardner, T.W., Eds.; Springer: New York, NY, USA, 2012; Chapter 31, pp. 613–627.
124. Galano, A.; Vargas, V.; Martinez, A. Carotenoids can act as antioxidants by oxidising the superoxide radical anion. *Phys. Chem. Chem. Phys.* **2010**, *12*, 193–200. [CrossRef]
125. Boehm, F.; Edge, R.; Truscott, T.G.; Witt, C. A dramatic effect of oxygen on protection of human cells against -radiation by lycopene. *FEBS Lett.* **2016**, *590*, 1086–1093. [CrossRef]
126. Land, E.J.; Lafferty, J.; Roach, A.C.; Sinclair, R.S.; Truscott, T.G. Absorption spectra of radical ions of polyenes of biological interest. *J. Chem. Soc. Faraday Trans.* **1977**, *73*, 416–429.
127. Edge, R.; Land, E.J.; McGarvey, D.J.; Burke, M.; Truscott, T.G. The reduction potential of the β-carotene$\bullet^{+}$/β-carotene couple in an aqueous micro-heterogeneous environment. *FEBS Lett.* **2000**, *471*, 125–127. [CrossRef]
128. Burke, M.; Edge, R.; Land, E.J.; McGarvey, D.J.; Truscott, T.G. One-electron reduction potentials of dietary carotenoid radical cations in aqueous micellar environments. *FEBS Lett.* **2001**, *500*, 132–136. [CrossRef]

129. Tinkler, J.H.; Tavender, S.M.; Parker, A.W.; McGarvey, D.J.; Mulroy, L.; Truscott, T.G. An investigation of carotenoid radical cations and triplet states by laser flash photolysis and time-resolved resonance Raman spectroscopy: Observation of competitive energy and electron transfer. *J. Am. Chem. Soc.* **1996**, *118*, 1756–1761. [CrossRef]
130. Cheng, H.; Han, R.-M.; Lyu, M.-K.; Zhang, J.-P.; Skibsted, L.H. Regeneration of β-carotene from the radical cation by tyrosine and tryptophan. *J. Phys. Chem. B* **2015**, *119*, 6603–6610. [CrossRef] [PubMed]
131. Chang, H.-T.; Cheng, H.; Han, R.-M.; Wang, P.; Zhang, J.-P.; Skibsted, L.H. Regeneration of β-carotene from radical cation by eugenol, isoeugenol, and clove oil in the Marcus theory inverted region for electron transfer. *J. Agric. Food Chem.* **2017**, *65*, 908–912. [CrossRef] [PubMed]
132. Mairanovsky, V.G.; Engovatov, A.A.; Ioffe, N.T.; Samokhvalov, G.I. Electron-donor and electron-acceptor properties of carotenoids: Electrochemical study of carotenes. *J. Electroanal. Chem.* **1975**, *66*, 122–137. [CrossRef]
133. Focsan, A.L.; Pan, S.; Kispert, L.D. Electrochemical study of astaxanthin and astaxanthinn-octanoic monoester and diester: Tendency to form radicals. *J. Phys. Chem. B* **2014**, *118*, 2331–3229. [CrossRef] [PubMed]
134. Ding, R.; Grant, J.L.; Metzger, R.M.; Kispert, L.D. Carotenoid radical cations produced by the interaction of carotenoids with iodine. *J. Am. Chem. Soc.* **1988**, *92*, 4600–4606. [CrossRef]
135. Edge, R.; El-Agamey, A.; Land, E.J.; Navaratnam, S.; Truscott, T.G. Studies of carotenoid one-electron reduction radicals. *Arch. Biochem. Biophys.* **2007**, *458*, 104–110. [CrossRef]
136. Edge, R.; Land, E.J.; McGarvey, D.; Mulroy, L.; Truscott, T.G. Relative one- electron reduction potentials of carotenoid radical cations and interactions of carotenoids with the vitamin E radical cation. *J. Am. Chem. Soc.* **1998**, *120*, 4087–4090. [CrossRef]
137. Boehm, F.; Edge, R.; Land, E.J.; McGarvey, D.J.; Truscott, T.G. Carotenoids enhance vitamin E antioxidant efficiency. *J. Am. Chem. Soc.* **1997**, *119*, 621–622. [CrossRef]
138. Rao, A.V.; Agarwal, S. Role of lycopene as an antioxidant carotenoid in the prevention of chronic diseases: A review. *Nutr. Res.* **1999**, *19*, 305–323. [CrossRef]
139. Edge, R.; Truscott, T.G. Singlet oxygen and free radical reactions of retinoids and carotenoids—A Review. *Antioxidants* **2018**, *7*, 5. [CrossRef]
140. Hill, T.J.; Land, E.J.; McGarvey, D.J.; Schalch, W.; Tinkler, J.H.; Truscott, T.G. Interactions between carotenoids and the CCl_3O_2• radical. *J. Am. Chem. Soc.* **1995**, *117*, 8322–8326. [CrossRef]
141. Edge, R. Radiolytic and Photolytic Production of Free Radicals and Reactive Oxygen Species: Interactions with Antioxidants and Biomolecules. In *Applied Photochemistry*; Evans, R., Douglas, P., Burrow, H., Eds.; Springer: Dordrecht, The Netherlands, 2013; Chapter 8, pp. 305–330.
142. Halliwall, B.; Gutteridge, J.M.C. Role of free radicals in human disease: An overview. In *Methods in Enzymology, Vol 186 Oxygen Radicals in Biological Systems, Part B Oxygen Radicals and Antioxidants*; Academic Press: San Diego, CA, USA, 2000; pp. 1–85.
143. Edge, R.; Land, E.J.; Rozanowska, M.; Sarna, T.; Truscott, T.G. Carotenoid radical – melanin interactions. *J. Phys. Chem. B* **2000**, *104*, 7193–7196. [CrossRef]
144. Rock, C.L. Relationship of Carotenoids to Cancer. In *Carotenoids in Health and Disease*; Krinsky, N.I., Mayne, S.T., Sies, H., Eds.; Marcel Dekker: New York, NY, USA, 2004; Chapter 17; pp. 373–407.
145. Anderson, H.J.; Chen, H.; Pellet, L.J.; Tappel, A.L. Ferrous-iron-induced oxidation in chicken liver slices as measured by hemichrome formation and thiobarbituric acid-reactive substances: Effects of dietary vitamin E and beta-carotene. *Free Radic. Biol. Med.* **1993**, *15*, 37–48. [CrossRef]
146. Truscott, T.G. β-carotene and disease: A suggested pro-oxidant and antioxidant mechanism and speculations concerning its role in cigarette smoking. *J. Photochem. Photobiol. B* **1996**, *35*, 233–235. [CrossRef]
147. Edge, R.; Truscott, T.G. Carotenoids: Free radical reactions. *Spectrum* **2000**, *13*, 12–20.

2

Determinants and Suitability of Carotenoid Reflection Score as a Measure of Carotenoid Status

Elaine Rush [1,2,*], Isaac Amoah [1,2], Tung Diep [1,2] and Shabnam Jalili-Moghaddam [1]

1 Faculty of Health and Environmental Studies, Auckland University of Technology, Auckland 1142, New Zealand; isaac.amoah@aut.ac.nz (I.A.); tung.diep@aut.ac.nz (T.D.); shabnam.jalili@aut.ac.nz (S.J.-M.)
2 Riddet Centre of Research Excellence, Palmerston North 0632, New Zealand
* Correspondence: elaine.rush@aut.ac.nz

Abstract: Carotenoids, orange-coloured pigments found in vegetables, fruit, eggs and dairy foods, act as antioxidants and vitamin A precursors in the human body. Skin carotenoid concentration is a biomarker of vegetable and fruit intake. The aim was to identify determinants of skin carotenoid concentration by measuring "Veggie Meter™" carotenoid reflection spectroscopy scores (CRS) from the fingertip of adults with a range of ages, ethnicity and body size. Frequencies of daily intake of vegetables and fruit and weekly intake of pumpkin and carrot, dark green leafy vegetables (DGLV), eggs (yolk), and dairy were determined from a self-completed food-frequency-questionnaire. A total of 571 (324 Women, 247 Men) adults, aged 16 to 85 years, completed measurements. The CRS ranged from 83 to 769, with a median of 327. Women and men did not score differently. For all participants there were negative correlations of CRS with weight ($r = -0.312$) and BMI ($r = -0.338$) and positive correlations with weekly intakes of DGLV ($r = 0.242$) and carrots and pumpkin ($r = 0.202$). Based on a review of health outcomes associated with plasma carotenoids, 82% of the participants in the current study are at moderate risk, or more, of negative health outcomes. Determinants of carotenoid status were body size, intake of DGLV, carrots and pumpkin, and ethnicity.

Keywords: vegetable and fruit intake; carotenoids; biomarker; Veggie Meter™

---

1. Introduction

A recent systematic review and meta-analysis [1] of 95 prospective studies has established a strong association between the reported consumption of vegetables and fruits with reduced incidence of chronic diseases, including diabetes, hypertension, coronary heart diseases and cancers. Globally, food-based dietary guidelines [2] encourage an increase in the quantity and variety of vegetables and fruit consumed because they are micronutrient-dense, rich in fibre and contain many phytochemicals with health-promoting bioactivity. The consumption of more vegetables than fruits is encouraged. The measurement errors in self-reports of dietary intakes, including fruits and vegetables, are additive and it is important to validate reports with the use of biomarkers [3].

Carotenoids, including beta carotene, alpha carotene, lycopene, lutein and xanthophylls are orange pigments ubiquitous in vegetables. Fruits [4] and some animal products such as eggs and dairy contribute provitamin A, antioxidant and chemoprotective components to the diet. Carotenoids are found mainly in vegetables [5,6]. For example, carrot, kale, spinach and pumpkin are good sources of beta carotene, corn contains lutein, and tomato is a good source of lycopene [7].

In New Zealand there is the ability to grow and market vegetables and fruits throughout the year. Yet, in the annual health survey only one third of respondents report that they consume 3 or more servings of vegetables plus 2 or more servings of fruit each day [8]. In addition, the same survey based on measures of height and weight records that the prevalence in adults of obesity and overweight is 34% and 31% respectively. Overweight and obesity are forms of malnutrition and may coexist with micronutrient deficiencies. While the frequency of vegetable and fruit intake is subjectively assessed by the Ministry of Health every year, these reports of vegetable and fruit intake have not been validated with a biomarker.

Concentrations of carotenoids in plasma are well established as biomarkers of vegetable and fruit intake [9–11]. Noninvasive point-of-care determination of carotenoid concentration is of benefit to individuals and health professionals. Advantages are convenience, less expense and time and the immediate opportunity to discuss the measurement with the individual. One such test for carotenoids is a measure of skin colour, also shown to be a valid and reliable biomarker for vegetable and fruit intakes [12,13]. Skin colour measurement by reflection spectroscopy is the principle of the "Veggie Meter™", a relatively small, portable instrument that interfaces with a dedicated laptop computer. The tip of the finger is pressed lightly over the head of a white light probe to momentarily remove the blood from the finger-tip, and the reflected light is then measured. This relatively rapid measurement, less than 15 s, enables immediate feedback and interpretation of the measurement to the individual. The device has been used to evaluate carotenoid reflection scores (CRS) of participants in the United States of America [14] and Japan [15] but not in New Zealand.

This study aimed to profile and identify determinants of fingertip CRS in women and men of five ethnic groups with a range of age, body size and self-reported intake of foods including vegetables and fruits containing carotenoids.

2. Materials and Methods

2.1. Setting and Participants

This cross-sectional study of members of diverse community groups selected to represent a convenience sample that varied by age, ethnicity and socioeconomic status determined by geographic location. For a prediction equation with three predictors and based on a moderate effect size of 0.15, a power of 0.80, and a probability level of 0.05, it was determined that the minimum sample size would be 76. Thirteen sites in Auckland and Hamilton, New Zealand responded to an invitation to take part. In all, 44% of participants were from 9 workplaces, 39% staff and students from the three campuses of the Auckland University of Technology and 17% from community groups such as Rotary Clubs. The Auckland University of Technology Ethics Committee provided ethical approval 18/420. Inclusion criteria were that participants were aged 16 years or more and able to give informed consent. Intentionally, to increase the diversity of the participants there were no further exclusion criteria. The main benefit to the participants was an immediate measurement of carotenoid status and general education about vegetable and fruit consumption. A total of 571 participants were measured by researchers with expertise in nutrition. All participants provided informed signed consent before taking part. Age, gender, smoking status, self-identified ethnic group and their self-reported height and weight were provided on a one-page questionnaire which also included questions about diet and supplement use.

2.2. Measurement of Carotenoid-Containing Food Intake

A 6-item food frequency questionnaire asked two questions from the annual national health survey about how many servings of vegetables and fruit were eaten in one day [16]. Daily servings of vegetables and fruit were summed. Specific questions concerning how many servings of carrot and pumpkin, dark green leafy vegetables, eggs (yolk) and dairy foods were eaten in one week were asked. These specific foods were selected because they are the most frequently consumed foods in the New Zealand diet that are significant sources of carotenoids [7].

2.3. Measurement of Skin Carotenoid Concentration

Pressure-mediated "Veggie Meter™" CRS (Longevity Link Corporation, Salt Lake City, UT, USA) were determined. The various carotenoid compounds—beta-carotene, lycopene, lutein, zeaxanthin, beta-crytoxanthin—and all isomers of these compounds generate a very similar yellow coloration that can be detected and quantified by the Veggie Meter. The manufacturer instructions were followed and the surface of the contact lens was regularly cleaned with an optical cloth. The instrument was calibrated prior to any measurements and every hour using the dark and white reference wedges provided by the manufacturer. After firmly wiping the fat pad at the tip of the right-hand index finger with a water-moistened swab, the finger-tip was dried and inserted into the finger port so that the tip was pressed over the contact lens. The finger was held gently in place by a spring-loaded clip. The CRS was recorded as the average of three consecutive measurements for each participant. The finger was removed from the port between measurements to allow reperfusion. If the average score was less than 250 or there was any irregularity, the measurements were repeated.

In a separate study, from 10 participants on three different occasions, blood was sampled at the same time as the CRS measurement, with the same Veggie Meter used for this study. Plasma carotenoids were measured by spectroscopy (Cary 400, Agilent Technologies, Victoria, Australia) at the Christchurch Health Laboratories (CHL). They reported plasma carotenoid concentration in μmol/L; laboratory reference range 1.5 to 3.0 μmol/L. Regression of the CRS against the plasma measure resulted in the equation: CHL concentration μmol/L = 0.0055 × CRS + 0.0197, SEE = 0.439 r^2 = 0.72. The equivalent reference range for the CRS was therefore 286 to 480. However, given the relatively wide 95% CI of the mean at these values, the "healthy" reference range for communication with the participants was set at 250 to 530 and we termed this a screening test. In other words, if the CRS was less than 250, we actively encouraged consumption of more vegetables and fruit, and if more than 530 we endorsed that they were eating, and should continue to eat, plenty of carotenoid-containing foods.

2.4. Statistical Analysis

Categorical variables are reported as count and prevalence (%). Where more than one ethnic group was identified by a participant, ethnic group was prioritized in the order Maori, Pacific, Asian (China and South East Asia); South Asian, European and other (Middle Eastern, African, Latin American). Continuous variables were checked for normality and are reported as mean, standard deviation and range. Comparisons by gender, ethnicity and age were assessed by unpaired t-test and ANOVA. Correlation was determined by visual inspection of scatter plots and Pearson r. Determinants of the CRS, previously identified by simple correlation, were entered stepwise, forward and backward into multiple regression to find the best combination of predictors. The absence of collinearity was confirmed by Variance Inflation Factors < 2. A regression equation was derived where CRS = β1 × determinant1 + β2 × determinant2 + β3 × determinant3. The β coefficients are the degree of change of CRS for one unit of change for the variable. The change in R^2, the multiple correlation coefficient of determination, was used to determine how much variance in the dependent variable (CRS) was accounted for with the addition of each determinant. Analyses were performed with IBM SPSS statistics software (version 25.0, IBM Corp., Armonk, New York, NY, USA).

3. Results

3.1. Participant Characteristics and Carotenoid Reflection Scores

In total, 571 participants were measured—324 women and 247 men. Of these, 6.7% self-identified their priority ethnicity as Maori, 14.7% as Pacific, 17.3% as Asian, 12.6% as South Asian, 41.0% as European, and 7.7% as other (Middle Eastern, African, Latin American). The average age was 39 ± 17 (mean ± SD, range 16 to 85) years; weight 76 ± 20 (range 41 to 170) kg; height 170 ± 10 (range 140 to 200) cm; and body mass index (BMI) 26 ± 6 (range 15 to 59) kg·m^{-2}. Twenty-seven participants did not provide their height or weight due to an omission in the questionnaire. These participants were

European, 13 years older and had higher scores (60 units) than those that provided weight and height. Seven percent (40/571) of the participants reported that they currently smoked tobacco.

Applying the cutoffs based on the screening test criteria, one out of five (21.4%) had a low CRS (<250), one out of three (32.2%) <280, with one out of 14 (7.1%) scoring higher that than 530 (Figure 1). Older participants (>40 years) had CRS 21 units higher than younger participants (95% CI 40, $p = 0.033$) (Table 1). By ethnicity, Pacific CRS were significantly lower than all other groups and Asian significantly higher than all groups except for "other". There were no differences by gender within ethnic groups (Table 1).

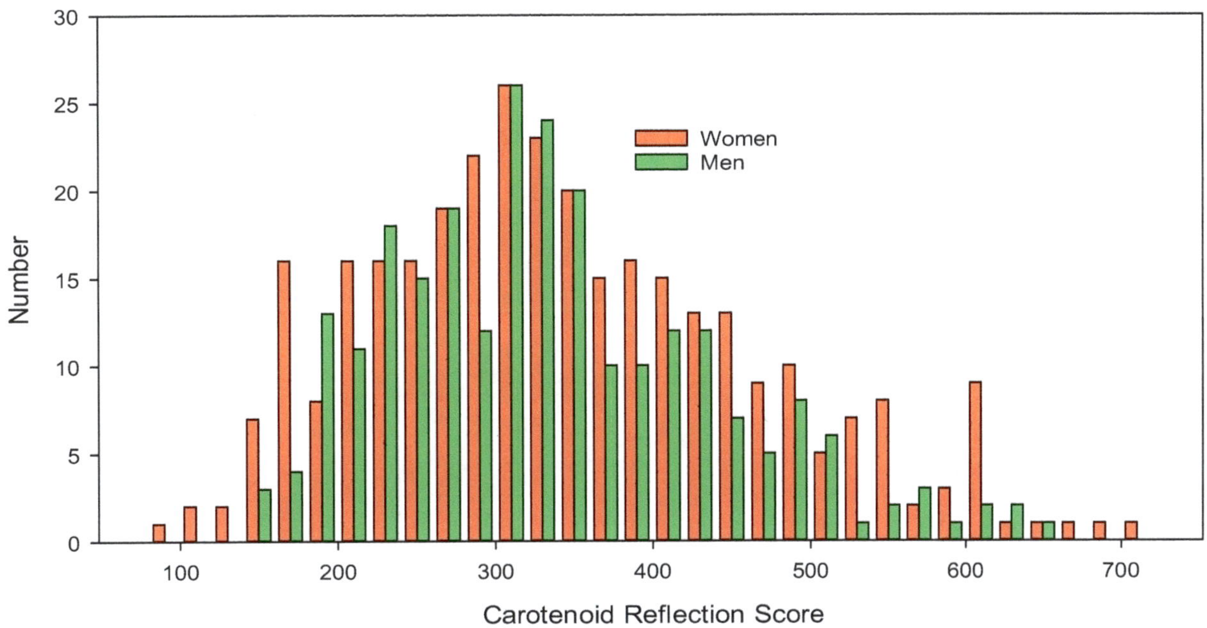

Figure 1. Histogram of carotenoid reflection scores in the study population.

Table 1. Carotenoid reflectance scores of participants by age, ethnicity and gender.

		Carotenoid Reflection Scores			
Characteristic	***N* (Women, Men)**	**All**	**Women**	**Men**	**Difference Women − Men (95% CI)**
All	571 (324, 247)	342 ± 116	345 ± 124	336 ± 105	10 (−9, 29)
Age ≤ 40 years	334 (201, 133)	333 ± 119	338 ± 122	325 ± 114	13 (−13, 39)
>40 years	237 (125, 122)	354 ± 111 [1]	358 ± 125	349 ± 93	9 (−20, 37)
Ethnicity					
Māori	38 (25, 13)	315 ± 110	293 ± 117	360 ± 83	−66 (−140, 8)
Pacific	84 (42, 42)	257 ± 85 [2]	247 ± 84	267 ± 87	−20 (−58, 17)
Asian	99 (62, 37)	388 ± 115	400 ± 119	367 ± 105	32 (−14, 80)
South Asian	72 (37, 35)	341 ± 113	340 ± 110	343 ± 118	−3 (−58, 50)
European	234 (137, 97)	352 ± 111	359 ± 115	341 ± 112	17 (−11, 46)
Other	44 (23, 21)	367 ± 126	367 ± 157	367 ± 84	0 (−78, 78)

N number, mean ± SD carotenoid reflection score, [1] $p < 0.03$ for difference by age independent t test. [2] $p < 0.001$ by ethnicity ANOVA.

3.2. Carotenoid Food Intake

Slightly more than half (53.3%) reported consuming 3 or more servings of vegetables a day and 61.6% 2 or more fruit a day, with 39.4% reporting 3 or more vegetables plus two or more fruit a day (i.e., 5+ a day). Women reported consuming around 0.5 servings a day of vegetables, and 0.5 servings of dark green leafy vegetables weekly more than men (Table 2). By ethnicity, Europeans reported almost one more serving a day of fruit plus vegetables than Pacific, Asian and South Asian but were not different to Maori or Other ethnic groups ($p = 0.015$, ANOVA) (Figure 2A). Weekly consumption of dark green leafy vegetables was reported as 4.0 ± 2.0 by Asian which was 0.5, 0.8, 1.4, 1.1 and 1.6 servings higher than European, "Other", Maori, South Asian and Pacific respectively (Figure 2B).

Table 2. Reported number of servings consumed each day or week of foods containing carotenoids.

Food Frequency	All (Range)	Women (Range)	Men (Range)	Difference (95% CI)	p [1]
Vegetables/day	2.8 ± 1.4 (0,7)	3.0 ± 1.6 (0,7)	2.5 ± 1.3 (0,6)	0.5 (0.3, 0.8)	<0.001
Fruit/day	2.1 ± 1.4 (0,7)	2.2 ± 1.4 (0,7)	2.0 ± 1.3 (0,7)	0.2 (−0.1, 0.4)	0.181
Fruit + vegetables/day	4.9 ± 2.4 (0,14)	5.2 ± 2.5 (0,14)	4.6 ± 2.2 (0,11)	0.7 (0.3, 1.0)	0.001
Dark green leafy vegetables/week	3.2 ± 2.8 (0,7)	3.5 ± 2.0 (0,7)	3.0 ± 2.0 (0,7)	0.5 (0.2, 0.8)	0.003
Carrots/pumpkin/week	2.7 ± 1.8 (0,7)	2.7 ± 1.7 (0,7)	2.6 ± 1.8 (0,7)	0.0 (−0.3, 3.0)	0.770
Eggs/week	2.6 ± 1.8 (0,7)	2.4 ± 2.4 (0,7)	2.8 ± 2.5 (0,7)	−0.4 (−0.8, 0.0)	0.078
Dairy/week	4.6 ± 2.2 (0,7)	4.5 ± 2.3 (0,7)	4.7 ± 2.2 (0,7)	−0.2 (−0.6, 0.2)	0.345

Mean ± SD, [1] Independent t test equal variances not assumed.

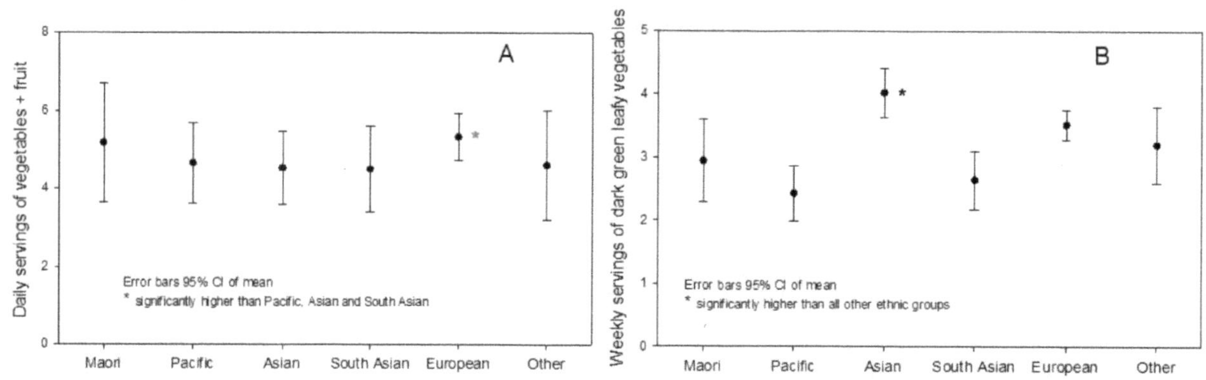

Figure 2. Comparison by ethnicity of (**A**) daily vegetable and fruit intake and (**B**) weekly dark green leafy vegetable intake.

3.3. Associations between Carotenoid Reflection Score and Determinants

For all participants there were moderate to strong negative correlations of CRS with weight and BMI and positive correlations with age, vegetables, fruit and vegetables plus fruit intakes and weekly intake of dark green leafy vegetables and carrots and pumpkin (Table 3). Fruit (but not vegetables) were a determinant for men but not women and carrots and pumpkin were a determinant for men but not women.

Table 3. Correlation of carotenoid reflection scores with participant characteristics and diet.

	Pearson Correlation Coefficient, r (95% CI)		
Determinant	**All**	**Women**	**Men**
Age	0.146 (0.065, 0.225) ***	0.164 (0.056, 0.268) **	0.130 (0.005, 0.251)
Weight	−0.312 (−0.384, −0.236) ***	−0.397 (−0.485, −0.301) ***	−0.251 (−0.364, −0.130) ***
Height	−0.078 (−0.159, 0.004)	−0.078 (−0.185, 0.031)	−0.067 (−0.190, 0.058)
BMI	−0.338 (−0.409, −0.263) ***	−0.393 (−0.481, −0.297) ***	−0.248 (−0.362, −0.127) ***
Vegetables/day	0.231 (0.152, 0.307) ***	0.273 (0.169, 0.371) ***	0.142 (0.017, 0.262) *
Fruits/day	0.169 (0.088, 0.248) ***	0.089 (−0.020, 0.196)	0.303 (0.185, 0.412) ***
Vegetables plus fruit/ day	0.243 (0.164, 0.319) ***	0.227 (0.121, 0.328) ***	0.265 (0.145, 0.377) ***
Dark green leafy veg/week	0.242 (0.187, 0.340) ***	0.266 (0.162, 0.364) ***	0.199 (0.076, 0.316) **
Carrots/pumpkin/week	0.203 (0.123, 0.280) ***	0.138 (0.029, 0.243)	0.302 (0.184, 0.411) ***
Eggs/week	0.067 (−0.015, 0.148)	0.054 (−0.055, 0.162)	0.096 (−0.029, 0.218)
Dairy/week	0.055 (−0.027, 0.136)	0.024 (−0.085, 0.133)	0.112 (−0.013, 0.234)

* $p < 0.05$, ** $p < 0.01$ and *** $p < 0.001$ denote statistically significant difference.

3.4. Predictors of Carotenoid Reflection Score

Based on the statistically significant correlations in Table 3, determinants of CRS were examined systematically by stepwise regression. Body weight and vegetable intake as predictors were excluded from the model as they exhibited collinearity with BMI and dark green leafy vegetable intakes respectively. There was overlap in the general questions about vegetables and fruits and the specific questions concerning dark green leafy vegetables and carrots and pumpkin, so vegetable and fruit intakes was were excluded from the model. The best model had four predictors that explained a total of 16.2% of the variation (Table 4). Body mass index explained 10.9% of the variation with each unit of increase of BMI associated with a reduction in the CRS of 5.4 units. Weekly intake of dark green leafy vegetables explained an additional 2.9%, with 1 serving a week adding 6.7 units to the CRS. One serving a week of carrots or pumpkin added 9.4 units to the CRS. Asian ethnicity added 17 units. Therefore, determinants of an increased CRS were a smaller body size, weekly intake of dark green leafy vegetables, carrots and pumpkin and Asian ethnicity.

While smoking tobacco was not a predictor in the above model, there was a difference between smoking or not. Smokers' mean CRS was 274 ± 116 (n = 40) and non-smokers 346 ± 115 (n = 531). On average, smokers were 72 score units (95% CI 34, 110), $p < 0.001$) lower than non-smokers.

Of the 571 participants there were 10 couples living in the same house, for 7/10 the man had a higher score but overall this was not significantly different.

Table 4. Multiple regression analysis with carotenoid reflection score as the independent variable.

Independent Variable	Regression Coefficient, β	SE, β	[a] R^2 (P)
Constant	439.660	24.940	(<0.001)
BMI, kg/m^2	−5.440	0.878	0.109 (<0.001)
Dark green leafy vegetables/week	6.670	2.504	0.138 (<0.001)
Carrots/pumpkin/week	9.380	2.738	0.154 (0.001)
Ethnic group [b]	16.981	7.029	0.162 (0.016)

[a] Adjusted for the number of predictors. [b] Ethnic group codes as European 0, Asian 1 and all other groups −1.

4. Discussion

To our knowledge, this is the first relatively large, multi-ethnic study to measure and validate carotenoid status using Veggie Meter™ carotenoid reflection scores. The most important finding is that body size, measured both as weight and BMI, was the strongest determinant of carotenoid status. We also show a relatively high prevalence of low carotenoid status, with no overall difference between women and men that decreases with age. The highest scores for Asian and lowest for Pacific are of importance alongside the observation that Asian participants reported the highest intake of green leafy vegetables and Pacific the lowest. Each of these findings will be discussed in turn.

Very few studies have used the Veggie Meter™ to assess CRS. Only one study in Japan [15], with 985 participants, mean age 69 years, has reported a negative correlation (r = −0.087) of CRS with BMI, a surrogate measure of body fatness, over a similar range to that in this study. We add to evidence for a negative association with BMI and the strength of our association was higher (r = −0.338) for all participants, and was present for women and men when analysed separately. Height was not correlated with CRS. Explanations for this association with body composition include that carotenoids are fat soluble and the concentration in body tissues will depend on both the amount (dose) ingested and absorbed [17] and also the volume of distribution. Larger people will have more absolute fat mass and higher body fat percentage. Also, excess body weight is associated with inflammation, which may deplete carotenoid stores [18] through oxidation. Finally, while servings were not quantified, a person weighing 100 kg with the same percentage body fat as a person weighing 50 kg will require twice the dose of carotenoids to achieve the same tissue concentration. No allowance for body size is made with generalized vegetable and fruit guidelines, yet we agree with others [19] that carotenoid requirements may be dependent on body composition.

It was not surprising that CRS scores of this study population were relatively low considering the low reported intake of vegetables and fruit in this study. Only 39.2% met the guideline of both 3+ vegetables and 2+ fruit a day. This is the same as the 2018, 2019 National Health Survey [8] which reports 39.4% of the New Zealand population meeting the guideline. The same survey shows that men eat less vegetables and fruit than women, with higher intakes of vegetables for Maori and European than Pacific and Asian ethnicities. However, the Ministry includes South Asian within the group Asian. We show a difference in diet between Asian and South Asian reflecting known differences in dietary patterns [20], otherwise our findings for vegetable and fruit intake are similar to the national survey.

Compared with the small number of other studies that have used the Veggie Meter™ technique, our mean CRS value of 346 is higher than that recorded in a diverse community sample in Eastern North Carolina USA of ~240 in African American and Non-African American (n = 469) [21] and 57 from an eye clinic in Utah, USA [14] with mean CRS of 297, but similar to a Japanese study where the mean CRS was 342 [15]. While we show no significant difference in CRS between men and women, the Japanese [15] study demonstrated that Japanese women scored higher than men (382 vs. 315).

A review of mostly prospective studies of health outcomes in relation to plasma carotenoids proposed a carotenoid health-based index for significant positive health outcomes including metabolic syndrome and cancer. Derived from our validation equation, the equivalent CRS score for their cut-point criteria of very high risk of <1 μM is 180, high risk 1–1.5 μM is 270, moderate risk 1.5–2.5 μM is 450, low risk 2.5–4 μM is 730. This means that 82% of the participants in the current study are at moderate risk or more of negative health outcomes. This lends support to strengthening the vegetable and fruit guideline to more than 3 vegetables a day and to encourage increased intake of a variety of dark green leafy and orange vegetables.

The difference in CRS observed by age may be related to higher socioeconomic status for the older people and therefore an ability to afford to purchase or grow greater quantities and more diverse vegetables and fruit and also time and ability to cook and prepare meals. Older participants were also more likely to be European.

Women reported that they consumed more vegetables and more dark green leafy vegetables than men. Women and men reported the same intake of carrots and pumpkins but only in men was intake significantly correlated with the CRS. This may relate to differences, by gender, in dietary recall, over and under-reporting and body size. The collinearity of the dietary questions infers that those who report that they eat more vegetables also report that they eat more fruit and within vegetables more carrot, pumpkin and dark green leafy vegetables are reported. In the multiple regression, gender was not a significant predictor. Another explanation is that women, in general, have a higher proportion of body fat than men. Carotenoids are fat soluble and therefore the same intake would result in more dilution in the fat for women than for men. In future studies it would be important to have a measure of body fat and to explore a gender difference in dose–response further.

A major omission of the dietary questions was not asking a question about tomato consumption, which would be a measure of the carotenoid lycopene. On the other hand, we did show that reported vegetable intake, dark green leafy vegetables and orange vegetables (carrot and pumpkin) was positively associated with CRS. We also did not formally ask about or record any digestive problems which could impair absorption of carotenoids because this was not part of the ethical approval. The representativeness of the study population was limited. Strengths of this work are the wide age range, diverse settings and the comparison of the five main ethnic groups living in Auckland, New Zealand. We also demonstrated the feasibility of using the Veggie Meter in the workplace at the same time as providing encouragement for the individual to increase intake and for the employer to support this.

5. Conclusions

Future investigations should include targeted interventions, children, members of the same household, a more objective measure of body fat, include tomatoes in the questionnaire and ask about digestive problems.

A considerable body of evidence exists that supports the contention that a diverse variety of and more vegetables should be consumed every day for health. The quantity should be in proportion to body size. Nationally, New Zealand, as a primary producer, exports a large quantity of premium quality fruit and vegetables [22], which implies that there is not a shortage of supply. This important public health issue has long term implications for prevention of non-communicable diseases and calls for action to improve access to vegetables and fruit. One way this could be done is to remove the goods and services tax from vegetables and fruit. Food-based dietary guidelines need to emphasise the importance of the diversity of vegetables and fruits required and consider serving size guidelines that take into account that larger people should consume a greater volume of vegetables than smaller individuals. Vegetable and fruit preferences of men and women and by ethnic group differ and dietary advice to improve carotenoid status should be tailored to gender and ethnicity.

Determinants of carotenoid status were body size, intake of DGLV, carrots and pumpkin, and ethnicity.

Author Contributions: Conceptualization E.R.; methodology, E.R., S.J.-M.; validation I.A. and E.R.; formal analysis, E.R.; investigation, I.A., T.D.; data curation, S.J.-M.; writing—original draft preparation, E.R.; writing—review and editing, all authors.; project administration, S.J.-M.; funding acquisition, E.R. All authors have read and agreed to the published version of the manuscript.

Acknowledgments: We gratefully acknowledge the participation of the participants and the managers of their workplaces for allowing access and time for the measurements.

References

1. Aune, D.; Giovannucci, E.; Boffetta, P.; Fadnes, L.T.; Keum, N.; Norat, T.; Greenwood, D.C.; Riboli, E.; Vatten, L.J.; Tonstad, S. Fruit and vegetable intake and the risk of cardiovascular disease, total cancer and all-cause mortality-a systematic review and dose-response meta-analysis of prospective studies. *Int. J. Epidemiol.* **2017**, *46*, 1029–1056. [CrossRef] [PubMed]
2. Food and Agricultural Organisation of the United Nations. Food-based Dietary Guidelines. Available online: http://www.fao.org/nutrition/nutrition-education/food-dietary-guidelines/en/ (accessed on 14 September 2019).
3. Naska, A.; Lagiou, A.; Lagiou, P. Dietary assessment methods in epidemiological research: Current state of the art and future prospects. *F1000Reserch* **2017**, *6*, 926. [CrossRef] [PubMed]
4. Shashirekha, M.N.; Mallikarjuna, S.E.; Rajarathnam, S. Status of bioactive compounds in foods, with focus on fruits and vegetables. *Crit. Rev. Food Sci. Nutr.* **2015**, *55*, 1324–1339. [CrossRef] [PubMed]
5. Moran, N.E.; Mohn, E.S.; Hason, N.; Erdman, J.W., Jr.; Johnson, E.J. Intrinsic and Extrinsic Factors Impacting Absorption, Metabolism, and Health Effects of Dietary Carotenoids. *Adv. Nutr.* **2018**, *9*, 465–492. [CrossRef] [PubMed]
6. Elvira-Torales, L.I.; Garcia-Alonso, J.; Periago-Caston, M.J. Nutritional Importance of Carotenoids and Their Effect on Liver Health: A Review. *Antioxidants* **2019**, *8*, 229. [CrossRef] [PubMed]
7. New Zealand Institute for Plant and Food Research Limited; Ministry of Health (New Zealand). New Zealand Food Composition Database. Available online: https://www.foodcomposition.co.nz/ (accessed on 7 November 2019).
8. Ministry of Health. New Zealand Health Survey 2018/19. Available online: https://minhealthnz.shinyapps.io/nz-health-survey-2017-18-annual-data-explorer (accessed on 19 November 2019).
9. Bationo, J.F.; Zeba, A.N.; Abbeddou, S.; Coulibaly, N.D.; Sombier, O.O.; Sheftel, J.; Bassole, I.H.N.; Barro, N.; Ouedraogo, J.B.; Tanumihardjo, S.A. Serum Carotenoids Reveal Poor Fruit and Vegetable Intake among Schoolchildren in Burkina Faso. *Nutrients* **2018**, *10*, 1422. [CrossRef] [PubMed]
10. Couillard, C.; Lemieux, S.; Vohl, M.C.; Couture, P.; Lamarche, B. Carotenoids as biomarkers of fruit and vegetable intake in men and women. *Br. J. Nutr.* **2016**, *116*, 1206–1215. [CrossRef] [PubMed]

11. Campbell, D.R.; Gross, M.D.; Martini, M.C.; Grandits, G.A.; Slavin, J.L.; Potter, J.D. Plasma carotenoids as biomarkers of vegetable and fruit intake. *Cancer Epidemiol. Biomark. Prev.* **1994**, *3*, 493–500.
12. Ashton, L.M.; Pezdirc, K.B.; Hutchesson, M.J.; Rollo, M.E.; Collins, C.E. Is Skin Coloration Measured by Reflectance Spectroscopy Related to Intake of Nutrient-Dense Foods? A Cross-Sectional Evaluation in Australian Young Adults. *Nutrients* **2017**, *10*, 11. [CrossRef] [PubMed]
13. Pezdirc, K.; Hutchesson, M.J.; Williams, R.L.; Rollo, M.E.; Burrows, T.L.; Wood, L.G.; Oldmeadow, C.; Collins, C.E. Consuming High-Carotenoid Fruit and Vegetables Influences Skin Yellowness and Plasma Carotenoids in Young Women: A Single-Blind Randomized Crossover Trial. *J. Acad. Nutr. Diet.* **2016**, *116*, 1257–1265. [CrossRef] [PubMed]
14. Ermakov, I.V.; Ermakova, M.; Sharifzadeh, M.; Gorusupudi, A.; Farnsworth, K.; Bernstein, P.S.; Stookey, J.; Evans, J.; Arana, T.; Tao-Lew, L.; et al. Optical assessment of skin carotenoid status as a biomarker of vegetable and fruit intake. *Arch. Biochem. Biophys.* **2018**, *646*, 46–54. [CrossRef] [PubMed]
15. Obana, A.; Gohto, Y.; Gellermann, W.; Ermakov, I.V.; Sasano, H.; Seto, T.; Bernstein, P.S. Skin Carotenoid Index in a large Japanese population sample. *Sci. Rep.* **2019**, *9*, 9318. [CrossRef] [PubMed]
16. Ministry of Health. *Content Guide 2017/18: New Zealand Health Survey*; Ministry of Health: Wellington, New Zealand, 2018.
17. Priyadarshani, A.M. A review on factors influencing bioaccessibility and bioefficacy of carotenoids. *Crit. Rev. Food Sci. Nutr.* **2017**, *57*, 1710–1717. [CrossRef] [PubMed]
18. Calder, P.C.; Albers, R.; Antoine, J.M.; Blum, S.; Bourdet-Sicard, R.; Ferns, G.A.; Folkerts, G.; Friedmann, P.S.; Frost, G.S.; Guarner, F.; et al. Inflammatory disease processes and interactions with nutrition. *Br. J. Nutr.* **2009**, *101* (Suppl. 1), 1–45. [CrossRef] [PubMed]
19. Bonet, M.L.; Canas, J.A.; Ribot, J.; Palou, A. Carotenoids in adipose tissue biology and obesity. In *Carotenoids in Nature*; Strange, C., Ed.; Springer: Berlin, Germany, 2016; Volume 79, pp. 377–414.
20. Devi, A.; Rush, E.; Harper, M.; Venn, B. Vitamin B12 Status of Various Ethnic Groups Living in New Zealand: An Analysis of the Adult Nutrition Survey 2008/2009. *Nutrients* **2018**, *10*, 181. [CrossRef] [PubMed]
21. Jilcott Pitts, S.B.; Jahns, L.; Wu, Q.; Moran, N.E.; Bell, R.A.; Truesdale, K.P.; Laska, M.N. A non-invasive assessment of skin carotenoid status through reflection spectroscopy is a feasible, reliable and potentially valid measure of fruit and vegetable consumption in a diverse community sample. *Public Health Nutr.* **2018**, *21*, 1664–1670. [CrossRef] [PubMed]
22. New Zealand Horticulture; Plant and Food Research. Fresh Facts. Available online: https://www.freshfacts.co.nz/files/freshfacts-2018.pdf (accessed on 19 November 2019).

3

Can Lycopene Impact the Androgen Axis in Prostate Cancer?: A Systematic Review of Cell Culture and Animal Studies

Catherine C. Applegate [1], Joe L. Rowles III [1] and John W. Erdman, Jr. [1,2,*]

[1] Division of Nutritional Sciences, University of Illinois at Urbana-Champaign, Urbana, IL 61801, USA; cca2@illinois.edu (C.C.A.); jrowles2@illinois.edu (J.L.R.)

[2] Department of Food Science and Human Nutrition, University of Illinois at Urbana-Champaign, Urbana, IL 61801, USA

* Correspondence: jwerdman@illinois.edu;

Abstract: First-line therapy for advanced or metastatic prostate cancer (PCa) involves the removal of tumor-promoting androgens by androgen deprivation therapy (ADT), resulting in transient tumor regression. Recurrent disease is attributed to tumor adaptation to survive, despite lower circulating androgen concentrations, making the blockage of downstream androgen signaling a chemotherapeutic goal for PCa. Dietary intake of tomato and its predominant carotenoid, lycopene, reduce the risk for PCa, and preclinical studies have shown promising results that tomato and lycopene can inhibit androgen signaling in normal prostate tissue. The goal of this systematic review was to evaluate whether mechanistic evidence exists to support the hypothesis that tomato or lycopene interact with the androgen axis in PCa. Eighteen studies ($n = 5$ in vivo; $n = 13$ in vitro) were included in the final review. A formal meta-analysis was not feasible due to variability of the data; however, the overall estimated directions of effect for the compared studies were visually represented by albatross plots. All studies demonstrated either null or, more commonly, inhibitory effects of tomato or lycopene treatment on androgen-related outcomes. Strong mechanistic evidence was unable to be ascertained, but tomato and lycopene treatment appears to down-regulate androgen metabolism and signaling in PCa.

Keywords: prostate cancer; tomato; lycopene; androgen; cell culture; animal

---

1. Introduction

Despite average annual declines in incidence, prostate cancer (PCa) remains the most commonly diagnosed male cancer in the United States, with an estimated three million men currently living with PCa [1]. It is well-understood that primary PCa growth is strongly dependent upon the activity of androgens within the prostate gland, as evidenced by the observed rise of androgen-regulated prostate-specific antigen (PSA) in the serum of men diagnosed with PCa [2]. First-line therapy for advanced or metastatic disease involves androgen suppression through androgen deprivation therapy (ADT) [3]. ADT results in castrate levels of androgens in the bloodstream and subsequent success of initial tumor regression; however, the return of castration-resistant disease inevitably occurs within a few years after ADT and is thought to be the result of adaptive or persistent intratumoral androgen production, metabolism, and signaling [4]. While the mechanisms of androgen metabolism and signaling leading to prostate carcinogenesis and continued tumor growth are still under investigation, the blockade of androgen signaling, in addition to ADT, has been identified as a target goal for chemotherapy.

Abundant epidemiological evidence indicates that tomato consumption and blood levels of the predominant carotenoid found in tomatoes, lycopene, are inversely associated with PCa risk [5–9].

Additional evidence suggests that tomato and lycopene interact with the androgen axis to reduce blood levels of PSA [10,11], as well as reduce the risk of advanced stage, lethal PCa [8,12,13]. Animal and cell culture studies reveal an interaction between lycopene and androgen status and signaling, further indicating a potential protective role of tomato and lycopene intake for PCa patients.

Androgens, such as testosterone and dihydrotestosterone (DHT), are male sex hormones required for prostate differentiation and the maintenance of prostate structure and function throughout the lifespan [14]. Once delivered to the prostate from the testes via the bloodstream, androgens can either be converted to more active forms or metabolized to less active forms by a variety of hydroxysteroid dehydrogenase (HSD) enzymes. For example, testosterone is a potent ligand for the androgen receptor (AR), but is converted to DHT by two isoforms of 5-α-reductase (SRD5A1 and SRD5A2). DHT has a higher affinity for binding to the AR, which leads to AR nuclear translocation, DNA binding, and the transcription of genes related to growth and survival pathways [15].

Our laboratory has previously shown that castrated male F344 rats accumulated two times more lycopene in the liver than intact rats or castrated rats treated with testosterone repletion [16,17]. We have also shown that short-term tomato or tomato carotenoid feeding led to significant decreases of serum testosterone in rats, with carotenoid intake interacting with castration to further decrease serum testosterone [18]. In addition, both castration and carotenoid intake resulted in the regulation of prostatic androgen-related enzyme gene expression. Expression of HSD17β4 was significantly higher after castration, as well as between castrated rats fed tomato or lycopene diets when compared to castrated or intact, control-fed rats. HSD17β4 activity results in the metabolism of more potent androgens to less potent forms, and HSD17β4 silencing has been shown to increase AR nuclear localization and PSA expression [19]. This upregulation of HSD17β4 may indicate a switch from androgen signaling propagation to androgen deactivation. Modulation of androgen-related enzyme gene expression by tomato and lycopene is supported by the observed upregulation of HSD17β4 and downregulation of SRD5A2 in the prostate of Copenhagen rats supplemented with lycopene [20]. Supplementation with lycopene also decreased the prostatic expression of steroid target genes prostatic steroid binding chains C1 and C3, cystatin-related protein 2, and seminal vesicle secretion protein IV. In addition, lycopene supplementation of human primary prostatic epithelial cells (PrE) reduced the expression of AR chaperone heat shock protein 90 (HSP90) and protein DJ1, a positive regulator of AR-dependent transcription [21].

These results support the hypothesis that lycopene metabolism is affected by androgen status and that tomato and lycopene interact with the androgen axis in the normal prostate by modulating the expression of genes involved in androgen metabolism and signaling. As such, we hypothesized that tomato and lycopene could similarly interact with the androgen axis during PCa. Because interference with androgen signaling is a critical chemotherapeutic goal for PCa treatment, the primary objective of this review was to systematically evaluate whether mechanistic evidence exists to support a role for tomato or lycopene interaction with the androgen axis during PCa. To accomplish this objective, we included animal and cell culture studies exploring this relationship and evaluated the overall strength and comparability of the evidence. This study is novel in that there is a general dearth of systematic reviews of animal and cell culture studies, and, to our knowledge, no studies currently exist to mechanistically evaluate the relationship between tomato or lycopene and the androgen axis during PCa. While strong mechanistic evidence was unable to be ascertained, the results showed that tomato and lycopene appeared to down-regulate androgen metabolism and signaling in PCa tissues.

2. Materials and Methods

2.1. Study Selection Criteria

Currently, no validated guidelines or tools exist for conducting systematic reviews or for evaluating the validity and quality of mechanistic studies. As part of an effort to utilize a cohesive and standardized set of guidelines for systematically reviewing evidence from cell culture and animal studies, this systematic review was conducted in accordance with the framework outlined by the

World Cancer Research Fund (WCRF) International/University of Bristol (UoB) [22]. In addition, care was taken to follow PRISMA reporting guidelines as closely as possible [23].

Cell culture and animal studies that met the following criteria were included in this systematic review: (a) evaluated the relationship between tomatoes and/or their primary bioactive, lycopene, and androgen metabolism, androgen signaling, or androgen-mediated outcomes in PCa through cell culture studies evaluating direct androgen endpoints in PCa cell lines, cell culture studies comparing androgen-sensitive versus androgen-insensitive PCa cell lines, or animal studies evaluating direct androgen endpoints in experimental animal models of PCa (carcinogen-induced, xenograft, transplantable, or transgenic); (b) methodology was documented in replicable detail; (c) used whole tomato, tomato extract, or lycopene as a single supplement; (d) were written in English; and (e) were peer-reviewed original research articles or theses.

2.2. Literature Search

We conducted a comprehensive literature search of PubMed, Web of Science, and the Cochrane Library using a combination of the following keywords and their variants: tomato, lycopene, testosterone, androgen, dihydrotestosterone, DHT, prostate specific antigen, PSA, prostate cancer, and prostate neoplasm (up to 23 January 2019). Titles and abstracts of articles that were identified by the search results were screened against the study selection criteria. Full texts of potentially relevant articles identified by abstract screening were further reviewed for study inclusion or exclusion. To minimize the risk of excluding potentially relevant studies, we also conducted a reference list search (i.e., backward search) and cited reference search (i.e., forward search) from studies meeting the study selection criteria. Studies identified through this process were further screened and evaluated using the afore-mentioned criteria. We repeated reference searches on all newly identified studies until no further relevant studies were found. Two authors (CCA and JLR3) individually determined the inclusion/exclusion of all studies retrieved in full text, and discrepancies were resolved through discussion.

2.3. Data Extraction and Quality Assessment

Data extraction was performed according to study type (animal or cell culture) using the recommendations set forth by the WCRF/UoB framework as a guide [22]. The following information was extracted from each animal study: animal model, housing conditions and dietary information for experimental and control groups, experimental design (investigator blinding, randomization or grouping of animals, etc.), duration of follow-up, androgen-related outcomes analyzed, results of androgen-related outcomes, sample size, and p-values. The following information was extracted from each cell culture study: names of cell lines, whether cell lines were established patient-derived tumor cell lines or freshly isolated primary cells, whether cell lines were authenticated, culture conditions, treatment regime (dose and length of treatment), details of laboratory procedures, outcomes analyzed, results, sample size, and p-values.

There is a lack of validated quality assessment (QA) tools to evaluate the risk of bias associated with animal and cell culture studies. QA of animal studies was performed using the SYstematic Review Centre for Laboratory animal Experimentation (SYRCLE) risk of bias tool [24] adapted from the established and validated Cochrane tool [25] for human study risk of bias assessment. Risk of bias was determined to be "high," "low," or "unclear." Total scores were not evaluated using the SYRCLE tool to avoid inappropriate weighting of each category. QA of cell culture studies was performed using the criteria recommended by the WCRF/UoB framework (score range 0–6; a score of 0 was assigned for each parameter not fulfilled or not reported) [22]. Based on the score, studies were rated as low (0–2), moderate (3–4), or high (5–6) quality. QA scores were utilized to provide a measure of the strength of the evidence and to determine if a risk of bias was present for each study, but were not used to determine the inclusion of studies. QA scores were considered when making conclusions about whether the included studies supported the biological plausibility of the causal pathway being investigated.

2.4. *Albatross Plot Generation*

The extreme degree of variation between the methodologies and outcome measures of animal and cell culture studies prevented statistical analysis via a meta-analysis. Due to this variation, outcome measures were grouped according to indirect or direct androgen-related outcomes. In lieu of a meta-analysis, albatross plots for each outcome measure were generated to both graphically represent the data and create an effect estimate for each outcome category measured. An albatross plot, as described by Harrison et al. [26], scatters the *p*-values of each study according to their sample size and according to the observed direction of the effect (positive or negative). In the absence of exact *p*-values provided, the most conservative *p*-value was assigned to that outcome (e.g., if given $p < 0.05$, set $p = 0.05$; if no *p*-value given for a non-significant association [e.g., $p > 0.05$], set $p = 1$). If studies included multiple *p*-values for different outcomes, all *p*-values were included as separate data points. The contour lines extending over the plots represent estimated effect sizes (represented as standardized mean differences [SMD]) to allow for the estimation of the magnitude of treatment effects for individual studies and for their association as a whole. Visual inspection of the albatross plots was used to determine an overall estimated effect for each outcome. Because study outcomes were grouped according to indirect or direct androgen-related outcomes and albatross plots only provide an estimate of the effect of tomato or lycopene for these categories, the results provided by the plots are representative of this estimate, rather than a true statistical analysis. Albatross plots were generated using STATA/IC V14.2 (StataCorp LP, College Station, TX, USA).

3. Results

3.1. *Literature Search*

In total, 326 studies were identified from the library search engines. After duplicate removal and adding studies identified from reference lists, 192 studies remained for abstract screening. Subsequently, 28 studies were found to contain potentially relevant information to be further evaluated by full text review. Inclusion was determined according to the afore-mentioned inclusion criteria, with a resulting 18 studies included in the final review. Ten studies were excluded because they did not discuss PCa ($n = 2$), did not evaluate direct androgen outcomes or compare androgen-sensitive vs. androgen-insensitive PCa cell lines ($n = 7$), or did not evaluate lycopene as a single supplement ($n = 1$). Of the 18 included studies, five were animal studies [27–31] and 13 were cell culture studies [32–44] (Figure 1).

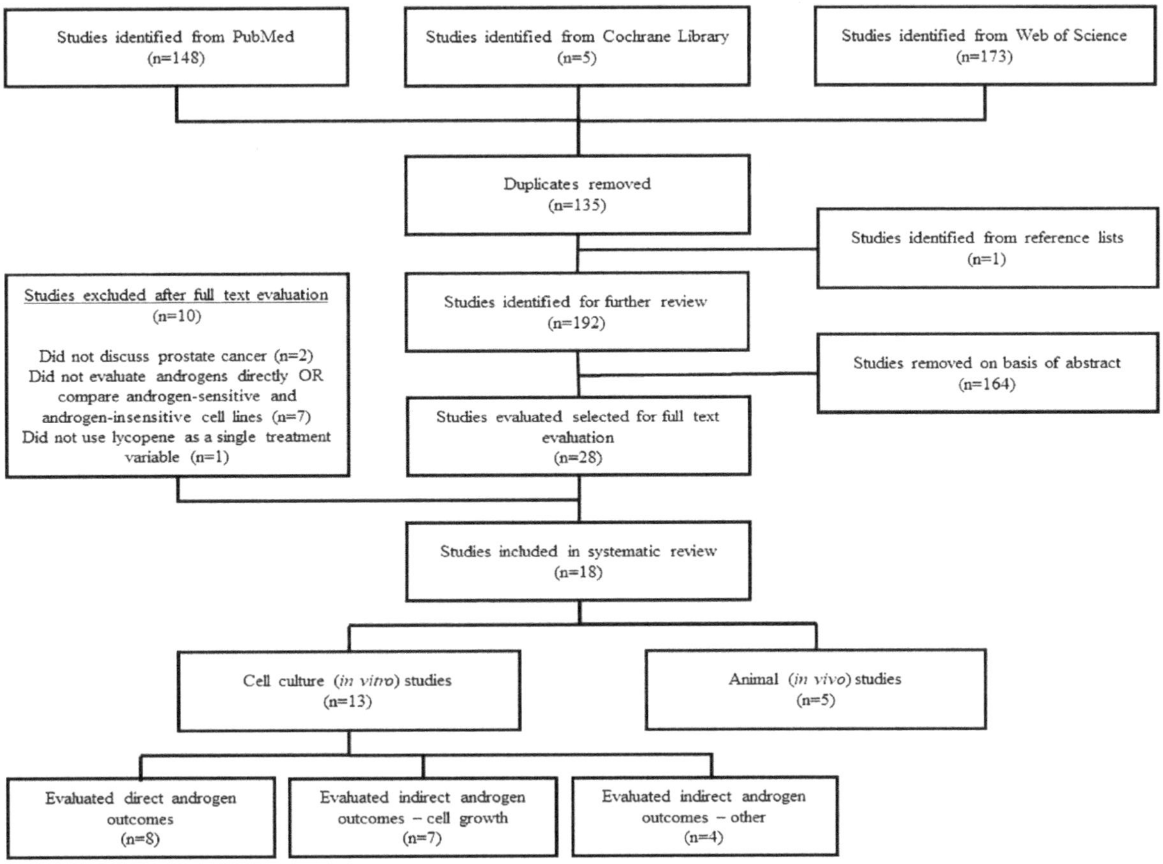

Figure 1. Literature search and study selection flow chart.

3.2. Study Characteristics

Of the five animal studies, three studies utilized rats (transplantable tumor models) [27,29,30] and two studies used mice (n = 1 xenograft model [28] and n = 1 transgenic model [31]). Animal study characteristics and results are summarized in Table 1. Of the 13 cell culture studies, 11 [32–34,36–40,42–44] used patient-derived PCa tumor cell lines, one [35] used primary PCa tumor cell lines, and one [41] used rat-derived PCa tumor cell lines. The cell culture studies were further stratified according to lycopene interaction with the androgen axis, as follows: (a) nine studies [32–34,36,40–44] evaluated androgen-related outcomes pertaining to indirect lycopene interaction with the androgen axis by comparing differential effects of lycopene between androgen-sensitive (AS) and androgen-insensitive (AI) PCa cell lines (indirect androgen outcomes); and (b) eight studies [32–39] evaluated androgen-related outcomes pertaining to direct lycopene interaction with androgen signaling, androgen metabolism, or androgen-regulated gene expression (direct androgen outcomes). Due to a range of indirect androgen outcomes reported, this group was further subdivided into studies that measured (i) growth [32,33,36,40–43] or (ii) other [32,34,40,43,44]. Cell culture study characteristics and results are summarized in Table 2.

QA of animal studies was carried out using the SYRCLE tool [24] and for cell culture studies using the criteria recommended by the WCRF/UoB framework [22]. The SYRCLE tool resulted in a largely unclear risk of bias for all animal studies (Appendix A, Table A1). The recommended criteria used to evaluate the quality of cell culture studies were vague, resulting in 10 cell culture studies considered to be high quality (5–6) [33–37,40–44] and three studies considered to be moderate quality (3–4) [32,38,39] (Appendix A, Table A2).

Table 1. Characteristics of included animal studies.

Author, Year	Animal Model	Baseline Diet(s)	Dietary Tomato and/or Lycopene Content *	Length of Intervention	Primary Findings
Canene-Adams, 2009 [27]	Dunning R3327-H transplantable tumors (Copenhagen rats)	AIN-93G-based diets fed; *ad libitum*	10% TP (providing 13 nmol lycopene/g diet and resulting in 511 nmol/g serum lycopene), 23 nmol/g diet supplemental lycopene beadlet (252 nmol/g serum lycopene), or 224 nmol/g diet supplemental lycopene beadlet (884 nmol/g serum lycopene)	18 weeks after tumor transplantation	No differences in serum testosterone or DHT between rats fed tomato, lycopene, or control diets
Limpens, 2006 [28]	Xenograft using PC-346C cells (athymic mice)	821077 CRM(P) low (but adequate) vitamin E rodent diet; *ad libitum*	5 or 50 mg/kg BW lycopene (from LycoVit) oral gavage = 0.5–1.5 mg lyco/day	42 days after tumor inoculation	No differences in plasma PSA between mice given control or lycopene gavages (PSA levels were proportional to tumor size regardless of intervention)
Lindshield, 2010 [29]	Dunning R3327-H transplantable tumors (Copenhagen rats)	AIN-93G-based diets; *ad libitum*	250 mg/kg diet supplemental lycopene beadlet = 5 mg lyco/day	18 weeks after tumor transplantation	No differences in serum testosterone or DHT between rats fed lycopene or control diets
Siler, 2004 [30]	MayLyLu Dunning transplantable tumors (Copenhagen rats)	Kliba #2019 with added coconut fat (6%), <5 ppm vitamin E, reduced (but adequate) vitamin A, and devoid of phytosterols; did not indicate if *ad libitum*	200 ppm lycopene (1.02 μM plasma lycopene)	4 weeks on diet prior to tumor transplantation, then 18 additional days	Lycopene supplementation reduced tumor expression levels of *SRD5A1* and androgen-target genes (*cystatin related proteins 1* and *2*; *prostatic spermine binding protein*; *prostatic steroid-binding protein C1*, *C2*, and *C3*; *probasin*) (only fold reductions reported—no other statistical values reported)
Wan, 2014 [31]	Transgenic (TRAMP mice)	AIN-93G -based diets; did not indicate if *ad libitum*	10% TP (providing 384 mg lycopene/kg diet) or 462 mg/kg diet supplemental lycopene beadlet (0.36 μM plasma lycopene) = 3–4 mg lyco/day	4 weeks diet prior to surgery, then 12 additional days	Reduced prostatic expression of genes related to androgen metabolism by tomato feeding (*SRD5A2* ($p = 0.04$), *Pxn* ($p = 0.04$), and *Srebf1* ($p = 0.05$)) and lycopene supplementation (*SRD5A1*, $p = 0.03$)

* All treatments can lead to blood levels of lycopene within a physiological range (~1 μM). Abbreviations: TRAMP (transgenic adenocarcinoma of the mouse prostate); TP (tomato powder); BW (body weight); DHT (dihydrotestosterone); PSA (prostate-specific antigen); SRD5A1 and 2 (5 α-reductase type 1 and 2); Pxn (paxillin); Srebf1 (sterol regulatory element binding transcription factor 1).

Table 2. Characteristics of included cell culture studies.

Author, Year	Cell Line(s)	Culture Conditions *†	Lycopene Dose(s) δ	Direct Androgen Outcomes: Primary Findings	Indirect Androgen Outcomes: Primary Findings	
					Growth	Other
Fu, 2014 [44]	LNCaP, PC-3	RPMI1640, 10% FBS	0, 5, 10, 20, 40 μM			10 μM lycopene inhibited GSTP1 methylation ($p < 0.05$), increased *GSTP1* gene expression ($p < 0.05$), and reduced *DNMT3A* gene expression ($p < 0.01$) in PC-3 but not LNCaP cells
Gong, 2016 [40]	LNCaP, C4-2, PC-3, DU145	RPMI1640, 10% FBS	1 μM		1 μM lycopene inhibited growth of LNCaP ($p < 0.05$) but not in C4-2, PC-3, or DU145 cells	1 μM lycopene induced *BCO2* gene expression in LNCaP ($p < 0.05$) but not DU145 cells
Gunasekera, 2007 [41]	AT3, DTE	RD (50% RPMI1640 + 50% DMEM), 2% FBS	0.02, 0.2, 5, 10, 20 μM		0.2 μM lycopene inhibited growth of AT3 ($p < 0.0001$) but not DTE cells	
Ivanov, 2007 [32]	LNCaP, PC-3	RPMI1640 or DMEM, 10% FBS	0.01–10 μM (cell proliferation) 0.2, 0.4 μM (protein expression) 0–100 μM (androgen responsiveness)	Lycopene did not inhibit reporter activity of ARE-Luc transfected LNCaP cells at any concentration (no statistical values reported)	0.2–0.8 μM lycopene inhibited growth of LNCaP and PC-3 cells ($p < 0.05$)	0.2–0.8 μM lycopene inhibited Akt phosphorylation, cyclins D1 and E, and CDK2 in LNCaP and PC-3 cells (no statistical values reported)
Linnewiel-Hermoni, 2015 [33]	LNCaP, PC-3, DU145	RPMI1640 or DMEM, 10% FCS, 10^{-9} DHT (for growth, stripped of steroid hormones prior to treatment)	1–5 μM (cell proliferation) 8 μM (ARE-Luc) 2.5 μM (PSA)	8 μM lycopene inhibited DHT-induced reporter activity of ARE-Luc transfected LNCaP cells ($p < 0.01$); non-significant decrease of DHT-induced PSA secretion by LNCaP cells treated with 2.5 μM lycopene	1–5 μM lycopene inhibited DHT-induced growth of LNCaP cells ($p < 0.01$)	
Liu, 2006 [34]	LNCaP, PC-3, DU145	RPMI1640 or Ham's F12K or EMEM, 10% FBS	1–1.48 μM	1.48 μM lycopene did not directly bind to the AR (no statistical values reported)		Uptake is highest in LNCaP ($p < 0.001$) with 1.48 μM lycopene compared to PC-3 or DU145 cells
Liu, 2008 [35]	6S, 6S + NPE	DMEM, 5% FBS	0.3, 1 μM	0.3, 1 μM lycopene increased CM-mediated cell death and reduced *IGF-I* gene expression of 6S + NPE cells in the presence of DHT ($p < 0.01$); lycopene reduced DHT-induced total ($p < 0.05$) and nuclear ($p < 0.01$) AR protein expression in 6S cells		

Table 2. *Cont.*

Author, Year	Cell Line(s)	Culture Conditions *†	Lycopene Dose(s) δ	Direct Androgen Outcomes: Primary Findings	Indirect Androgen Outcomes: Primary Findings	
					Growth	Other
Peternac, 2008 [36]	LNCaP, C4-2	T medium (80% DMEM + 20% Ham's F12K) + 10% FCS	0.04, 0.4, 4 μg/mL (equivalent to 0.075, 0.75, and 7.5 μM)	Lycopene did not reduce PSA gene or protein expression in LNCaP or C4-2 cells at any concentration	Lycopene inhibited growth of LNCaP (0.04, 0.4, 4 μg/mL) and C4-2 (0.4, 4 μg/mL) cells ($p < 0.05$)	
Rafi, 2013 [37]	PC-3	RPMI1640, 10% FBS	25 μM	25 μM lycopene led to fold reductions of kallikrein peptidase family proteins gene expression in PC-3 cells (only fold reductions reported—no other statistical values reported)		
Richards, 2003 [38]	LNCaP	Did not report cell culture conditions	1, 10 μM	1, 10 μM lycopene appeared to reduce PSA in LNCaP cells (no statistical values reported)		
Tang, 2005 [42]	LNCaP, PC-3, DU145	DMEM + Ham's F12K, 10% FBS	Up to 50 μM		10–50 μM lycopene more potently inhibited growth of PC-3 and DU145 cells ($p < 0.01$) compared to LNCaP cells	
Tang, 2011 [43]	LNCaP, LAPC-4, PC-3, 22Rv1, DU145	RPMI1640, 10% FBS	1 μM		1 μM lycopene appeared to reduce growth of all cell lines (no statistical values reported)	1 μM lycopene more potently reduced Akt phosphorylation in DU145 (by 60%) than LNCaP (by 20%) cells (no statistical values reported)
Zhang, 2010 [39]	LNCaP	RPMI1640, no other conditions reported	0.5, 5, 10, 15 μM	0.5–15 μM lycopene appeared to reduce reporter activity and ARE protein expression in ARE-Luc transfected LNCaP cells (no statistical values reported)		

* All studies reported standard incubator conditions (5% CO_2, 37 °C) unless otherwise stated. † Media does not contain added androgens unless otherwise stated; FBS and FCS supply castrate levels of androgens. δ Compare to reference of ~1 μM in human plasma. Abbreviations: GSTP1 (glutathione *S*-transferase Pi 1); DNMT3A (DNA methyltransferase 3A); BCO2 (β-carotene 9′,10′-oxygenase 2); ARE (androgen receptor element); Luc (luciferase); CDK2 (cyclin-dependent kinase 2); DHT (dihydrotestosterone); PSA (prostate-specific antigen); AR (androgen receptor); CM (camptothecin); IGF-I (insulin-like growth factor-I).

3.3. Animal Studies

Animal studies did not compare differences between AS or AI PCa. As such, only animal studies measuring direct androgen outcomes were included in this review. Of the five animal studies included, one study [28] measured the effect of lycopene supplementation on plasma PSA levels, and two studies [27,29] measured whether lycopene or tomato feeding impacted serum testosterone or DHT. Limpens et al. [28] tested the effects of low- and high-dose lycopene supplementation on PSA levels in a xenograft PCa model. After 42 days of daily oral gavage, plasma PSA values did not differ between dietary treatments, suggesting that PSA levels were proportional to tumor size, regardless of dietary intervention. Canene-Adams et al. [27] analyzed the effect of a 10% tomato powder (TP) diet and two different supplemental doses of lycopene (similar dose to the lycopene content of the TP diet and a dose 10-fold higher) on serum testosterone and DHT levels in the Dunning R3327-H transplantable prostate adenocarcinoma model after 18 weeks of tumor growth. None of the interventions had any effect on serum testosterone or DHT levels. Using the same model, Lindshield et al. [29] similarly saw no effect of lycopene supplementation on serum testosterone or DHT levels.

Siler et al. [30] observed reductions in the expression of genes involved in androgen metabolism (SRD5A1) and signaling (cystatin related proteins 1 and 2; prostatic spermine binding protein; prostatic steroid-binding protein C1, C2, and C3; and probasin) in MayLyLu Dunning transplantable tumors with dietary lycopene intake. Only fold-changes in gene expression with no statistical measurements were reported; however, consistent with these results, Wan et al. [31] confirmed that tomato feeding and lycopene supplementation similarly impacted androgen-related gene expression in the prostate of the transgenic mouse model (TRAMP) at early stages of prostate carcinogenesis. Tomato and lycopene diets both decreased the expression of genes related to androgen metabolism (SRD5A2 by tomato and SRD5A1 by lycopene), while the tomato diet reduced the expression of androgen co-regulators paxillin (pxn) and sterol regulatory element binding transcription factor 1 (srebf1).

An albatross plot (Figure 2) was generated for these animal studies to integrate the data, and visual inspection of the plot provided an estimated standardized effect for tomato or lycopene intake on androgen-related outcomes. The effects given were not intended to be precise, as they only provide estimates of the treatment magnitude of effect. The overall SMD of −0.4 (range: 0 to −1.25) represented a reduction in androgen-related outcome measures by exposure to tomato or lycopene. Three studies [27–29] showed no effects (assigned $p = 1$) of tomato or lycopene on androgen-related outcomes and as such, cluster at the center (null) line of the plot. The remaining two studies [30,31] showed inverse associations, with SMDs of between −0.5 and −1 and between −1 and −1.5, indicating a reduction in androgen-related outcome measures by exposure to tomato or lycopene. It is important to note that no studies reported an increase in androgen levels or androgen-regulated gene expression with tomato or lycopene exposure, suggesting that neither tomato nor lycopene propagate androgen production or signaling.

3.4. Cell Culture Studies

We present the results of cell culture studies here as reported by the original studies with the caveat that care must be taken when interpreting results involving cell culture treatment with lycopene, as antioxidants such as lycopene are extremely labile and are readily oxidized in cell culture [45]. For this reason, lycopene source, purity, storage, delivery vehicle, air and light exposure, and length of time in culture can substantially affect the initial lycopene integrity. These factors vary by study, creating the immediate limitation that the observed results could be due in part to the oxidation products of lycopene, rather than solely to the parent compound.

In general, cell culture studies supported the wide breadth of existing in vivo evidence that tomato and lycopene inhibit PCa tumor growth. Cell culture studies also provide some support for the limited in vivo evidence that tomato and lycopene down-regulate the expression of genes related to androgen signaling and metabolism. The included studies provided mixed evidence to indicate that lycopene interacts with AS and AI PCa cell lines in a differential manner (indirect androgen outcomes) and that lycopene directly interacts with the androgen axis (direct androgen outcomes), as detailed below. Study results provided limited insight into the specific mechanisms by which lycopene might interact with the androgen axis.

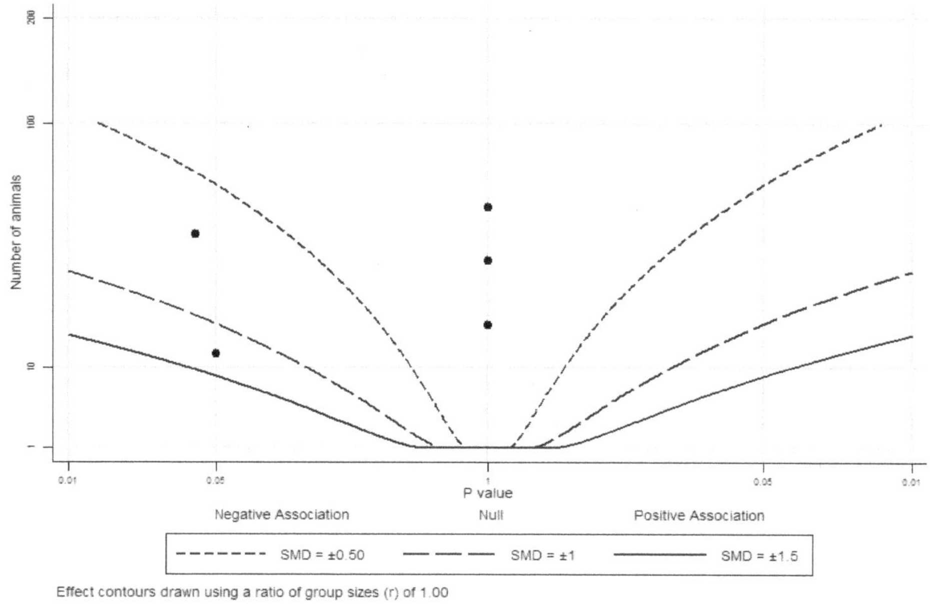

Figure 2. Albatross plot for animal studies. Each point represents a single study, with the effect estimate (represented as a p-value), plotted against the total given sample size (n) included within each study. Contour lines are standardized mean differences (SMD). p-values reported as <0.05 were plotted as 0.05 as a conservative estimate, while non-significant (null) p-values were plotted as 1.

3.4.1. Influence of Lycopene on Indirect Androgen Outcomes: Comparison of Androgen-Sensitive vs. Androgen-Insensitive Cell Lines

The limited pool of mechanistic studies makes it difficult to conclude if or how lycopene may directly interact with the androgen axis in PCa to exert growth inhibitory effects. In an effort to glean some insight into this question, it is important to consider how lycopene may impact human PCa cells of differing androgen-responsiveness. To this end, studies that evaluated the differences in outcomes between AS and AI cell lines were included as an indicator of how androgen signaling may influence lycopene activity. Appendix A Table A3 outlines the differences between each cell line in the included cell culture studies, which may impact the observed results.

(i) Cell Growth

Seven studies [32,33,36,40–43] evaluated the relationship between PCa cell growth and lycopene treatment. Despite large variation in study methodologies and lycopene doses, all seven studies demonstrated lycopene inhibition of PCa cell growth. All six studies [32,33,36,40,42,43] utilizing human PCa cells lines reported that lycopene treatment inhibited the growth of AS cell lines (LNCaP, LAPC-4), with three studies [33,36,40] reporting greater growth inhibition of an AS cell line (LNCaP) when compared to AI cell lines (C4-2, PC-3, DU145), one study [32] reporting growth inhibition regardless of androgen sensitivity, and two studies [42,43] reporting greater growth inhibition in AI cell lines (PC-3, DU145) than what was observed in an AS cell line (LNCaP). The single study [41] comparing an AS rat-derived PCa cell line (DTE) with its AI daughter cell line (AT-3) reported that lycopene inhibited AI cell growth, but not AS cell growth.

Gong et al. [40] showed that cell growth was reduced by lycopene and its metabolite, apo-10′-lycopenal, in AS LNCaP cells, but not in AI DU145, PC-3, or C4-2 cells. Peternac et al. [36] also found that lycopene inhibited cell proliferation in LNCaP cells and, to a slightly lesser extent, C4-2 cells. Comparably, Linnewiel-Hermoni et al. [33] showed that DHT-induced growth of LNCaP cells and serum-induced (castrate levels of androgens) growth of DU145 and PC-3 cells were inhibited by lycopene treatment, with LNCaP cells exhibiting a more profound response.

Ivanov et al. [32] observed that physiological doses of lycopene (0.2–0.8 μM) resulted in the dose-responsive inhibition of cell proliferation in both LNCaP and PC-3 cells. However, lycopene was observed to exert these effects in each cell line at different mitotic phases, with LNCaP cells mainly undergoing G_0/G_1 cell cycle arrest and subsequent apoptosis and PC-3 cells mainly undergoing S and G_2/M cell cycle arrest without an observed increase in the apoptotic index.

Tang et al. [42] (2005) observed that LNCaP cells resisted apoptosis by high-dose (up to 50 μM) lycopene, while PC-3 and DU145 cells were very responsive to apoptosis by high-dose lycopene. Tang et al. [43] (2011) tested the effects of lycopene on the growth inhibition of PCa cell types with varying androgen sensitivity (LAPC-4, LNCaP, 22Rv1, PC-3, DU145) and found DU145 cells to be the most inhibited by a physiological dose of lycopene (1 μM). Interestingly, PC-3 cells were completely unaffected by lycopene treatment, while LNCaP cells were only marginally affected. AI DU145 cells were not compared with AS LNCaP cells, but both Tang et al. [42] (2005) and Tang et al. [43] (2011) observed that DU145 cells mainly underwent cell cycle arrest at G_0/G_1, which contrasts with the S and G_2/M cell cycle arrest in PC-3 cells observed by Ivanov et al. [32]. The degree of androgen-insensitivity of DU145 cells is greater than that of PC-3 cells, making it possible that the level of androgen insensitivity affects at which stage of the cell cycle lycopene may interfere. More likely, these differing results best serve to highlight the inherent variability of cell culture studies, with different treatment variables potentially impacting outcomes.

Finally, Gunasekera et al. [41] showed significant concentration-dependent decreases of the cell proliferation of malignant, rat-derived, AI AT-3 cells, with lycopene concentrations as low as 0.2 μM and up to 10 μM when compared to the control treatment, with no effect on cell proliferation of AS DTE parent tumor cells by any concentration of lycopene.

An albatross plot summarizing the effects of lycopene on cell growth is presented in Figure 3A. The overall SMD of −2 (range: −0.6–<−2) indicates a reduction in cell growth by lycopene exposure. Two studies [33,36] showed reduced growth with smaller effect estimates (SMDs between −0.5 and −1), two studies [40,43] showed SMDs between −1 and −2, and three studies [32,41,42] showed an SMD < −2.

(ii) Other Outcomes

As introduced in the previous section, Ivanov et al. [32] observed that while physiological doses of lycopene inhibited cell proliferation in both AS LNCaP and AI PC-3 cells at different phases of the cell cycle, lycopene treatment led to similar dose-responsive changes in protein expression, regardless of androgen sensitivity. These effects were not differentially mediated by proteins involved in cell growth pathways in AS and AI cells; protein expression of cyclins D1 and E, cyclin-dependent kinase 2 (CDK2), and Akt phosphorylation were similarly inhibited by lycopene treatment in both cell types.

Tang et al. [43] (2011) attributed the growth inhibitory effects of lycopene in AI DU145 cells when compared to other AS and AI cell types to a correlation with higher levels of insulin-like growth factor-I receptor (IGF-IR) present in cells. The reported order of lycopene leading to the most growth inhibition to the least growth inhibition in cell types was: DU145 > LAPC-4 > 22Rv1 > LNCaP > PC-3; the order of highest to lowest IGF-IR expression in each cell type was: DU145 > PC-3 > LNCaP > 22Rv1 > LAPC-4. However, to determine this correlation, the group used calculated IC_{50} values (reported to be ordered as: LAPC-4 > LNCaP > 22Rv1 > PC-3 > DU145), but did not directly measure lycopene uptake into the cells. Liu et al. [34] (2006) showed lycopene uptake to be much higher in LNCaP cells when compared to PC-3 or DU145 cells (2.5× and 4.5× higher, respectively) at a physiological concentration (1.48 μM). Because lycopene uptake differs between cell lines, using the IC_{50} values calculated from lycopene treatment effects on growth inhibition alone may not be the most appropriate approach. Lycopene was also found to inhibit Akt phosphorylation to a greater extent in DU145 cells (60%) than in LNCaP cells (20%). Because LNCaP cells have a phosphatase and tensin homolog (PTEN) mutation that may lead to enhanced Akt phosphorylation by phosphatidylinositol 3-kinase (PI3K) rather than IGF-IR, the greater inhibition of Akt phosphorylation by lycopene in the DU145 cells may be attributed to lycopene inhibition of the IGF-IR pathway.

Gong et al. [40] showed that lycopene uptake, lycopene cleaving enzyme β-carotene 9′,10′-oxygenase (BCO2) gene expression, and lycopene-induced BCO2 expression were greater in LNCaP cells than in DU145 cells; transfection with either a wild-type (active) or mutant (inactive) BCO2 expression vector led to reduced cell growth in each cell line with or without lycopene treatment. Increased BCO2 expression (wild-type or mutant) also inhibited nuclear factor-κB (NF-κB) luciferase reporter activity by hindering NF-κB p65 subunit nuclear translocation and DNA binding in response to lycopene treatment. Constitutive NF-κB signaling is observed in AI cells lines and is associated with enhanced cell proliferation. These results show that both wild-type (active) BCO2 and mutant (inactive) BCO2 inhibit proliferation, indicating that the anti-proliferative effects of BCO2 are independent of its enzymatic (lycopene cleavage) functions and instead rely on some structural element of BCO2. However, the cellular uptake of lycopene and lycopene-induced expression of BCO2 are dependent on androgen sensitivity, suggesting that lycopene may be less effective at reducing AI cell growth.

Fu et al. [44] compared the effects of lycopene on the methylation and expression of an enzyme involved in detoxification reactions and tumor suppression, glutathione *S*-transferase Pi (GSTP1), in PC-3 and LNCaP cell lines. Treatment of PC-3 cells with 10 μM lycopene significantly reduced levels of GSTP1 promoter methylation, significantly increased the mRNA and protein expression of GSTP1, and significantly decreased the protein expression of DNA methyltransferase 3A (DNMT3A) when compared to control cells. Increasing lycopene treatment to 40 μM showed no additional inhibition of DNMT3A protein expression than the inhibition observed at a dose of 10 μM. Alternatively, LNCaP cells treated with lycopene showed no changes in GSTP1 methylation or expression.

The albatross plot presented in Figure 3B shows a reduction in other androgen-mediated outcomes by lycopene exposure with an SMD of <-3, and one study [40] with an SMD ≈ -2.

3.4.2. Influence of Lycopene on Direct Androgen Outcomes

Liu et al. [34] (2006) reported that lycopene uptake was much higher in AS LNCaP cells when compared to AI PC-3 or DU145 cells. To evaluate whether this higher uptake resulted in direct lycopene binding to the AR, LNCaP cells were transfected with a plasmid containing the ligand-binding domain of L701H, the T877A double mutant, cortisone/cortisol-responsive AR with a broader ligand specificity (AR^{ccr}). No direct lycopene binding to the AR occurred, but subcellular fractionation revealed the majority of lycopene to localize within the nuclear membranes and nuclear matrix. Therefore, these data suggest that because lycopene uptake followed the order of AR expression in AS and AI cell lines, lycopene uptake and storage may be mediated by androgen signaling by some mechanism not involving direct binding to the AR.

As discussed in the previous section, Ivanov et al. [32] showed that physiological doses of lycopene decreased cell proliferation in both LNCaP and PC-3 cells at different phases of the cell cycle. These effects were not shown to rely on androgen signaling directly, as the transfection of LNCaP cells with a luciferase-containing androgen response element (ARE) reporter (ARR3-Luc) exhibited no effect of lycopene treatment on androgen-stimulated expression of the gene construct.

Linnewiel-Hermoni et al. [33] showed that DHT-induced growth of LNCaP cells and serum-induced growth of DU145 and PC-3 cells were inhibited by lycopene treatment. To determine whether these effects may be mediated by direct androgen responsiveness, LNCaP cells were transfected with a PSA enhancer luciferase reporter gene construct containing six AREs. Physiological levels of lycopene were not tested, but a high lycopene concentration (8 μM) was found to significantly lower the reporter activity after DHT treatment. Similarly, DHT-induced PSA secretion by LNCaP cells was reported to be ~40% reduced by a more physiological, albeit still high, dose of lycopene (2.5 μM), but statistical analysis did not indicate a significant reduction.

Zhang et al. [39] measured the effect of 0.5–15 μM lycopene on LNCaP cells transfected with a luciferase-containing ARE reporter. The authors reported that lycopene inhibited ARE reporter activity and ARE protein expression in a dose-dependent manner, but failed to include a statistical analysis. Visually, it appears as though 5 μM lycopene acted similarly to 15 μM lycopene, but effects were seen with doses as low as 0.5 μM lycopene. The three studies (Ivanov et al. [32], Linnewiel-Hermoni et al. [33], and Zhang et al. [39]) using luciferase-containing ARE reporters in LNCaP cells show some conflicting evidence. However, it could be insinuated that lycopene effects were directly related to the ARE rather than the AR, mainly at supraphysiological doses of lycopene.

Liu et al. [35] co-cultured primary human prostate cancer stromal (6S) cells with primary normal prostatic epithelial (NPE) cells to determine the effects of DHT on camptothecin (CM)-induced cell death by DNA fragmentation. DHT treatment increased the mRNA expression of IGF-I in 6S cells, which then led to the rescue of CM-induced NPE cell death. Treatment of this co-culture with physiological doses of lycopene (0.3 and 1 μM) inhibited the pro-survival effects of DHT in a dose-responsive manner, potentially due to the administration of lycopene decreasing DHT-induced IGF-I gene expression in 6S cells. Furthermore, lycopene treatment inhibited DHT-induced AR expression in both whole cell lysates and nuclear extracts of 6S cells.

Peternac et al. [36] found that lycopene inhibited cell proliferation in both AS LNCaP and AI C4-2 cell lines. However, these growth effects were not directly related to AR activation, as lycopene had no effect on PSA mRNA or protein levels in either cell line.

Rafi et al. [37] showed that while strictly androgen-regulated genes were largely unaffected in PC-3 cells treated with supraphysiological doses of lycopene (25 μM), some genes within the kallikrein-related peptidase family did show a fold-reduction in expression (klk1, 5, 9, 10, 14). These genes are regulated by members of the steroid hormone family and their expression is typically associated with carcinogenesis, so a slight reduction in gene expression by lycopene treatment may indicate some interference with steroid hormone-regulated gene activation.

Richards et al. [38] measured the effects of low (physiological)- (1 μM) and high-dose (10 μM) lycopene on the PSA secretion of LNCaP cells. While the results showed that PSA protein levels were decreased by about 50% in both treatment groups compared to the control group at all time points, the authors did not report any statistical values or make any comment about the treatments. They also failed to report cell incubation conditions and the mode of delivery of lycopene. Therefore, while these results suggesting that lycopene treatment had direct effects on PSA secretion of LNCaP cells appear promising at first glance, closer inspection revealing the lack of methodological and statistical reporting creates uncertainty when considering the accuracy of the results (refer to Appendix A Table A2 for study quality assessment).

The albatross plot presented in Figure 3C shows the overall effect estimate as an SMD of −2 (range: 0–<−3), indicating a reduction in direct androgen-mediated outcomes by lycopene exposure. Three studies [32,34,36] showed no effects (assigned $p = 1$) of lycopene on androgen-related outcomes and cluster at the center (null) line of the plot. Three studies [33,35,38] showed SMDs between −0.75 and −1.5, two studies [35,37] showed SMDs between −1.5 and −3, and one study [39] showed an SMD < −3. It is important to note that similar to the effect estimates seen in the animal studies, no cell culture studies reported an increase in androgen-regulated gene activity or expression with lycopene exposure, despite a wide range of effect sizes, suggesting that lycopene has either a neutral or muting impact on androgen signaling.

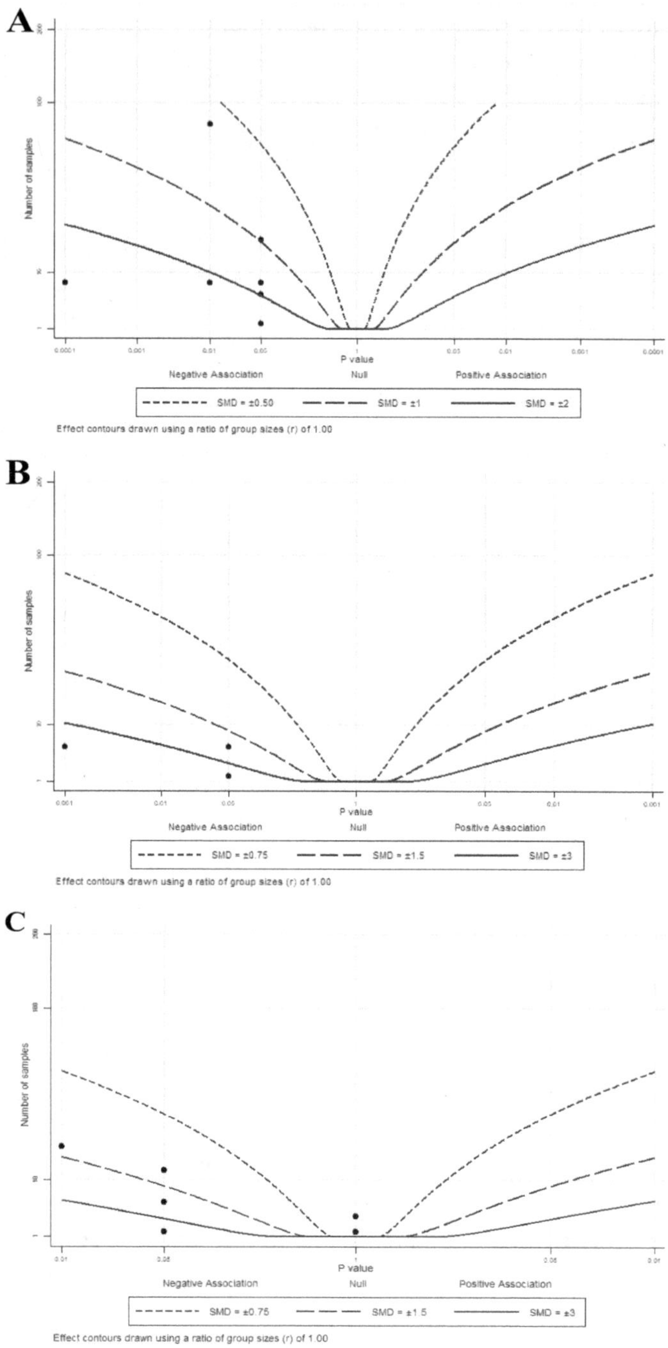

Figure 3. Albatross plots for each outcome of cell culture studies: (**A**) indirect effects (growth); (**B**) indirect effects (other); and (**C**) direct effects. Each point represents a single study, with the effect estimate (represented as a p-value), plotted against the total given sample size (n) included within each study. Contour lines are standardized mean differences (SMD). p-values reported as <0.05 were plotted as 0.05 as a conservative estimate, while non-significant (null) p-values were plotted as 1.

4. Discussion

This systematic review sought to determine whether there was any mechanistic evidence to demonstrate that lycopene directly interacts with the androgen axis during PCa. To our knowledge, this is the first systematic review synthesizing evidence to support the biological plausibility of a role for lycopene interaction with the androgen axis in PCa, a disease state in critical need of the identification of potential therapeutic interventions. The choice to conduct a systematic review was made in accordance with a growing need for the systematic evaluation of preclinical research to determine the strength of the evidence associated with a given topic. In addition, this systematic examination of all available evidence was intended to eliminate the risk of bias incurred by preparing a narrative review. In the absence of validated methods for performing systematic reviews of cell culture and animal studies, we used the guidelines recently set forth by the WCRF/UoB [22]. These guidelines serve as a good starting point for conducting mechanistic systematic reviews and meta-analyses; however, the suggested QA tool provides limited criteria for the critical evaluation of cell culture studies, leading to an inappropriate distribution of high range scores, highlighting a need for validated tools to assess the quality of these studies.

Unfortunately, performing a meta-analysis to statistically analyze the results was not feasible due to the inherent variability in the design and outcomes measured for the included studies. As such, data were grouped according to categories of androgen-related outcomes and graphically presented using albatross plots, a novel method described by Harrison et al. [26] by which to provide estimated SMDs of effects of the available data in the absence of sufficient homogenous data to perform a true meta-analysis. Because insufficient data were available to perform this statistical analysis and because reported outcomes were grouped according to their relationship with the androgen axis, it is important to note that these plots are not intended to provide an exact statistical evaluation of lycopene treatment on the androgen axis. Considering these limitations, the effect estimates shown are largely shifted to the left of the plots, suggesting that tomato or lycopene treatment decreased the effects of androgen signaling or metabolism for almost all outcomes measured. Therefore, while we were not able to determine mechanistically how lycopene interacts with the androgen axis during PCa, we have presented some proposed pathways by which lycopene exerts its anti-androgenic effects (Figure 4). These effects are complex and differ in lycopene uptake and growth pathway activation, depending on model used (animal or cell type), cell metabolism, and androgen signaling and metabolism.

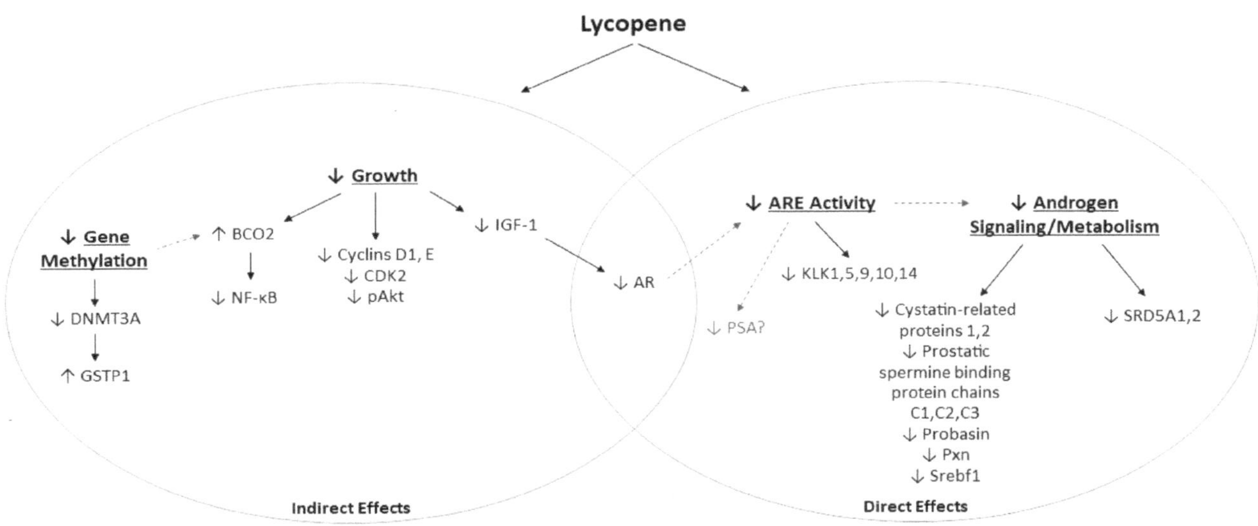

Figure 4. Summary of potential mechanisms by which lycopene may interact with the androgen axis in PCa. Solid lines represent outcomes reported by the reviewed studies, and dashed lines represent potential connections.

Based on the results of the limited animal studies available for inclusion in this systematic review, there was no evidence that tomato or lycopene intake impact circulating PSA, testosterone, or DHT during PCa. Previous research by our laboratory has shown reductions in serum testosterone by tomato and lycopene intake in a non-PCa rat model [18]. However, while previously thought to be a biomarker for advancing or aggressive PCa, discordance between circulating and intraprostatic levels of androgens, as well as observed adaptive changes in intratumoral steroidogenesis and metabolism, have made serum androgens unreliable markers of disease status [46–48]. Instead, changes in intratumoral androgen signaling may be a better indicator of androgen activity than serum testosterone or DHT levels. In accordance with this, there was evidence that tomato and lycopene intake decreased the expression of genes involved in androgen signaling (cystatin-related proteins 1 and 2; prostatic spermine binding protein; prostatic steroid-binding protein C1, C2, and C3; probasin; pxn; and srebf1) and metabolism (SRD5A1 and SRD5A2).

Results from cell culture studies were varied and provided weak mechanistic evidence to demonstrate that lycopene interacts with the androgen axis during PCa. To allow for all possible evidence to be considered, studies comparing differences in cell growth, gene, or protein expression in AS versus AI PCa cell lines were included. Overall, the results showed that cell growth was inhibited by lycopene, regardless of androgen sensitivity. However, the extent to which physiological levels of lycopene inhibit cell growth may be greater in AS cell lines than AI cell lines. In general, AS cell lines more readily accumulate lycopene than AI cell lines [34,40], as shown in Appendix A Table A3. This difference in lycopene accumulation may contribute to the differences seen in gene expression between the two cell types. AI cells express lower levels of the lycopene metabolizing enzyme, BCO2, which assists in inhibiting tumor promoting NF-κB signaling, independent of its lycopene metabolizing function. However, BCO2 is also inducible by lycopene [40], so the lower lycopene uptake by AI cell types may result in attenuated growth inhibitory effects by BCO2. IGF-1 expression was also shown to be higher in AI cells when compared to AS cells, with lycopene treatment resulting in the inhibition of IGF-1 expression and a resultant decrease in total and nuclear AR expression. Proteomic comparisons between AS and AI cells showed differences in the expression of proteins involved in metabolism, with AI cells exhibiting enhanced glycolysis [49]. Comparisons also revealed AI cells to have decreased poly[ADP-ribose] polymerase 1 (PARP-1) expression when compared to their AS counterparts; PARP-1 plays a role in promoting AR transcriptional activity, with a reduction of PARP-1 correlating with a reduced dependence on androgen signaling in AI cells. Combined, these results suggest that androgen signaling and cellular metabolism interact in PCa cells, with changes in lycopene uptake and metabolism, thereby having the potential to influence androgen signaling.

In addition to its growth inhibitory effects, DNA methylation was inhibited by lycopene in AI cells but not AS cells. DNA hypermethylation is an epigenetic modification that occurs more frequently as PCa progresses [50]. One such example of DNA hypermethylation occurs with GSTP1, a detoxifying enzyme with tumor suppressive activity. GSTP1 promoter hypermethylation and accompanying gene silencing have been consistently detected in more than 90% of PCa cases, with more advanced cases exhibiting higher levels of GSTP1 promoter methylation [51]. Lycopene treatment resulted in reduced GSTP1 methylation and associated suppression of DNA methylating enzyme DNMT3A expression in DU145 cells, but not LNCaP cells. Interestingly, Gong et al. [40] showed that the inhibition of methyltransferase activity resulted in a robust increase of BCO2 expression in all cell lines. This suggests that lycopene may have multiple beneficial effects in both cell types, regardless of androgen sensitivity.

When considering all available studies evaluating lycopene effects on PSA secretion, there is weak evidence, at best, to indicate that lycopene has a direct effect on PSA secretion. A meta-analysis to determine if clinical evidence shows an association between tomato or lycopene intake and PSA levels in humans is currently in progress by our laboratory. Despite a lack of evidence showing a direct impact of lycopene treatment on PSA levels, some evidence exists to suggest that while lycopene does not directly associate with the AR, it may reduce ARE activity. However, this may be at levels higher than the normal physiologic intake of lycopene. Reduction of ARE activity may be associated with lycopene accumulation in the nucleus, which could point to lycopene interference with AR co-regulators and subsequent DNA binding and expression. In addition, both in vivo and in vitro evidence has shown that lycopene influences the expression of genes associated with androgen signaling and metabolism. Combined, these data suggest that because lycopene uptake follows the order of AR expression in AS and AI cell lines, lycopene uptake may be mediated by androgen signaling through mechanisms independent of direct AR binding.

This review is novel in topic and sought to incorporate the use of standardized guidelines recommended for conducting a preclinical systematic review with the addition of quantitative estimates of effects using albatross plots. However, this review presents some limitations. First, few studies mechanistically evaluating the effects of lycopene or tomato intervention on endpoints directly related to androgen status, signaling, or metabolism exist. While cell culture studies measuring endpoints comparing AS and AI cell lines were included for a consideration of the potential differences of lycopene treatment with varying androgen sensitivity, these studies do not directly link lycopene to androgen signaling and must be considered separately from the studies evaluating the effects of lycopene treatment on direct androgen endpoints.

Second, the variability of study design and outcome measurement creates difficultly in comparing animal and cell culture studies. Models used must be carefully evaluated and follow the general progression of human disease. While extremely useful for studying mechanistic outcomes, cell culture models are generally not considered to mimic human disease progression. Cancer, particularly PCa, is considered to be a heterogenous disease. Multiple cell types expressing different mutations are available and considered within this review (e.g., LNCaP, PC-3, DU145), but these single cell lines only represent a small subset of individual tumor phenotypes and do not account for cell interaction with the surrounding tumor microenvironment. In addition, differences between cell culture medium, lycopene dose and delivery method, length of treatment, and laboratory tests conducted may significantly contribute to differences in the overall outcomes. Animal models are a step-up in study design, but only models mimicking the human progression of disease (i.e., tumors originate from the animal) are considered to be high quality models. To this end, only one of the five included studies used a transgenic animal model of PCa (TRAMP), while all others used some form of transplantable tumor model. Furthermore, differences in laboratory tests conducted and outcomes reported for both cell culture and animal studies necessitated the grouping of outcomes by indirect or direct interaction with the androgen axis. As a result, these groupings only served to create estimations of the effects of lycopene treatment on each outcome category, rather than a true statistical evaluation of the effects.

Finally, as previously discussed, lycopene is a potent antioxidant and, as such, is unstable when isolated and exposed to light and air, making it a difficult compound to work with in vitro [45]. Lycopene source, purity, storage, delivery vehicle, air and light exposure, and length of time in culture are all factors that vary by study. These factors can result in oxidation of the parent compound, making study outcomes the result of these oxidized lycopenoids. Studies generally addressed this issue by confirming cellular lycopene uptake, lycopene stability after media culture, or simply by refreshing cell media and treatment daily. However, the labile nature of lycopene and the inherent variability in the study methodology pose major limitations when considering results from cell culture studies.

To address these limitations, future studies should be designed specifically to probe the hypothesis that physiologically relevant doses of lycopene can impact the androgen axis by measuring changes related to androgen activity, signaling, or metabolism. Studies evaluating the effect of lycopene on androgen concentrations, androgen metabolizing enzyme activity, and androgen-regulated gene activity (such as PSA) in animal models, as well as cell lines representative of varying stages of PCa, would result in valuable additions to strengthen the current literature. In the interest of enabling systematic reviews of preclinical research to identify potential mechanisms whereby lycopene can modulate androgen status, future studies should also take care to report a detailed and comprehensive methodology and experimental results.

The reviewed evidence shows that lycopene potentially reduces androgen metabolism and signaling in PCa, thereby reducing the effects of one of the main factors driving PCa growth and progression. While the current pool of research is promising, there is a general lack of preclinical and clinical research relating to the effects or mechanisms of lycopene or other compounds present in tomatoes on androgens, their metabolites, and their downstream effectors at different stages of PCa. Androgen signaling is an important chemotherapeutic target for advanced PCa because intratumoral signaling persists, despite the removal of androgens through ADT. Regular and feasible dietary intake of tomatoes has been shown to reduce the risk for PCa. The mechanisms behind this risk reduction are unclear; however, a reduction of androgen signaling would suggest an important role for tomato and tomato carotenoids at all stages of PCa growth and progression. Therefore, it is essential to identify how simple and widely accepted dietary interventions such as increased tomato intake may act as adjuvant therapies to attenuate the adverse effects of persistent androgen signaling on tumor growth and, as a result, on patient outcome. Future research is needed to fill the large gap that still exists in the literature pertaining to the mechanisms by which tomatoes or lycopene may work to modulate androgen status and androgen signaling during various stages of PCa development and progression.

Author Contributions: Conceptualization, methodology design, data curation, and validation, C.C.A., J.L.R., and J.W.E.; investigation and formal analysis, C.C.A.; writing—original draft preparation, C.C.A.; writing—review and editing, C.C.A, J.L.R., and J.W.E. All authors approved the manuscript.

Acknowledgments: We would like to thank Sean Harrison for his extensive knowledge, patience, and kind guidance in the use and creation of the albatross plots.

Appendix A

Table A1. Quality assessment of included animal studies (SYRCLE tool) [24].

Author, Year	Selection Bias			Performance Bias		Detection Bias		Attrition Bias [8]	Reporting Bias [9]	Other Bias [10]
	Sequence Generation [1]	Baseline [2]	Allocation Concealment [3]	Random Housing [4]	Blinding [5]	Random Outcome Assessment [6]	Blinding [7]			
Canene-Adams, 2009 [27]	Unclear	Low	Unclear	Low	Unclear	Unclear	Unclear	Low	Low	Low
Limpens, 2006 [28]	Low	Low	Unclear	Low	Unclear	Unclear	Low	Low	Low	Low
Lindshield, 2010 [29]	Unclear	Low	Unclear	Low	Unclear	Unclear	Unclear	Low	Low	Low
Siler, 2004 [30]	Low	Low	Unclear	Low	Unclear	Unclear	Unclear	Low	Low	Low
Wan, 2014 [31]	Low	Low	Unclear	Low	Unclear	Unclear	Unclear	Low	Low	Low

Studies are given a risk of bias of either "high" (disagreement with parameters), "low" (agreement with parameters), or "unclear" (unclear is parameters were met/unmet) based on the following parameters: [1] random allocation of animals; [2] similarity of baseline characteristics; [3] allocation blinding; [4] random housing distribution within the room; [5] investigator blinding; [6] random animal selection for outcome assessment; [7] outcome assessor blinding; [8] incomplete outcome data addressed; [9] free from selective outcome reporting; [10] free from any other potential sources of bias (e.g., contamination, funding sources, unit of analysis errors). No summary score is given to avoid assigning weights to each category.

Table A2. Quality assessment of included cell culture studies (adapted from WCRF/UoB recommendations) [22].

Author, Year	Source [1]	Experimental Conditions				Selective Reporting [6]	Total
		Culture Conditions [2]	Replicates [3]	Controls [4]	Multiple Cell Lines [5]		
Fu, 2014 [44]	1	1	0	1	1	1	5
Gong, 2016 [40]	1	1	1	1	1	1	6
Gunasekera, 2007 [41]	1	1	1	1	1	1	6
Ivanov, 2007 [32]	1	1	0	1	1	0	4
Linnewiel-Hermoni, 2015 [33]	1	1	1	1	1	1	6
Liu, 2006 [34]	1	1	1	0	1	1	5
Liu, 2008 [35]	1	1	1	1	1	1	6
Peternac, 2008 [36]	1	1	1	1	1	1	6
Rafi, 2013 [37]	1	1	1	1	0	1	5
Richards, 2003 [38]	1	0	1	1	0	0	3
Tang, 2005 [42]	1	1	1	1	1	1	6
Tang, 2011 [43]	1	1	1	1	1	0	5
Zhang, 2010 [39]	1	1	0	1	0	0	3

Studies are given a score of 0 or 1 for each of the following parameters (a score of 0 was given for a lack of criteria fulfillment or failure to report): [1] cell lines are independently validated; [2] comparable culture conditions to other studies; [3] experiment performed in replicate(s); [4] appropriate controls included; [5] more than one cell line used; [6] all experimental results are reported (a score of 0 was given for missing statistical data).

Table A3. Characteristics of prostate cancer cell lines.

Cell Line	Source	Androgen Receptor Expression	Androgen Sensitivity (AS or AI)	Other Characteristics
LNCaP [52]	Human PCa left supraclavicular lymph node metastasis	AR+	AS	Broad AR ligand-specificity; PTEN mutation [52]
C4-2 [53]	Human PCa (subline of LNCaP cells derived from prostate epithelial cells of mouse xenograft cultured from osteosarcoma of mouse xenograft)	AR+ †	AI	High EGFR expression (5–10-fold higher) when compared to parental LNCaP cell line
LAPC-4 [54,55]	Human PCa (subline of LNCaP cells derived from mouse xenograft)	AR+	AS	
22Rv1 [56]	Human PCa (derived from prostate epithelial cells of muse xenograft after castration-induced regression and relapse of the parental, androgen-dependent CWR22 xenograft)	AR+	AS	Express AR splice variants, making this line potentially AI
PC-3 [57]	Human PCa bone metastasis	AR– †	AI	Low SRD5A activities; PTEN deletion [52]
DU145 [57]	Human PCa brain metastasis	AR-	AI	High IGF-I expression [58]
6S [35]	Primary human PCa stromal cells	AR+	AS	
DTE [59]	Rat PCa (Dunning-R3327 tumors)	AR+	AS	
AT-3 [59]	Rat PCa (derived from castration selection of parental DTE Dunning-R3327 tumors)	AR-	AI	Low SRD5A activities
Order of AR expression *		LNCaP > LAPC-4 > ? 22Rv1 > ? C4-2 > PC-3 > DU145		
Order of lycopene uptake [34,40] *		LNCaP > PC-3 > DU145 > C4-2		

* Comparison between all cell lines not reported. Question marks indicate suggested order of AR expression. † Potentially weak AR expression; variable results reported. ? Direct comparisons of AR expression levels between LAPC-4, C4-2, and 22Rv1 cell not reported. Abbreviations: AS (androgen-sensitive); AI (androgen-insensitive); AR (androgen receptor); PTEN (phosphatase and tensin homolog); EGFR (epidermal growth factor receptor); SRD5A (5α-reductase); IGF-I (insulin-like growth factor-I).

References

1. Negoita, S.; Feuer, E.J.; Mariotto, A.; Cronin, K.A.; Petkov, V.I.; Hussey, S.K.; Benard, V.; Henley, S.J.; Anderson, R.N.; Fedewa, S.; et al. Annual Report to the Nation on the Status of Cancer, part II: Recent changes in prostate cancer trends and disease characteristics. *Cancer* **2018**, *124*, 2801–2814. [CrossRef] [PubMed]
2. Pezaro, C.; Woo, H.H.; Davis, I.D. Prostate cancer: Measuring PSA. *Intern. Med. J.* **2014**, *44*, 433–440. [CrossRef] [PubMed]
3. Huggins, C.; Stevens, R.E., Jr.; Hodges, C.V. Studies on prostatic cancer: II. the effects of castration on advanced carcinoma of the prostate gland. *Arch. Surg.* **1941**, *43*, 209–223. [CrossRef]
4. Tilki, D.; Evans, C.P. The changing landscape of advanced and castration resistant prostate cancer: Latest science and revised definitions. *Can. J. Urol.* **2014**, *21*, 7–13. [PubMed]
5. Rowles, J.L., 3rd; Ranard, K.M.; Applegate, C.C.; Jeon, S.; An, R.; Erdman, J.W., Jr. Processed and raw tomato consumption and risk of prostate cancer: A systematic review and dose-response meta-analysis. *Prostate Cancer Prostatic. Dis.* **2018**, *21*, 319–336. [CrossRef] [PubMed]
6. Rowles, J.L., 3rd; Ranard, K.M.; Smith, J.W.; An, R.; Erdman, J.W., Jr. Increased dietary and circulating lycopene are associated with reduced prostate cancer risk: A systematic review and meta-analysis. *Prostate Cancer Prostatic. Dis.* **2017**, *20*, 361–377. [CrossRef] [PubMed]
7. Xu, X.; Li, J.; Wang, X.; Wang, S.; Meng, S.; Zhu, Y.; Liang, Z.; Zheng, X.; Xie, L. Tomato consumption and prostate cancer risk: A systematic review and meta-analysis. *Sci. Rep.* **2016**, *6*, 37091. [CrossRef] [PubMed]
8. Zu, K.; Mucci, L.; Rosner, B.A.; Clinton, S.K.; Loda, M.; Stampfer, M.J.; Giovannucci, E. Dietary lycopene, angiogenesis, and prostate cancer: A prospective study in the prostate-specific antigen era. *J. Natl. Cancer Inst.* **2014**, *106*, djt430. [CrossRef] [PubMed]
9. Wang, Y.; Cui, R.; Xiao, Y.; Fang, J.; Xu, Q. Effect of carotene and lycopene on the risk of prostate cancer: A systematic review and dose-response meta-analysis of observational studies. *PLoS ONE* **2015**, *10*, e0137427. [CrossRef]
10. Paur, I.; Lilleby, W.; Bohn, S.K.; Hulander, E.; Klein, W.; Vlatkovic, L.; Axcrona, K.; Bolstad, N.; Bjoro, T.; Laake, P.; et al. Tomato-based randomized controlled trial in prostate cancer patients: Effect on PSA. *Clin. Nutr.* **2017**, *36*, 672–679. [CrossRef] [PubMed]
11. Zhang, X.; Yang, Y.; Wang, Q. Lycopene can reduce prostate-specific antigen velocity in a phase II clinical study in Chinese population. *Chin. Med. J.* **2014**, *127*, 2143–2146. [PubMed]
12. Wang, Y.; Jacobs, E.J.; Newton, C.C.; McCullough, M.L. Lycopene, tomato products and prostate cancer-specific mortality among men diagnosed with nonmetastatic prostate cancer in the Cancer Prevention Study II Nutrition Cohort. *Int. J. Cancer* **2016**, *138*, 2846–2855. [CrossRef] [PubMed]
13. Key, T.J.; Appelby, P.N.; Travis, R.C.; Albanes, D.; Alberg, A.J.; Barricarte, A.; Black, A.; Boeing, H.; Bueno-de-Mesquita, H.B.; Chan, J.M.; et al. Carotenoids, retinol, tocopherols, and prostate cancer risk: A pooled analysis of 15 studies. *Am. J. Clin. Nutr.* **2015**, *102*, 1142–1157. [CrossRef] [PubMed]
14. Schrecengost, R.; Knudsen, K.E. Molecular pathogenesis and progression of prostate cancer. *Semin. Oncol.* **2013**, *40*, 244–258. [CrossRef] [PubMed]
15. Cai, C.; Balk, S.P. Intratumoral androgen biosynthesis in prostate cancer pathogenesis and response to therapy. *Endocr. Relat. Cancer* **2011**, *18*, R175–R182. [CrossRef] [PubMed]
16. Boileau, T.W.M.; Clinton, S.K.; Erdman, J.W., Jr. Tissue lycopene concentrations and isomer patterns are affected by androgen status and dietary lycopene concentration in male F344 rats. *J. Nutr.* **2000**, *130*, 1613–1618. [CrossRef] [PubMed]
17. Boileau, T.W.M.; Clinton, S.K.; Zaripheh, S.; Monaco, M.H.; Donovan, S.M.; Erdman, J.W., Jr. Testosterone and food restriction modulate hepatic lycopene isomer concentrations in male F344 rats. *J. Nutr.* **2001**, *131*, 1746–1752. [CrossRef] [PubMed]
18. Campbell, J.K.; Stroud, C.K.; Nakamura, M.T.; Lila, M.A.; Erdman, J.W., Jr. Serum testosterone is reduced following short-term phytofluene, lycopene, or tomato powder consumption in F344 rats. *J. Nutr.* **2006**, *136*, 2813–2819. [CrossRef] [PubMed]
19. Ko, H.-K.; Berk, M.; Chung, Y.-M.; Willard, B.; Bareja, R.; Rubin, M.; Sboner, A.; Sharifi, N. Loss of an androgen-inactivating and isoform-specific HSD17B4 splice form enables emergence of castration-resistant prostate cancer. *Cell Rep.* **2018**, *22*, 809–819. [CrossRef] [PubMed]

20. Herzog, A.; Siler, U.; Spitzer, V.; Seifert, N.; Denelavas, A.; Hunziker, P.B.; Hunziker, W.; Goralczyk, R.; Wertz, K. Lycopene reduced gene expression of steroid targets and inflammatory markers in normal rat prostate. *FASEB J.* **2005**, *19*, 272–274. [CrossRef] [PubMed]
21. Qiu, X.; Yuan, Y.; Vaishnav, A.; Tessel, M.A.; Nonn, L.; van Breemen, R.B. Effects of lycopene on protein expression in human primary prostatic epithelial cells. *Cancer Prev. Res.* **2013**, *6*, 419–427. [CrossRef] [PubMed]
22. Lewis, S.J.; Gardner, M.; Higgins, J.; Holly, J.M.P.; Gaunt, T.R.; Perks, C.M.; Turner, S.D.; Rinaldi, S.; Thomas, S.; Harrison, S.; et al. Developing the WCRF International/University of Bristol methodology for identifying and carrying out systematic reviews of mechanisms of exposure-cancer associations. *Cancer Epidemiol. Biomark. Prev.* **2017**, *26*, 1667–1675. [CrossRef] [PubMed]
23. Moher, D.; Liberati, A.; Tetzlaff, J.; Altman, D.G.; Group, P. Preferred reporting items for systematic reviews and meta-analyses: The PRISMA statement. *J. Clin. Epidemiol.* **2009**, *62*, 1006–1012. [CrossRef] [PubMed]
24. Hooijmans, C.R.; Rovers, M.M.; de Vries, R.B.M.; Leenaars, M.; Ritskes-Hoitinga, M.; Langendam, M.W. SYRCLE's risk of bias tool for animal studies. *BMC Med. Res. Methodol.* **2014**, *14*, 43. [CrossRef] [PubMed]
25. Higgins, J.P.T.; Altman, D.G.; Gøtzsche, P.C.; Jüni, P.; Moher, D.; Oxman, A.D.; Savović, J.; Schulz, K.F.; Weeks, L.; Sterne, J.A.C. The Cochrane Collaboration's tool for assessing risk of bias in randomised trials. *BMJ* **2011**, *343*, d5928. [CrossRef] [PubMed]
26. Harrison, S.; Jones, H.E.; Martin, R.M.; Lewis, S.J.; Higgins, J.P.T. The albatross plot: A novel graphical tool for presenting results of diversely reported studies in a systematic review. *Res. Synth. Methods* **2017**, *8*, 281–289. [CrossRef] [PubMed]
27. Canene-Adams, K.; Lindshield, B.L.; Wang, S.; Jeffery, E.H.; Clinton, S.K.; Erdman, J.W., Jr. Combinations of tomato and broccoli enhance antitumor activity in dunning r3327-h prostate adenocarcinomas. *Cancer Res.* **2007**, *67*, 836–843. [CrossRef] [PubMed]
28. Limpens, J.; Schroder, F.H.; de Ridder, C.M.A.; Bolder, C.A.; Wildhagen, M.F.; Obermuller-Jevic, U.C.; Kramer, K.; van Weerden, W.M. Combined lycopene and vitamin E treatment suppresses the growth of PC-346C human prostate cancer cells in nude mice. *J. Nutr.* **2006**, *136*, 1287–1293. [CrossRef] [PubMed]
29. Lindshield, B.L.; Ford, N.A.; Canene-Adams, K.; Diamond, A.M.; Wallig, M.A.; Erdman, J.W., Jr. Selenium, but not lycopene or vitamin E, decreases growth of transplantable dunning R3327-H rat prostate tumors. *PLoS ONE* **2010**, *5*, e10423. [CrossRef] [PubMed]
30. Siler, U.; Barella, L.; Spitzer, V.; Schnorr, J.; Lein, M.; Goralczyk, R.; Wertz, K. Lycopene and Vitamin E interfere with autocrine/paracrine loops in the Dunning prostate cancer model. *FASEB J.* **2004**, *18*, 1019–1021. [CrossRef] [PubMed]
31. Wan, L.; Tan, H.L.; Thomas-Ahner, J.M.; Pearl, D.K.; Erdman, J.W., Jr.; Moran, N.E.; Clinton, S.K. Dietary tomato and lycopene impact androgen signaling and carcinogenesis-related gene expression during early TRAMP prostate carcinogenesis. *Cancer Prev. Res.* **2014**, *7*, 1228–1239. [CrossRef] [PubMed]
32. Ivanov, N.I.; Cowell, S.P.; Brown, P.; Rennie, P.S.; Guns, E.S.; Cox, M.E. Lycopene differentially induces quiescence and apoptosis in androgen-responsive and -independent prostate cancer cell lines. *Clin. Nutr.* **2007**, *26*, 252–263. [CrossRef] [PubMed]
33. Linnewiel-Hermoni, K.; Khanin, M.; Danilenko, M.; Zango, G.; Amosi, Y.; Levy, J.; Sharoni, Y. The anti-cancer effects of carotenoids and other phytonutrients resides in their combined activity. *Arch. Biochem. Biophys.* **2015**, *572*, 28–35. [CrossRef] [PubMed]
34. Liu, A.; Pajkovic, N.; Pang, Y.; Zhu, D.; Calamini, B.; Mesecar, A.L.; van Breemen, R.B. Absorption and subcellular localization of lycopene in human prostate cancer cells. *Mol. Cancer Ther.* **2006**, *5*, 2879–2885. [CrossRef] [PubMed]
35. Liu, X.X.; Allen, J.D.; Arnold, J.T.; Blackman, M.R. Lycopene inhibits IGF-I signal transduction and growth in normal prostate epithelial cells by decreasing DHT-modulated IGF-I production in co-cultured reactive stromal cells. *Carcinogenesis* **2008**, *29*, 816–823. [CrossRef] [PubMed]
36. Peternac, D.; Klima, I.; Cecchini, M.G.; Schwaninger, R.; Studer, U.E.; Thalmann, G.N. Agents used for chemoprevention of prostate cancer may influence PSA secretion independently of cell growth in the LNCaP model of human prostate cancer progression. *Prostate* **2008**, *68*, 1307–1318. [CrossRef] [PubMed]
37. Rafi, M.M.; Kanakasabai, S.; Reyes, M.D.; Bright, J.J. Lycopene modulates growth and survival associated genes in prostate cancer. *J. Nutr. Biochem.* **2013**, *24*, 1724–1734. [CrossRef] [PubMed]

38. Richards, L.T.R.; Benghuzzi, H.; Tucci, M.; Hughes, J. The synergistic effect of conventional and sustained delivery of antioxidants on LNCaP prostate cancer cell line. *Biomed. Sci. Instrum.* **2003**, *39*, 402–407. [PubMed]
39. Zhang, X.; Wang, Q.; Neil, B.; Chen, X.A. Effect of lycopene on androgen receptor and prostate-specific antigen velocity. *Chin. Med. J.* **2010**, *123*, 2231–2236. [CrossRef] [PubMed]
40. Gong, X.; Marisiddaiah, R.; Zaripheh, S.; Wiener, D.; Rubin, L.P. Mitochondrial beta-carotene 9′,10′ oxygenase modulates prostate cancer growth via NF-kappaB inhibition: A lycopene-independent function. *Mol. Cancer Res.* **2016**, *14*, 966–975. [CrossRef] [PubMed]
41. Gunasekera, R.S.; Sewgobind, K.; Desai, S.; Dunn, L.; Black, H.S.; McKeehan, W.L.; Patil, B. Lycopene and lutein inhibit proliferation in rat prostate carcinoma cells. *Nutr. Cancer* **2007**, *58*, 171–177. [CrossRef] [PubMed]
42. Tang, L.L.; Jin, T.Y.; Zeng, X.B.; Wang, J.S. Lycopene inhibits the growth of human androgen-independent prostate cancer cells in vitro and in BALB/c nude mice. *J. Nutr.* **2005**, *135*, 287–290. [CrossRef] [PubMed]
43. Tang, Y.; Parmakhtiar, B.; Simoneau, A.R.; Xie, J.; Fruehauf, J.; Lilly, M.; Zi, X. Lycopene enhances docetaxel's effect in castration-resistant prostate cancer associated with insulin-like growth factor I receptor levels. *Neoplasia* **2011**, *13*, 108–119. [CrossRef] [PubMed]
44. Fu, L.J.; Ding, Y.B.; Wu, L.X.; Wen, C.J.; Qu, Q.; Zhang, X.; Zhou, H.H. The effects of lycopene on the methylation of the GSTP1 promoter and global methylation in prostatic cancer cell lines PC3 and LNCaP. *Int. J. Endocrinol.* **2014**, *2014*, 620125. [CrossRef] [PubMed]
45. Lin, C.Y.; Huang, C.S.; Hu, M.L. The use of fetal bovine serum as delivery vehicle to improve the uptake and stability of lycopene in cell culture studies. *Br. J. Nutr.* **2007**, *98*, 226–232. [CrossRef] [PubMed]
46. Cook, M.B.; Stanczyk, F.Z.; Wood, S.N.; Pfeiffer, R.M.; Hafi, M.; Veneroso, C.C.; Lynch, B.; Falk, R.T.; Zhou, C.K.; Niwa, S.; et al. Relationships between circulating and intraprostatic sex steroid hormone concentrations. *Cancer Epidemiol. Biomark. Prev.* **2017**, *26*, 1660–1666. [CrossRef] [PubMed]
47. Izumi, K.; Shigehara, K.; Nohara, T.; Narimoto, K.; Kadono, Y.; Mizokami, A. Both high and low serum total testosterone levels indicate poor prognosis in patients with prostate cancer. *Anticancer Res.* **2017**, *37*, 5559–5564. [CrossRef] [PubMed]
48. Wang, K.; Chen, X.; Bird, V.Y.; Gerke, T.A.; Manini, T.M.; Prosperi, M. Association between age-related reductions in testosterone and risk of prostate cancer-an analysis of patients' data with prostatic diseases. *Int. J. Cancer* **2017**, *141*, 1783–1793. [CrossRef] [PubMed]
49. Shu, Q.; Cai, T.; Chen, X.; Zhu, H.H.; Xue, P.; Zhu, N.; Xie, Z.; Wei, S.; Zhang, Q.; Niu, L.; et al. Proteomic comparison and MRM-based comparative analysis of metabolites reveal metabolic shift in human prostate cancer cell lines. *J. Proteome Res.* **2015**, *14*, 3390–3402. [CrossRef] [PubMed]
50. Jerónimo, C.; Bastian, P.J.; Bjartell, A.; Carbone, G.M.; Catto, J.W.F.; Clark, S.J.; Henrique, R.; Nelson, W.G.; Shariat, S.F. Epigenetics in prostate cancer: Biologic and clinical relevance. *Eur. Urol.* **2011**, *60*, 753–766. [CrossRef] [PubMed]
51. Lin, X.; Tascilar, M.; Lee, W.-H.; Vles, W.J.; Lee, B.H.; Veeraswamy, R.; Asgari, K.; Freije, D.; van Rees, B.; Gage, W.R.; et al. GSTP1 CpG island hypermethylation is responsible for the absence of GSTP1 expression in human prostate cancer cells. *Am. J. Pathol.* **2001**, *159*, 1815–1826. [CrossRef]
52. Russell, P.J.; Kingsley, E.A. Human prostate cancer cell lines. *Methods Mol. Med.* **2003**, *81*, 21–39. [CrossRef] [PubMed]
53. Wu, H.C.; Hsieh, J.T.; Gleave, M.E.; Brown, N.M.; Pathak, S.; Chung, L.W. Derivation of androgen-independent human LNCaP prostatic cancer cell sublines: Role of bone stromal cells. *Int. J. Cancer* **1994**, *57*, 406–412. [CrossRef] [PubMed]
54. Klein, K.A.; Reiter, R.E.; Redula, J.; Moradi, H.; Zhu, X.L.; Brothman, A.R.; Lamb, D.J.; Marcelli, M.; Belldegrun, A.; Witte, O.N.; et al. Progression of metastatic human prostate cancer to androgen independence in immunodeficient SCID mice. *Nat. Med.* **1997**, *3*, 402–408. [CrossRef] [PubMed]
55. Hoefer, J.; Akbor, M.; Handle, F.; Ofer, P.; Puhr, M.; Parson, W.; Culig, Z.; Klocker, H.; Heidegger, I. Critical role of androgen receptor level in prostate cancer cell resistance to new generation antiandrogen enzalutamide. *Oncotarget* **2016**, *7*, 59781–59794. [CrossRef] [PubMed]
56. Sramkoski, R.M.; Pretlow, T.G., II; Giaconia, J.M.; Pretlow, T.P.; Schwartz, S.; Sy, M.-S.; Marengo, S.R.; Rhim, J.S.; Zhang, D.; Jacobberger, J.W. A new human prostate carcinoma cell line, 22R*v1*. *In Vitro Cell Dev. Biol. Anim.* **1999**, *35*, 403–409. [CrossRef] [PubMed]

57. Matsuoka, T.; Shigemura, K.; Yamamichi, F.; Fujisawa, M.; Kawabata, M.; Shirakawa, T. Detection of tumor markers in prostate cancer and comparison of sensitivity between real time and nested PCR. *Kobe J. Med. Sci.* **2012**, *58*, E51–E59. [PubMed]
58. Pietrzkowski, Z.; Mulholland, G.; Gomella, L.; Jameson, B.A.; Wernicke, D.; Baserga, R. Inhibition of growth of prostatic cancer cell lines by peptide analogues of insulin-like growth factor 1. *Cancer Res.* **1993**, *53*, 1102–1106. [PubMed]
59. Isaacs, J.T.; Isaacs, W.B.; Feitz, W.F.; Scheres, J. Establishment and characterization of seven dunning rat prostatic cancer cell lines and their use in developing methods for predicting metastatic abilities of prostatic cancers. *Prostate* **1986**, *9*, 261–281. [CrossRef] [PubMed]

4

Astaxanthin Prevents Alcoholic Fatty Liver Disease by Modulating Mouse Gut Microbiota

Huilin Liu [1], Meihong Liu [2,3], Xueqi Fu [1], Ziqi Zhang [4], Lingyu Zhu [4], Xin Zheng [4] and Jingsheng Liu [2,3,*]

1 School of Life Sciences, Jilin University, Changchun 130012, China; lhl14@mails.jlu.edu.cn (H.L.); fxq@jlu.edu.cn (X.F.)
2 College of Food Science and Engineering, Jilin Agricultural University, Changchun 130118, China; liumh@jlau.edu.cn
3 National Engineering Laboratory for Wheat and Corn Deep Processing, Changchun 130118, China
4 College of Animal Science and Technology, Jilin Agricultural University, Changchun 130118, China; zhangziqi@jlau.edu.cn (Z.Z.); zhulingyu@jlau.edu.cn (L.Z.); zhengxin@jlau.edu.cn (X.Z.)
* Correspondence: liujs1007@vip.sina.com;

Abstract: The development and progression of alcoholic fatty liver disease (AFLD) is influenced by the intestinal microbiota. Astaxanthin, a type of oxygenated carotenoid with strong antioxidant and anti-inflammatory properties, has been proven to relieve liver injury. However, the relationship between the gut microbiota regulation effect of astaxanthin and AFLD improvement remains unclear. The effects of astaxanthin on the AFLD phenotype, overall structure, and composition of gut microbiota were assessed in ethanol-fed C57BL/6J mice. The results showed that astaxanthin treatment significantly relieves inflammation and decreases excessive lipid accumulation and serum markers of liver injury. Furthermore, astaxanthin was shown to significantly decrease species from the phyla Bacteroidetes and Proteobacteria and the genera *Butyricimonas*, *Bilophila*, and *Parabacteroides*, as well as increase species from Verrucomicrobia and *Akkermansia* compared with the Et (ethanol)group. Thirteen phylotypes related to inflammation as well as correlated with metabolic parameters were significantly altered by ethanol, and then notably reversed by astaxanthin. Additionally, astaxanthin altered 18 and 128 KEGG (Kyoto Encyclopedia of Genes and Genomes) pathways involved in lipid metabolism and xenobiotic biodegradation and metabolism at levels 2 and 3, respectively. These findings suggest that *Aakkermansia* may be a potential target for the astaxanthin-induced alleviation of AFLD and may be a potential treatment for bacterial disorders induced by AFLD.

Keywords: astaxanthin; *Akkermansia*; alcoholic fatty liver disease; inflammation; gut microbiota

1. Introduction

According to the "Global Status Report on Alcohol and Health 2014" released by the World Health Organization (WHO), the use of alcohol has reached a detrimental level, resulting in more than 3 million deaths every year and accounting for 5.9% of all deaths worldwide. As the metabolism of alcohol in the organism mainly depends on the liver, the long-term consumption and over-consumption of alcohol leads to liver damage and triggers alcoholic fatty liver disease (AFLD) [1], thereafter causing health issues ranging from fatty liver to alcoholic hepatitis and even cirrhosis [2,3]. The first two phases can be reversible through alcohol abstinence and lifestyle intervention. Thus, the detection of potential functional ingredients for AFLD prevention is significant.

Astaxanthin is one of the major xanthophyll carotenoids in marine organisms, and is found in shrimp, crabs, fish, algae, yeast, and feathers of birds [4,5]. As astaxanthin cannot be synthesized in humans, its uptake fully depends on dietary sources. Astaxanthin-associated protection against aging as well as cardiovascular and cancerous diseases is attributed to its great antioxidative and anti-inflammatory activity [4]. In particular, it has been suggested that astaxanthin is protective against various types of liver damage [6,7], such as non-alcoholic fatty liver disease (NAFLD) [8–10] and liver fibrosis [11]; however, further investigation is required to determine the effect of astaxanthin on AFLD protection.

Previous studies have confirmed that gut microbiota imbalance is related to a variety of chronic diseases, such as obesity, cardiovascular disease, and cancer [12–14]. The relationship between gut microbiota and AFLD has become a topic of increasing concern to researchers. In healthy humans, the intestinal microbiota remains in symbiotic balance, but alcohol intake induces the modification of its composition, thereby inhibiting dominant intestinal bacteria and promoting a small amount of pathogenic bacteria overgrowth [15], resulting in the impairment of intestinal physiological function. The long-term intake of alcohol breaks the barrier function of the intestine and promotes the growth of intestinal pathogenic bacteria and harmful metabolites (such as lipopolysaccharides). These health-threatening components lead to the development of AFLD by invading into other tissues and organs through blood circulation [16,17]. *Akkermansia muciniphila* (*A. muciniphila*), which can degrade mucin and maintain intestinal barrier integrity, colonizes in the human gut mucus layer and is negatively associated with certain diseases like obesity, diabetes, inflammation, and metabolic disorders [18]. Long-term dietary intervention can restore the gut microbiota and improve intestinal physiological function [19]. The concentration of *A. muciniphila* can be increased through the ingestion of *Bifidobacteria*, fructo-oligosaccharides, short-chain carbohydrates, metformin, rhubarb extract, or specific antibiotics [18]. Bacterial imbalance is an important factor in inducing disease in AFLD patients. An increase in probiotics species and the inhibition of pathogenic bacteria may improve AFLD status.

Astaxanthin has been reported to prevent liver damage [6,20], but there has been little research on the effect of astaxanthin on AFLD. Studying intestinal microbiota regulation in AFLD may provide new insight into the pathogenesis and therapeutic target of AFLD. In the present study, we investigated whether astaxanthin can protect against alcohol-induced liver injury and its association with the intestinal microecology. We also determined the main influence of bacteria during the astaxanthin intervention.

2. Materials and Methods

2.1. Animal Experimentation

Male C57BL/6J mice (22 ± 2 g, six weeks old) were purchased from the Beijing Vital River Laboratory Animal Technology Co., Ltd. (Beijing, China) and housed individually in cages with a 12-h light/dark cycle at 23 ± 2 °C with full access to chow diet and water. All experiment protocols were approved by the Institutional Animal Care and Use Committee at the Jilin Institute of Traditional Chinese Medicine (approval number: SYXK (JI) 2015-0009).

The alcoholic liver disease (AFLD) mouse model was established using the modified Lieber–DeCarli liquid diet [21]. The 60 mice were randomly separated into five groups, each consisting of 12 mice. The first group was fed with a normal standard growth diet while the other four groups were fed high-fat liquid diets (35% fat, 18% protein, 47% carbohydrates, provided by TROPHIC Animal Feed High-Tech Co., Ltd., Nantong, China) for an acclimation period of two weeks acclimation. Then the four high-fat diet groups were fed with either only the high-fat liquid diet (Con), or combined with the astaxanthin (AST group, 50 mg/kg bw), ethanol-containing (Et group, 5% ethanol v/v, accounted for 36% of the total caloric intake), or ethanol plus astaxanthin (EtAST group) treatments for 12 weeks. Compositions of the diets are shown in Supplementary Table S1. The astaxanthin was purchased from Sigma-Aldrich (St. Louis, MO, USA; purity ≥97%, SML0982), isolated from *Blakeslea trispora* and dissolved in corn oil for utilization in this experiment. The dose selection of astaxanthin was chosen in accordance with previous research [22], while the amount of ethanol included increased over two weeks to reach a final concentration of 5% (*v*/*v*). Body weight gain and food intake were assessed once a week. The pair-fed control group (Con) was included in this model.

After 12 weeks of treatment, the fasted mice were euthanized and blood samples were collected. The feces in the colon were also harvested into 2-mL sterile tubes to assess the gut microbiota. The tissues were immediately removed and weighed, and the liver coefficient (liver weight/body weight) was calculated. The left lobe of the liver was instantly fixed in 10% buffered formalin for histology analysis with the rest of the tissues frozen in liquid nitrogen and stored at −80 °C until further use.

2.2. Biochemical Analyses

The serum was obtained from the collected blood by centrifugation at 5000 rpm for 10 min at 4 °C and stored at −80 °C. Plasma triacylglycerol (TG), total cholesterol (TC), high-density lipoprotein (HDL), low-density lipoprotein (LDL), aspartate aminotransferase (AST), and alanine aminotransferase (ALT) were measured by enzymatic colorimetric assays using commercial detection kits (Nanjing Jiancheng of Bioengineering Institute, Nanjing, China).

2.3. Hepatic Triglyceride Staining

The left lobe of the liver tissue was separated and rapidly fixed in 4% neutral buffered formalin solution for 24 h and then processed for paraffin embedding. Five-micrometer-thick paraffin sections were stained with hematoxylin and eosin (H&E) and oil-red solution. The liver steatosis status was examined under a light microscope (Olympus, Tokyo, Japan), and photographed at 200× magnification.

2.4. Quantification of Genes Expression in Liver Tissue

Total RNA was extracted and purified in the liver tissue using TRIzol reagent (TAKARA, Beijing, China. RNAiso Plus, Code No. 9108). The purity, concentration, and quality of RNA were measured. High-quality RNA was converted to cDNA using PrimeScript™ RT reagent Kit with gDNA Eraser (TAKARA, Beijing China. Code No. RR047A). The SYBR fluorescent dye method (TAKARA, Beijing China. Code No. RR420A) and Agilent Stratagene Mx3000P Real-Time PCR System (Santa Clara, CA, USA) were used to detect the gene expression. The primers used are shown in Supplementary Table S2. The data were calculated using the $2^{-\Delta\Delta Ct}$ relative quantification method and normalized to β-actin.

2.5. Fecal DNA Extraction

Total bacterial genomic DNA was extracted from the fecal material in the colon using Fast DNA SPIN extraction kits (MP Biomedicals, Santa Ana, CA, USA), following the manufacturer's instructions. The DNA yield was measured for quantity using a NanoDrop ND-1000 spectrophotometer (Thermo Fisher Scientific, Waltham, MA, USA) and the quality was analyzed by 0.8% agarose gel electrophoresis; the DNA was then stored at −20 °C until further analysis.

2.6. Amplification and Sequencing of the 16S rRNA Genes

The V3–V4 region of bacterial 16S rRNA genes was subjected to PCR amplification using the forward primer 5′-ACTCCTACGGGAGGCAGCA-3′ and the reverse primer 5′-GGACTACH VGGGTWTCTAAT-3′. The specific system was a 25-μL reaction including 5 μL of Q5 High-Fidelity DNA Polymerase (New England Biolabs (Beijing) Ltd., Beijing, China). PCR amplicons were purified with Agencourt AMPure Beads (Beckman Coulter, Indianapolis, IN, USA) and quantified using the PicoGreen dsDNA Assay Kit (Invitrogen, Carlsbad, CA, USA). The amplicons were pooled and normalized, and then paired-end 2 × 300 bp sequencing was performed using the Illumina

MiSeq platform with the MiSeq Reagent Kit v3 at Shanghai Personal Biotechnology Co., Ltd. (Shanghai, China).

Sequencing data for the 16S rRNA sequences have been deposited in the SRA database under GenBank accession NO. SRP148082.

2.7. Bioinformatics and Statistical Analysis

Sequence data were processed using Quantitative Insights into Microbial Ecology (QIIME, v1.8.0), as previously described [23]. The low-quality sequences, which had lengths of <150 bp and average Phred scores of <20, and contained ambiguous bases and mononucleotide repeats of >8 bp, were filtered with the following criteria. Paired-end reads were assembled using FLASH. The remaining high-quality sequences were clustered into operational taxonomic units (OTUs) at 97% sequence identity by UCLUST (Edgar 2010) [24]. OTU taxonomic classification was conducted by BLAST and the OTUs containing more than 99.999% of total sequences across all samples were reserved.

All results are presented as means ± standard deviation. Data were analyzed with SPSS 19.0 using one-way analysis of variance (ANOVA), and, when appropriate, using a two-tailed Student's *t*-test between different groups. Differences among groups were evaluated for significance with the comparable variances, followed by Tukey's and least significant difference (LSD) tests. $p < 0.05$ was considered statistically significant. GraphPad Prism 7.0 software (GraphPad Software, La Jolla, CA, USA) was used for graph-making.

Sequence data analysis was mainly performed using QIIME (v1.8.0, University of Colorado, Denver, CO, USA) and R packages (v3.2.0, Bell Labs Technology Showcase, Murray Hill, NJ, USA). The alpha diversity indices, Chao1 richness estimator, and the Shannon diversity index were calculated using the OTU table in QIIME. Beta diversity analysis was performed using UniFrac distance metrics and visualized by principle coordinate analysis (PCoA), and the unweighted pair-group method with arithmetic means (UPGMA) hierarchical clustering. The significance of microbiota structure differentiation among groups was assessed by PERMANOVA (permutational multivariate analysis of variance) and ANOSIM (analysis of similarities) using the R package "vegan". Taxa abundances at different taxonomies were statistically compared among groups by Metastats and visualized as box plots. Microbial functions were predicted by PICRUSt (phylogenetic investigation of communities by reconstruction of unobserved states), based on high-quality sequences.

3. Results

3.1. Astaxanthin Protects Mice from High-Fat Diet and Ethanol-Induced Liver Lesions

We investigated whether different diets affect the growth status of mice. The five groups have similar body weights at baseline which were still not significantly difference after 12 weeks of intervention (Figure 1A). On the other hand, compared with the Control (Con) group, the liver indices of mice in the ethanol group were significantly increased, and markedly reversed in the EtAST (ethanol plus astaxanthin treatments) group, which was not different from that of the Con group (Figure 1B). The light microscopy images of the liver slices, stained by Oil Red O, showed that lipid droplets increased in size and number in the Et group compared with those in the Con group. Astaxanthin intervention significantly relieved fat accumulation in the liver induced by ethanol. H&E staining showed the structure of hepatic lobules and neatly arranged normal liver cells in the normal diet (ND) group, which showed no obvious differences among the Con and AST groups. Ethanol supplementation markedly increased the amount of hepatic steatosis and the number of necrotic cells, which appeared in a large number of fat vacuoles within liver cells and significantly enlarged them. Hepatic steatosis caused by ethanol was reversed by astaxanthin intervention (Figure 1C).

There were no significant changes in the serum markers involved in lipid dysmetabolism and liver injury in normal and astaxanthin-supplied groups compared with those in the Con group.

However, the levels of ALT and AST were markedly increased in the Et group compared to the Con group, indicating the existence of liver damage, which affected cell membrane permeability and promoted ALT and AST overflow, suggesting that mice suffered significant alcoholic liver injuries. Moreover, 50 mg kg^{-1} astaxanthin treatment significantly decreased the levels of ALT, AST, TG, and LDL compared to the Et diet. However, there were no obvious differences in the levels when compared with the ND group. These results suggest that astaxanthin has the ability to alleviate lipid dysmetabolism and alcohol-induced liver injury (Figure 1D).

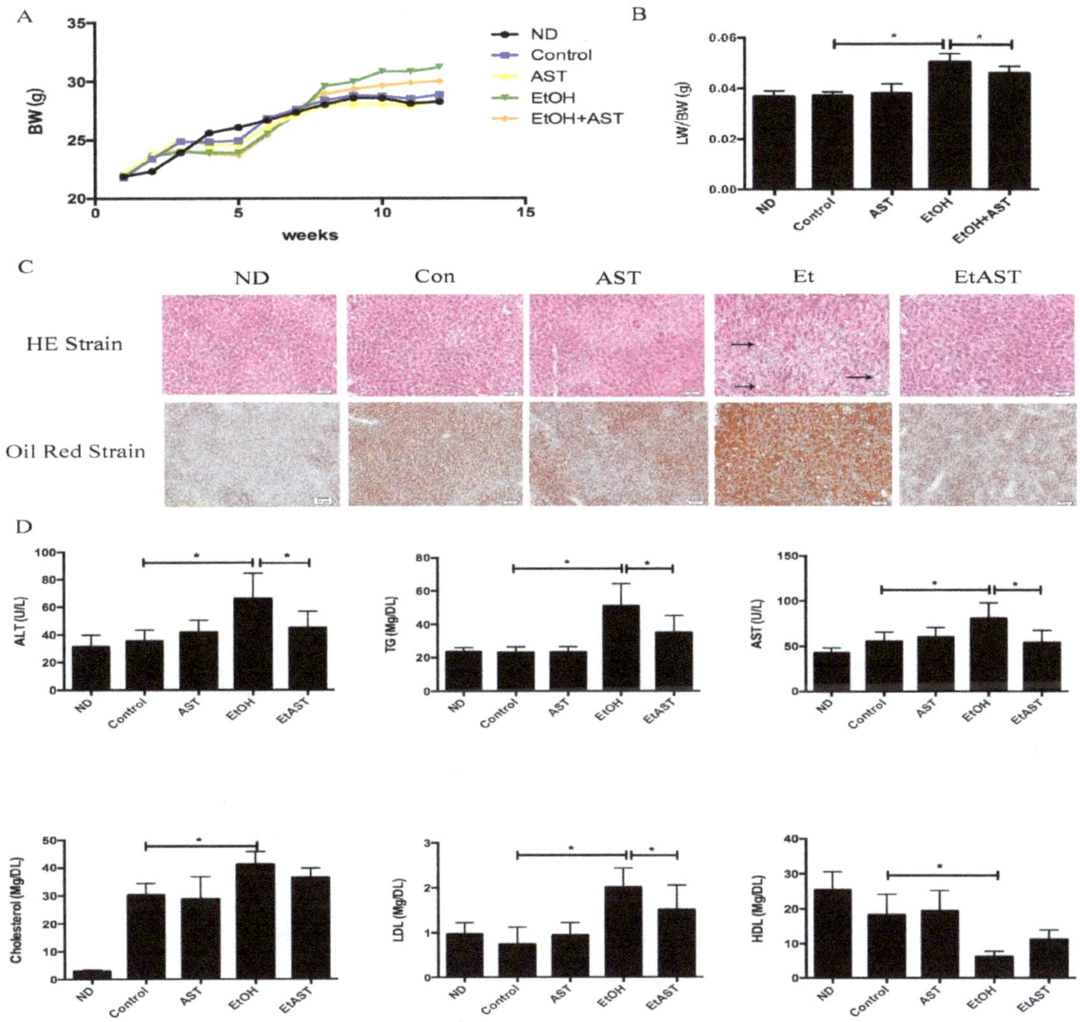

Figure 1. Effect of astaxanthin on body weight, pathological morphology, and serum markers involved in liver injury in ethanol diet-fed mice. C57BL/6J mice were fed the Lieber–DeCarli liquid diet containing 5% ethanol for 12 weeks ad libitum with or without 50 mg kg^{-1} of astaxanthin. Body weight was measured once a week (**A**). The liver index was represented by calculating liver weight/body weight (**B**). The statues of hepatic steatosis were checked by hematoxylin and eosin (H&E) staining and hepatic lipid accumulation was detected by Oil red O staining. The symbol $\rightarrow$ plays a indicate role to identify the fat vacuoles (**C**). The serum markers of liver injury were determined by the enzyme activities of alanine aminotransferase (ALT) and aspartate aminotransferase (AST). Lipid accumulation in the liver was reflected by the levels of hepatic markers, including plasma triacylglycerol (TG), low-density lipoprotein (LDL), high-density lipoprotein (HDL), and total cholesterol (TC) (**D**). ND: normal diet; Con: high-fat diet with 35% of total calories from fat; AST: high-fat diet + astaxanthin; Et: Lieber–DeCarli liquid ethanol diet with 35% of total calories from fat; EtAST: Lieber–DeCarli liquid ethanol diet with 35% of total calories from fat + astaxanthin. All values represent means $\pm$ SD. * $p < 0.05$ represents significant differences in each group compared with the ethanol (Et) group by ANOVA analysis.

3.2. Astaxanthin Can Relieve Liver Injury Through the Regulation of Inflammatory Genes Expression in Mice

To explore whether astaxanthin can reverse the development of AFLD that is associated with inflammatory responses, liver inflammatory gene expression in liver was measured. A high-fat diet did not promote inflammatory gene expression. However, as expected, the consumption of ethanol in a high-fat diet significantly induced the mRNA expression of interleukin-1 alpha (IL-1α), macrophage inflammatory protein 2 (MIP-2), interleukin-6 (IL-6), and tumor necrosis factor-alpha (TNF-α). However, these effects were markedly reversed by astaxanthin supplementation (Figure 2).

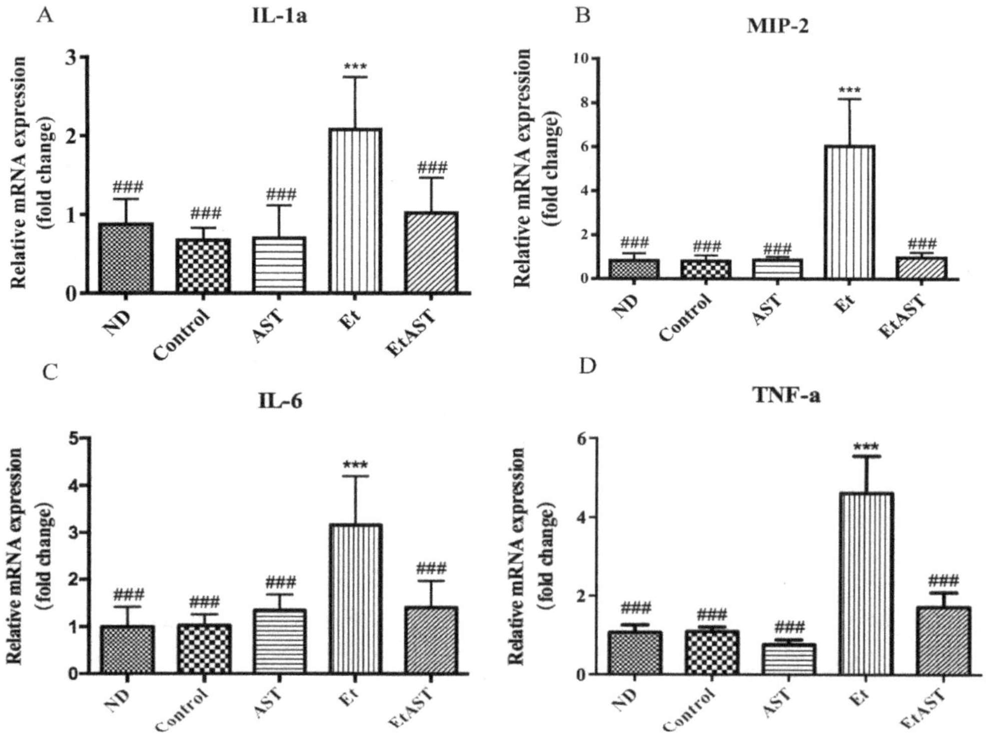

Figure 2. Effect of astaxanthin on inflammatory genes expression in alcoholic fatty liver disease (AFLD) mice. At the end of the experiment, total RNA was extracted from liver tissues. The mRNA expressions of interleukin-1 alpha (IL-1α) (**A**), macrophage inflammatory protein 2 (MIP-2) (**B**), interleukin-6 (IL-6) (**C**), and tumor necrosis factor-alpha (TNF-α) (**D**) were normalized to that of β-actin. Data are presented as means ± SD, $n = 6$. *** $p < 0.001$ compared with the control (Con) group, and ### $p < 0.001$ compared with the Et group.

3.3. Astaxanthin Alters the Profiles of Gut Microbiota in Ethanol-Fed Mice

The microbiota can influence the development and progression of AFLD. High-throughput 16S rRNA gene sequencing produced a total of 332,981 good-quality sequences from 15 samples (with 21,532 ± 231 sequences per sample) (Table S3). Rarefaction curves and rank abundance curves have shown that the most gut microbes in samples were captured based on the current sequencing depth and the data can be used for further analysis (Figure S1).

Next, we analyzed the gut bacterial community in mice affected by high-fat and/or ethanol exposure with or without astaxanthin. Alpha-diversity analysis indicated that the values of Chao1, abundance-based coverage estimator (ACE), and Shannon were significantly increased in the Con and Et groups compared to the ND group. After treatment with 50 mg kg^{-1} astaxanthin, the values were not influenced by the high-fat diet alone but markedly decreased when ethanol was added, and even improved relative to the normal group (Figure 3A–C). Furthermore, to investigate the similarities in gut microbial community structure among different samples, certain analyses were conducted. The PCoA plot indicated that the structure of gut microbiota in the Et group was statistically different from the ND along the PC1 axis (59.16% and 42.3% of overall variation based on weighted and unweighted UniFrac, respectively), and a significant structural shift was also shown for most of the astaxanthin-supplemented mice compared with those in the Et group (Figure 3D–F). As expected, the results of the unweighted pair group method with arithmetic mean (UPGMA) based on weighted and unweighted Unifrac also showed overt changes in the composition of gut microbiota in the EtAST group compared with the Et group (Figure S2), which is in line with the PCoA results, indicating that the microbial structure was disturbed by ethanol feeding, but remedied and returned to normal status by astaxanthin administration.

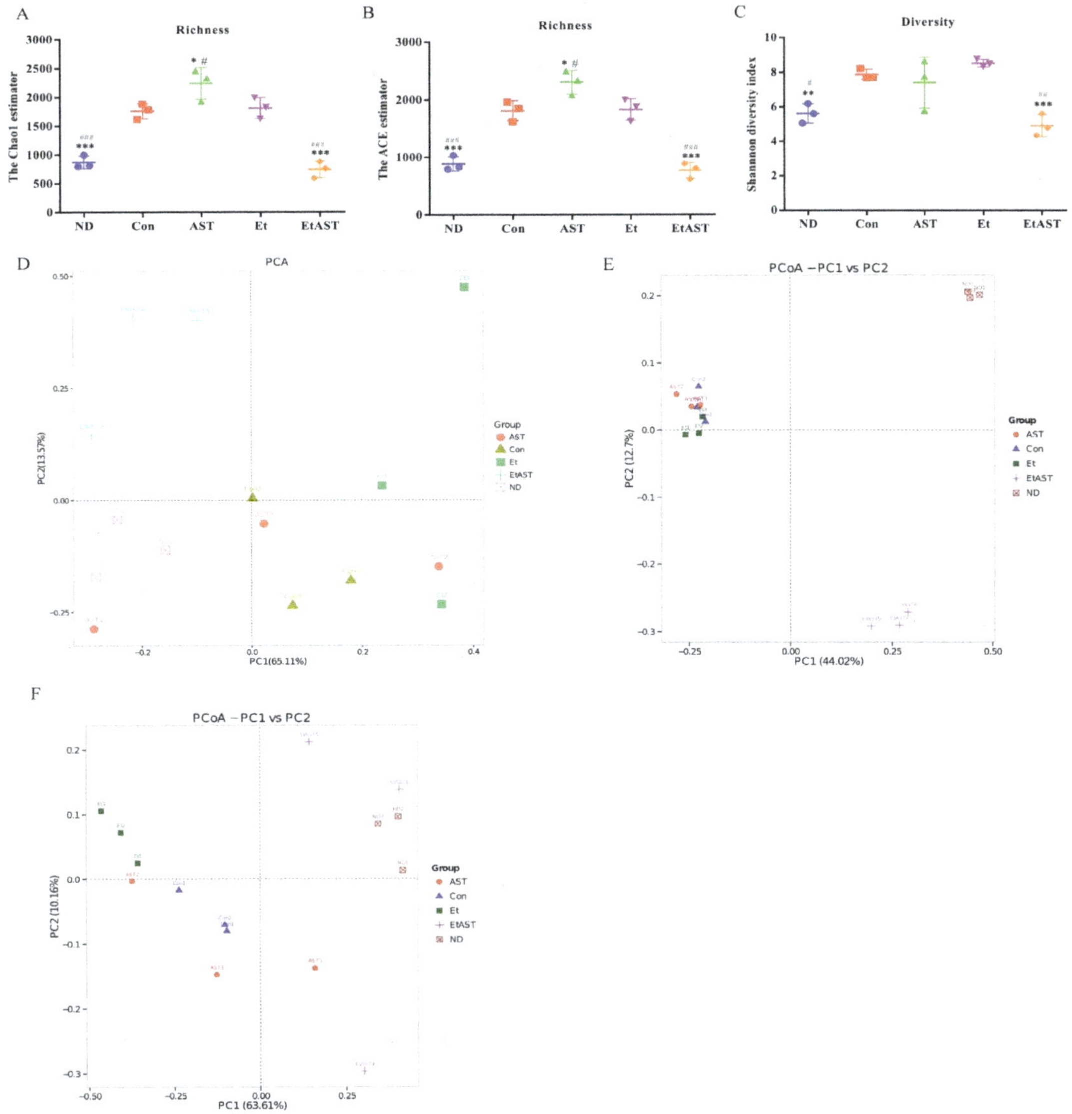

Figure 3. Astaxanthin treatment ameliorates the microbiota profiles affected by the ethanol diet. Bacterial genomic DNA was extracted from the feces collected at the end of week 12, and 16S rDNA sequence analysis was performed. Alpha diversity analysis, the Chao1 estimator (**A**), the ACE estimator (**B**), and the Shannon diversity index (**C**) were used for evaluation. To investigate the similarity of gut microbial community structure among different samples, we conducted beta-diversity analysis and PCA analysis (**D**), PCoA score plot based on unweighted UniFrac (**E**), and weighted UniFrac (**F**). ND: normal diet; Con: high-fat diet with 35% of total calories from fat; AST: high-fat diet + astaxanthin; Et: Lieber–DeCarli liquid ethanol diet with 35% of total calories from fat; EtAST: Lieber–DeCarli liquid ethanol diet with 35% of total calories from fat + astaxanthin. # represents $p < 0.05$, ## represents $p < 0.01$, and ### represents $p < 0.001$ compared with the Con group, * represents $p < 0.05$, ** represents $p < 0.01$, and *** represents $p < 0.001$ compared with the Et group.

3.4. Astaxanthin Regulates the Gut Microbiota Composition in Ethanol Feeding Mice

We detected nine bacterial phyla and 60 genera among the mice. The structure and composition of gut microbiota were significantly influenced by the high-fat plus ethanol diet. The results of the top 20 most abundant OTUs at all taxonomic levels in samples, as inferred by GraPhlAn, showed that *Firmicutes, Bacteroidetes, Proteobacteria,* and *Verrucomicrobia* were the most abundant phyla, and *Akkermansia, Bacteroides, Prevotella,* and *Paraprevotella* were the most abundant genera among the OTUs (Figure S3A). Additionally, the relative bacterial abundance in groups was reflected by the cladogram and linear discriminant analysis (LDA) score (Figure S3B,C). The taxonomic profiles indicated that the proportions of *Bacteroidetes* and *Proteobacteria* increased significantly, and the abundance of *Verrucomicrobia* decreased markedly in the Con group, especially in the Et group when compared with those of the ND group, while astaxanthin was shown to significantly reverse the tendency of this bacterial abundance, similar to the ND group (Figure 4A,B). Specifically, *Cyanobacteria* was completely depleted in both the Et and EtAST groups (Figure 4B). At the genus level, bacterial taxa displayed obvious changes in the heat maps, which were affected by different diets. The genera abundance, including *Akkermansia, Bacillus, Adlercreutzia, Lactococcus, Bacteroides, Butyricimonas, Parabacteroides,* and *Bilophila,* was significantly switched by ethanol feeding compared with the normal diet and partially reversed by the addition of astaxanthin (Figure S4). Astaxanthin treatment significantly decreased the *Butyricimonas, Bilophila,* and *Parabacteroides* concentrations relative to the Et group, and the abundance of *Akkermansia* decreased markedly in the Et group (3%) and recovered dramatically in the EtAST group (34%), while the abundance was similar to that of the ND group (38%, Figure 4D and Figure S5).

Next, we identified changes in the strain-specific key phenotypes which were affected by astaxanthin in the AFLD mice. The results showed that the abundance levels of 27 OTUs were markedly changed by ethanol supplementation (15 increased and 12 decreased OTUs) compared with those of the Con group, while astaxanthin intervention significantly altered 31 OTUs including enhanced or reduced abundance in 2 and 29 OTUs, respectively (EtAST group vs. Et group). Particularly, among the 43 OTUs, 13 were significantly increased or decreased by ethanol, and afterwards notably reversed by astaxanthin (Figure 4E), which including bacteria belonging to *Akkermansia_muciniphila,* species from *Butyricimonas, S24-7, Oscillospira, Clostridiales,* and *Bilophila.*

3.5. Associations of the Bacterial Abundance Altered by Astaxanthin with the AFLD Phenotype

To assess the relationships between OTUs and metabolic parameters altered by astaxanthin, Spearman's correlation coefficient was employed. Among the 43 OTUs that were altered in abundance by ethanol or astaxanthin shown in Figure 5, 33 OTUs were markedly correlated with at least one of the following metabolic parameters: AST, ALT, TG, LDL, liver weight/body weight (LW/BW). Thirty-eight of these OTUs were positively correlated with the abnormal parameters, and five OTUs were negatively correlated with abnormal parameters. The abundance levels of 20 OTUs were markedly changed by ethanol supplementation (15 increased and five decreased OTUs) compared with those of the Con group, while astaxanthin intervention significantly altered 27 OTUs, including enhanced and reduced abundances in two and 25 OTUs, respectively, compared with those of the Et group. Notably, 13 OTUs were significantly increased or decreased by ethanol and then markedly reversed by astaxanthin (Figure 5).

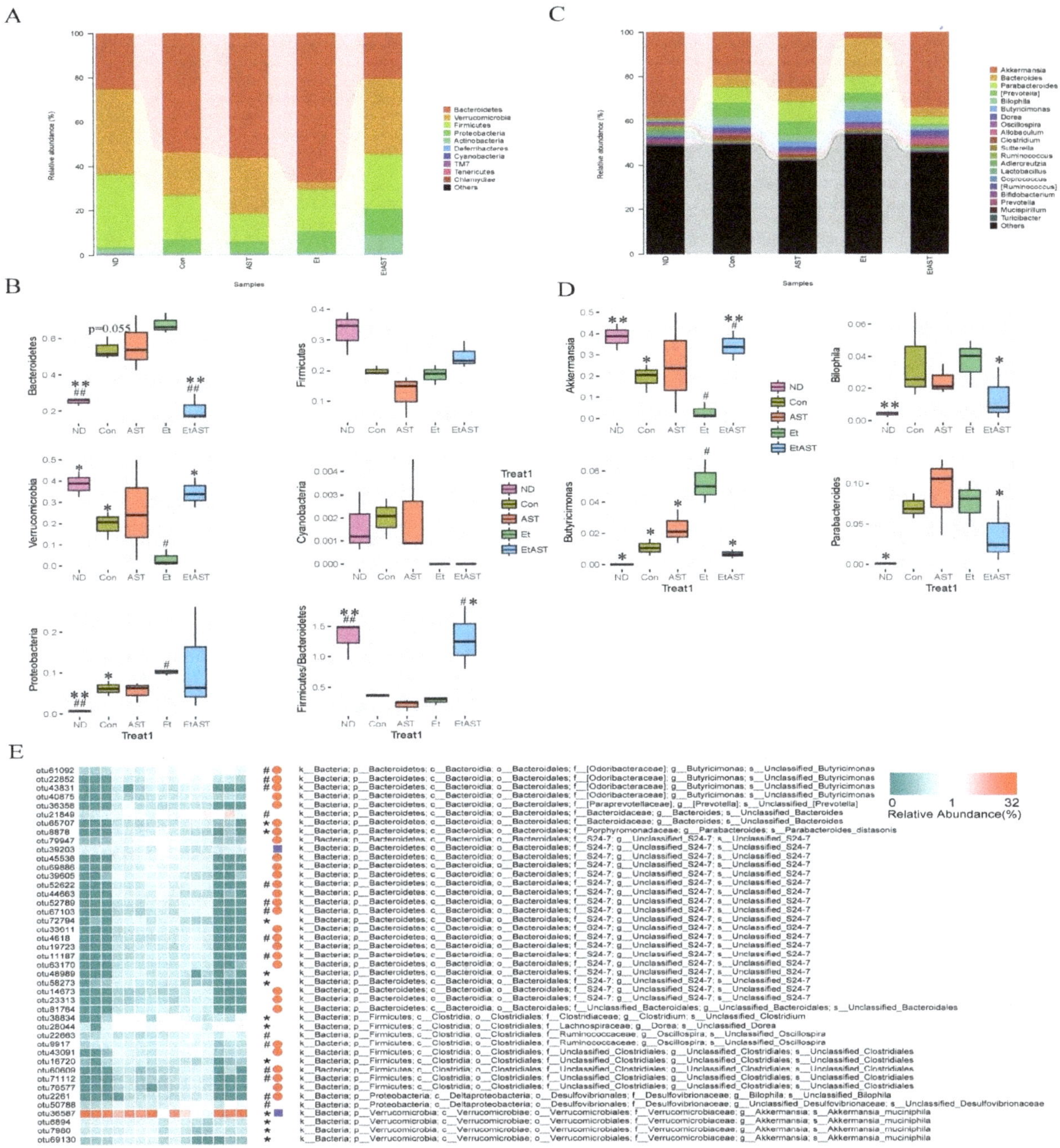

Figure 4. Bacterial community analysis and comparison. The composition and abundance distributions of each group at the phylum (**A**) and genus (**C**) levels were shown using QIIME software. At the phylum (**B**) and genus (**D**) levels, pairwise comparisons, conducted to determine the sequence amounts between two groups, were presented as pair-wise comparisons using Metastats analysis. # represents $p < 0.05$ and ## represents $p < 0.01$ compared with the Con group; * represents $p < 0.05$ and ** represents $p < 0.01$ compared with the Et group. A heat map of 43 operational taxonomic units (OTUs) which were altered in abundance by ethanol or astaxanthin is shown, based on the redundancy analysis (RDA) model. OTUs with a relative abundance greater than 0.1% in at least in one group were selected and used to analyze these differences. The red and green colors indicate the relative abundances of OTUs that were more or less abundant. The symbols represent the OTUs whose abundance were reduced and increased in the Et group relative to the Con group, while the circles in red and rectangles in blue represent the OTUs whose abundances were reduced and increased in the EtAST group relative to the Et group (**E**).

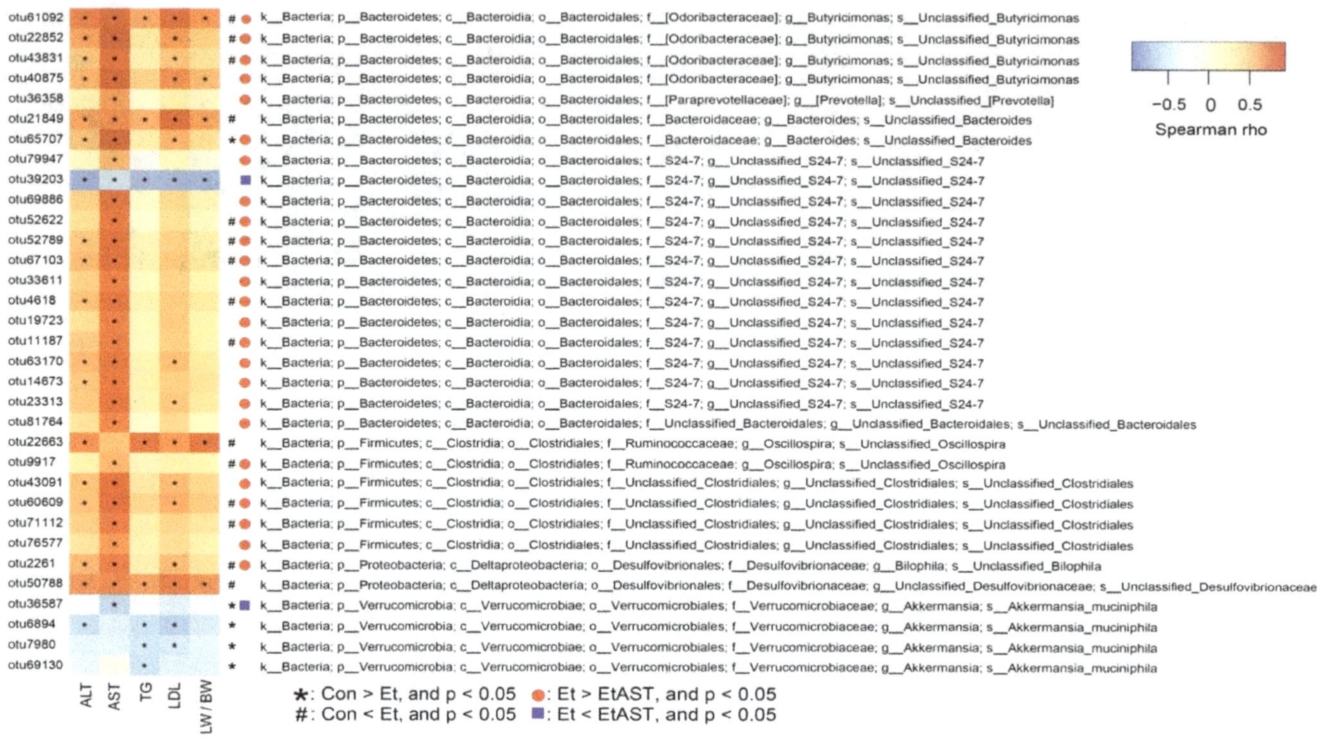

Figure 5. Heat map of 33 OTUs which were significantly associated with the AFLD disease phenotype altered by ethanol or astaxanthin as determined by Spearman's correlation coefficient. These 33 OTUs were selected from the 43 OTUs which had significant changes after ethanol or astaxanthin treatment. The red and blue colors indicate the relative abundance of OTUs that were more or less abundant. The symbols * and #, shown on the right-hand side of the map, represent the OTUs whose abundances were reduced and increased in the Et group relative to those of the Con group, while the red circles and blue rectangles represent the OTUs whose abundances were reduced and increased in the EtAST group relative to the Et group. The symbol * in the cells of the heat map represents the significant correlation between the corresponding metabolic parameters and OTU abundance.

3.6. Predicted Metabolic Functions of the Metagenome in Gut Microbiota

The PICRUSt analysis based on metagenomes was used to predict the metabolic function of gut microbiota that were influenced by astaxanthin in AFLD mice. The results revealed that 18 and 128 KEGG (Kyoto Encyclopedia of Genes and Genomes) pathways were changed in the EtAST group at levels 2 (Figure 6B) and 3 (Figure S6), respectively, among which seven were increased and 11 were decreased compared to the Et group at level 2. In particular, we found several interesting changes among the 128 altered KEGG pathways at level 3. Firstly, the biosynthesis processes of bacteria, such as nucleotide metabolism (level 2), was increased in the Et group compared to that in the Con group, including pyrimidine metabolism, energy metabolism, DNA replication proteins, and cytoskeleton proteins (level 3), while astaxanthin intervention significantly restrained these pathways. In addition, the metagenome of the EtAST group was enriched in the pathways related to lipid metabolism, including glycerophospholipid metabolism; arachidonic acid metabolism; the biosynthesis of unsaturated fatty acids; fatty acid elongation in mitochondria; fatty acid metabolism; the synthesis and degradation of ketone bodies; xenobiotic biodegradation and metabolism, including aminobenzoate degradation, atrazine degradation, caprolactam degradation, drug metabolism, cytochrome P450 and fluorobenzoate degradation; and amino acid metabolism, including tryptophan metabolism, lysine degradation, tyrosine metabolism, and phenylalanine metabolism.

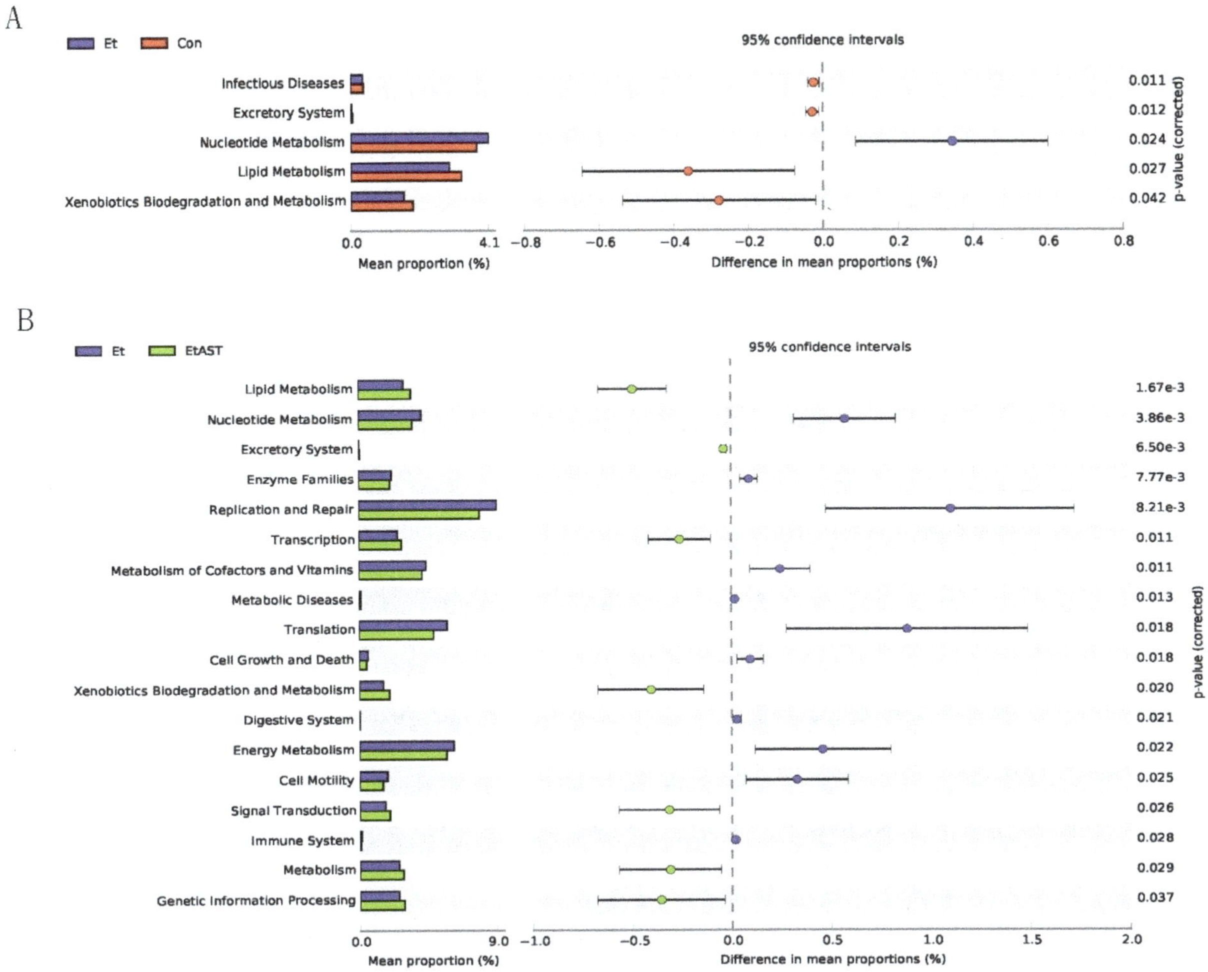

Figure 6. Predicted functions for the altered metagenome of gut microbiota in each group shown with KEGG (Kyoto Encyclopedia of Genes and Genomes) pathways. These data were obtained by PICRUSt. (**A**) A total of five markedly altered KEGG pathways at level 2 in the Et group compared with that in the Con group. (**B**) A total of 18 significantly changed the pathways through astaxanthin supplementation in alcoholic fatty liver disease (AFLD) mice.

4. Discussion

Increasing evidence indicates that the gut microbiota could significantly affect the emergence and development of AFLD [25,26]. Astaxanthin can prevent liver injury by suppressing inflammation, fibrosis [27], and fat accumulation [10,28]. However, previously, there was little evidence suggesting an effect of astaxanthin on AFLD protection. Here, we demonstrated that astaxanthin intervention can mitigate ethanol-induced hepatic steatosis through the reconstruction of the gut microbiota structure and a subsequent increased abundance of *Akkermansia*.

Organ dysfunction is mainly associated with prolonged excessive drinking, which leads to tissue injury-related conditions, such as AFLD, with initial symptoms like fatty liver, and may be responsible for the development of alcoholic hepatitis, liver fibrosis, and cirrhosis. Proper dietary habits can reverse the pathological state of fatty liver in the early stages [29]. Astaxanthin has been proven to protect against liver injury in mice suffering from NAFLD [27] and liver fibrosis in mice [7] due to its anti-inflammation and antioxidant ability. In addition, Zheng et al. has demonstrated that astaxanthin can protect against maternal ethanol-induced embryonic developmental retardation in C57BL/6J mice [22]. In the present study, we found that astaxanthin can protect against ethanol-induced liver injury in mice by alleviating lipid accumulation, inflammatory cell infiltration, and necrosis in the liver. Furthermore, we explored whether astaxanthin could reverse the AFLD development associated with inflammatory responses, and we detected inflammatory gene expression. Various inflammatory mediators and cytokines can be generated after the activation of inflammatory signaling, particularly the major inflammatory markers TNF-α and IL-6 [30]. IL-1α and MIP-2 are important pro-inflammatory cytokines [31,32] that are significantly induced by ethanol. Astaxanthin significantly decreased these mRNA expression level and partly protected the liver from inflammation and injury.

Increasing evidence indicates that the gut microbiota is responsible for the pathogenesis and development of liver disease. A large microbial ecosystem exists in the human gastrointestinal tract, which is associated closely with health and disease control [33]. The gut–liver circulation pathway plays a critical role in alcohol metabolism and is strongly regulated by the gut microbiota. It has been proven that dietary perturbations have dominant effects on the gut microbiota [34]. We further identified bacterial groups that are significantly affected by ethanol and astaxanthin supplementation. Phyla and genera imbalance are associated with health disorders. In this model of alcohol-induced liver injury, we found that several *Bacteroidetes*, including the genera *Bacteroides*, *Butyricimonas*, and *Parabacteroides*, were significantly increased. Consistent with our results, Llopis et al. reported that after five weeks' consumption of a diet including alcohol, *Bacteroides* was significantly more represented in severe alcoholic hepatitis mice relative to the control group [35]. Similarly, other studies have reported that the relative abundance of *Bacteroidetes* increases in alcohol-fed mice [36–38]. The phylum of *Bacteroidetes* is composed of three major classes of Gram-negative bacteria, normally resident in the intestines, mouth, upper respiratory tract, and genital tracts of humans and animals, which have been described as having both beneficial and detrimental features. *Bacteroidetes* can lead to endogenous infections due to a micro-ecological imbalance. In particular, *Bacteroides fragilis* can produce polysaccharide A to relieve colitis in animals [39]. However, it can also produce a toxin, which triggers a pro-carcinogenic effect, to induce colon tumorigenesis [40]. In addition, *Proteobacteria*, as pro-inflammatory intestinal microbes, can multiply in the gut in response to an imbalanced microbial composition and are associated with disease occurrence and development [41]. During this experiment, astaxanthin intervention was found to significantly reverse the ethanol-induced increases in *Bacteroidetes* and *Proteobacteria*, restoring their proportions to the levels of the ND group. This indicates that the protective effect of astaxanthin is likely associated with its anti-inflammatory activity.

Cyanobacteria was completely suppressed in mice after treatment with ethanol as compared to the ethanol-free treatment. Although the abundance of *Cyanobacteria* is extremely low in the microbiota, we focused on this phylum because *Cyanobacteria* is completely inhibited in the gut when the diet contains ethanol, either with or without astaxanthin. This phenomenon indicated that astaxanthin did not affect the action of alcohol.

Accumulating reports have focused on the beneficial effects of *Akkermansia* on host metabolism. *Akkermansia* is a dominant genus in *Verrucomicrobia* and can degrade intestinal mucin [42], increasing mucus thickness and enhancing gut barrier function, which correlates inversely with the incidence of inflammation [43] and metabolic syndrome [18]. Lack of *Akkermansia* has been determined to be an early marker of alcohol-induced gut dysbiosis [37]. Moreover, ethanol exposure reduces the abundance of *Akkermansia* in both mice and humans, and the status of AFLD can be improved by oral supplementation of the genus, directly demonstrating the protective effect of this bacterium in AFLD [44]. As a probiotic, the abundance of *Akkermansia* can be affected by the administration of specific dietary components [45]. In the current research, the abundance of *Akkermansia* in ethanol-exposed AFLD mice dramatically reduced, and astaxanthin intervention obviously recovered its abundance, to even higher than that of the ND group. Our data suggest that mice with AFLD might benefit from astaxanthin supplementation increasing *Akkermansia*. Studies have proved that *Akkermansia* can play a protective role in ethanol-induced liver injury as a result of its function of improving the gut barrier [46], and the present research requires the further investigation of astaxanthin barrier function in the future.

The different bacterial species in the same genus may reflect different responses by the same treatment. Thus, it is indispensable to identify changes in the microbiota at the species level. In the present study, among the 13 OTUs altered by ethanol and reversed by astaxanthin intervention, the proportions of *Akkermansia muciniphila* (OTU36578) were significantly decreased in the Et group, while they were enriched in the EtAST and ND groups. *Akkermansia muciniphila* is a species of the *Akkermansia* genus, and extensive research has shown that it can improve the status of obesity, diabetes, and inflammation [47]. On the other hand, the species from *Butyricimonas* (OTU 61092, OTU22852, and OTU43831), S24-7 (OTU52622, OTU52789, OTU67103, OTU4618, and OTU11187), *Oscillospira* (OTU9917), *Clostridiales* (OTU60609 and OTU71112), and *Bilophila* (OTU2261) were significantly increased by ethanol diet and markedly reversed by astaxanthin supplementation. It has been reported that the abundance of *Oscillospira* and *Clostridales* increased in inflammatory response and is associated with the barrier injury of intestinal mucosa [48,49]. Stanislawski et al. demonstrated that *Bilophila* was positively correlated with the fat fraction of the liver [50]. Our research found that astaxanthin treatment significantly decreased the levels of ALT, AST, TG, LDL, and the index of LW/BW, which were increased by ethanol diet. Among the 13 OTUs altered by ethanol and reversed by astaxanthin supplementation, Spearman's correlation analysis suggested that *Akkermansia muciniphila*, enriched in the EtAST group, was negatively associated with the AFLD phenotype. On the other hand, the 12 enriched OTUs in the Et group were positively associated with the AFLD phenotype. These results indicate that astaxanthin relieves the AFLD phenotype through its ability to enrich the bacteria responsible for intestinal integrity and anti-inflammation.

The typical characteristic of AFLD is excessive hepatic lipid accumulation. Therefore, lipid metabolic regulation plays an important role in the pathogenesis of metabolic disorders. In this study, the predicted metabolic function of the gut microbiota showed that the lipid metabolism pathway was increased after astaxanthin treatment, while further research proved that *Akkermansia* acts as a probiotic to promote lipid metabolism and avoid lipid excessive accumulation [51]. The results indicate that the inhibition by astaxanthin of excessive lipid accumulation in the liver may be associated with gut bacteria that promote lipid metabolism. In addition, astaxanthin increased the xenobiotic biodegradation and metabolism pathways. Xenobiotics are a kind of foreign chemical in living systems, which, after entering an organism, may induce adverse or even very serious consequences [52]. The liver is the major organ of metabolism, and astaxanthin supplementation can increase the abundance of bacteria that promote hepatic xenobiotic biodegradation and metabolism, resulting in detoxification and liver injury protection. However, the current findings need to be verified in larger samples.

Interestingly, astaxanthin was more effective in ameliorating alcohol-induced liver injury rather than that related to HFD. There is evidence that astaxanthin can protect against liver damage conditions like NAFLD and AFLD through multiple mechanisms, including antioxidant and anti-inflammatory effects [10,22,53]. In this research, mice in the Con group fed a high-fat diet did not show obvious inflammation, as measured by the liver index, histopathology, and liver gene expression. However, ethanol interference induced a marked inflammatory response which promoted astaxanthin to exert its anti-inflammatory effects to protect the liver from injury. This can also be explained from another aspect; specifically, astaxanthin will not disturb the metabolic balance under non-inflammatory conditions [54], which is consistent with the result that most responses in the AST group were similar to those in the Con group in our research. Future research should determine the content of astaxanthin in the mouse (liver and serum) and its feces.

5. Conclusions

Our research explored the protective effects of astaxanthin on AFLD injury mice and its regulation of gut microbiota. Astaxanthin has the ability to reverse the ethanol-induced liver weight ratio increase, hepatic inflammation, and lipid dysmetabolism. Furthermore, the overall structure and composition of the gut microbiota altered by ethanol feeding can be balanced by astaxanthin, particularly recovering the beneficial bacterium *Akkermansia*. Our results indicate that *Akkermansia* may be a potential target for the astaxanthin-related alleviation of AFLD, which provides further evidence for its molecular mechanism, and suggests that it could be used for the treatment of bacterial disorders induced by AFLD.

Supplementary Materials: , Table S1: Compositions of the diets (DOC); Table S2: Primer sequences used for q-PCR reactions (DOC); Table S3: The OTUs obtained from high-throughput 16S rRNA gene sequencing (XLS); Figure S1: Rationality of sequencing data was evaluated by rarefaction and rank abundance curve (DOC 359); Figure S2: Cluster analysis using the UPGMA method based on unweighted Unifrac and weighted Unifrac analysis (DOC); Figure S3: The overall classification levels based on GraphlAn and LEfSe analyses were used to visualize the taxonomy compositions and bacterial abundance; Figure S4: Heatmap of the abundance of bacteria at the genus level at different groups (DOC); Figure S5: Astaxanthin protect ethanol-induced *Akkermansia muciniphila* depletion (DOC); Figure S6: Predicted functions for the altered metagenome of gut microbiota (PDF).

Author Contributions: H.L., X.F., X.Z. and J.L. conceived and designed the experiments; H.L., Z.Z. and L.Z. performed the experiments; H.L. and M.L. analyzed the data; X.F., X.Z. and J.L. contributed reagents/materials/analysis tools; H.L. and M.L. wrote the paper. All authors reviewed the manuscript.

Acknowledgments: The sequencing service was provided by Personal Biotechnology Co., Ltd. of Shanghai, China. The program was supported by the National Natural Science Foundation of China–General program (grant number: 31672511).

Abbreviations

AST	astaxanthin
AFLD	alcoholic fatty liver disease
IL-1α	interleukin-1 alpha
MIP-2	macrophage inflammatory protein 2
ND	normal diet
Et	ethanol
ALT	alanine aminotransferase
TG	triacylglycerol
LDL	low-density lipoprotein
LW	liver weight
BW	body weight
Con	control
PCoA	principle coordinate analysis
OTUs	operational taxonomic units
KEGG	Kyoto Encyclopedia of Genes and Genomes

References

1. O'Shea, R.S.; Dasarathy, S.; McCullough, A.J. Alcoholic liver disease. *Hepatology* **2010**, *51*, 307–328. [CrossRef] [PubMed]
2. Menon, K.V.; Gores, G.J.; Shah, V.H. Pathogenesis, diagnosis, and treatment of alcoholic liver disease. *Mayo Clin. Proc.* **2001**, *76*, 1021–1029. [CrossRef] [PubMed]
3. MacSween, R.N.; Burt, A.D. Histologic spectrum of alcoholic liver disease. *Semin. Liver Dis.* **1986**, *6*, 221–232. [CrossRef] [PubMed]
4. Hussein, G.; Sankawa, U.; Goto, H.; Matsumoto, K.; Watanabe, H. Astaxanthin, a carotenoid with potential in human health and nutrition. *J. Nat. Prod.* **2006**, *69*, 443–449. [CrossRef] [PubMed]
5. Yuan, J.P.; Peng, J.; Yin, K.; Wang, J.H. Potential health-promoting effects of astaxanthin: A high-value carotenoid mostly from microalgae. *Mol. Nutr. Food Res.* **2011**, *55*, 150–165. [CrossRef] [PubMed]
6. Sila, A.; Kamoun, Z.; Ghlissi, Z.; Makni, M.; Nasri, M.; Sahnoun, Z.; Nedjar-Arroume, N.; Bougatef, A. Ability of natural astaxanthin from shrimp by-products to attenuate liver oxidative stress in diabetic rats. *Pharmacol. Rep.* **2015**, *67*, 310–316. [CrossRef] [PubMed]

7. Shen, M.; Chen, K.; Lu, J.; Cheng, P.; Xu, L.; Dai, W.; Wang, F.; He, L.; Zhang, Y.; Chengfen, W.; et al. Protective effect of astaxanthin on liver fibrosis through modulation of TGF-beta1 expression and autophagy. *Mediat. Inflamm.* **2014**, 954502. [CrossRef]
8. Kobori, M.; Takahashi, Y.; Sakurai, M.; Ni, Y.; Chen, G.; Nagashimada, M.; Kaneko, S.; Ota, T. Hepatic Transcriptome Profiles of Mice with Diet-Induced Nonalcoholic Steatohepatitis Treated with Astaxanthin and Vitamin E. *Int. J. Mol. Sci.* **2017**, *18*, 593. [CrossRef] [PubMed]
9. Takemoto, M.; Yamaga, M.; Furuichi, Y.; Yokote, K. Astaxanthin Improves Nonalcoholic Fatty Liver Disease in Werner Syndrome with Diabetes Mellitus. *J. Am. Geriatr. Soc.* **2015**, *63*, 1271–1273. [CrossRef] [PubMed]
10. Jia, Y.; Wu, C.; Kim, J.; Kim, B.; Lee, S.J. Astaxanthin reduces hepatic lipid accumulations in high-fat-fed C57BL/6J mice via activation of peroxisome proliferator-activated receptor (PPAR) alpha and inhibition of PPAR gamma and Akt. *J. Nutr. Biochem.* **2016**, *28*, 9–18. [CrossRef] [PubMed]
11. Ni, Y.; Nagashimada, M.; Zhuge, F.; Zhan, L.; Nagata, N.; Tsutsui, A.; Nakanuma, Y.; Kaneko, S.; Ota, T. Astaxanthin prevents and reverses diet-induced insulin resistance and steatohepatitis in mice: A comparison with vitamin E. *Sci. Rep.* **2015**, *5*, 17192. [CrossRef] [PubMed]
12. Battson, M.L.; Lee, D.M.; Weir, T.L.; Gentile, C.L. The gut microbiota as a novel regulator of cardiovascular function and disease. *J. Nutr. Biochem.* **2015**, *56*, 1–15. [CrossRef] [PubMed]
13. Koh, J.C.; Loo, W.M.; Goh, K.L.; Sugano, K.; Chan, W.K.; Chiu, W.Y.; Choi, M.G.; Gonlachanvit, S.; Lee, W.J.; Lee, W.J.; et al. Asian consensus on the relationship between obesity and gastrointestinal and liver diseases. *J. Gastroenterol. Hepatol.* **2016**, *31*, 1405–1413. [CrossRef] [PubMed]
14. Dao, M.C.; Clement, K. Gut microbiota and obesity: Concepts relevant to clinical care. *Eur. J. Intern. Med.* **2018**, *48*, 18–24. [CrossRef] [PubMed]
15. Chen, P.; Torralba, M.; Tan, J.; Embree, M.; Zengler, K.; Starkel, P.; van Pijkeren, J.P.; DePew, J.; Loomba, R.; Ho, S.B.; et al. FoutsandB. Schnabl. Supplementation of saturated long-chain fatty acids maintains intestinal eubiosis and reduces ethanol-induced liver injury in mice. *Gastroenterology* **2015**, *148*, 203–214. [CrossRef] [PubMed]
16. Leclercq, S.; De Saeger, C.; Delzenne, N.; de Timary, P.; Starkel, P. Role of inflammatory pathways, blood mononuclear cells, and gut-derived bacterial products in alcohol dependence. *Biol. Psychiatry* **2014**, *76*, 725–733. [CrossRef] [PubMed]
17. Lippai, D.; Bala, S.; Catalano, D.; Kodys, K.; Szabo, G. Micro-RNA-155 deficiency prevents alcohol-induced serum endotoxin increase and small bowel inflammation in mice. *Alcohol. Clin. Exp. Res.* **2014**, *38*, 2217–2224. [CrossRef] [PubMed]
18. Dao, M.C.; Everard, A.; Aron-Wisnewsky, J.; Sokolovska, N.; Prifti, E.; Verger, E.O.; Kayser, B.D.; Levenez, F.; Chilloux, J.; Hoyles, L. *Akkermansia muciniphila* and improved metabolic health during a dietary intervention in obesity: Relationship with gut microbiome richness and ecology. *Gut* **2016**, *65*, 426–436. [CrossRef] [PubMed]
19. Requena, T.; Martinez-Cuesta, M.C.; Pelaez, C. Diet and microbiota linked in health and disease. *Food Funct.* **2018**, *9*, 688–704. [CrossRef] [PubMed]
20. Chen, J.T.; Kotani, K. Astaxanthin as a Potential Protector of Liver Function: A. Review. *J. Clin. Med. Res.* **2016**, *8*, 701–704. [CrossRef] [PubMed]
21. Lieber, C.S.; DeCarli, L.M.; Sorrell, M.F. Experimental methods of ethanol administration. *Hepatology* **1989**, *10*, 501–510. [CrossRef] [PubMed]
22. Zheng, D.; Li, Y.; He, L.; Tang, Y.; Li, X.; Shen, Q.; Yin, D.; Peng, Y. The protective effect of astaxanthin on fetal alcohol spectrum disorder in mice. *Neuropharmacology* **2014**, *84*, 13–18. [CrossRef] [PubMed]
23. Caporaso, J.G.; Kuczynski, J.; Stombaugh, J.; Bittinger, K.; Bushman, F.D.; Costello, E.K.; Fierer, N.; Pena, A.G.; Goodrich, J.K.; Gordon, J.I.; et al. QIIME allows analysis of high-throughput community sequencing data. *Nat. Methods* **2010**, *7*, 335–336. [CrossRef] [PubMed]
24. Edgar, R.C. Search and clustering orders of magnitude faster than BLAST. *Bioinformatics* **2010**, *26*, 2460–2461. [CrossRef] [PubMed]
25. Neuman, M.G.; French, S.W.; Zakhari, S.; Malnick, S.; Seitz, H.K.; Cohen, L.B.; Salaspuro, M.; Voinea-Griffin, A.; Barasch, A.; Kirpich, I.A.; et al. Alcohol, microbiome, life style influence alcohol and non-alcoholic organ damage. *Exp. Mol. Pathol.* **2017**, *102*, 162–180. [CrossRef] [PubMed]
26. Scarpellini, E.; Forlino, M.; Lupo, M.; Rasetti, C.; Fava, G.; Abenavoli, L.; De Santis, A. Gut Microbiota and Alcoholic Liver Disease. *Rev. Recent Clin. Trials* **2016**, *11*, 213–219. [CrossRef] [PubMed]

27. Kim, B.; Farruggia, C.; Ku, C.S.; Pham, T.X.; Yang, Y.; Bae, M.; Wegner, C.J.; Farrell, N.J.; Harness, E.; Park, Y.K.; et al. Astaxanthin inhibits inflammation and fibrosis in the liver and adipose tissue of mouse models of diet-induced obesity and nonalcoholic steatohepatitis. *J. Nutr. Biochem.* **2017**, *43*, 27–35. [CrossRef] [PubMed]
28. Bhuvaneswari, S.; Arunkumar, E.; Viswanathan, P.; Anuradha, C.V. Astaxanthin restricts weight gain, promotes insulin sensitivity and curtails fatty liver disease in mice fed a obesity-promoting diet. *Process Biochem.* **2010**, *45*, 1406–1414. [CrossRef]
29. Bae, M.; Park, Y.K.; Lee, J.Y. Food components with antifibrotic activity and implications in prevention of liver disease. *J. Nutr. Biochem.* **2017**, *55*, 1–11. [CrossRef] [PubMed]
30. Fard, M.T.; Arulselvan, P.; Karthivashan, G.; Adam, S.K.; Fakurazi, S. Bioactive extract from Moringa oleifera inhibits the pro-inflammatory mediators in lipopolysaccharide stimulated macrophages. *Pharmacogn. Mag.* **2015**, *11*, 556–563.
31. Malik, A.; Kanneganti, T.D. Function and regulation of IL-1alpha in inflammatory diseases and cancer. *Immunol. Rev.* **2018**, *281*, 124–137. [CrossRef] [PubMed]
32. Qin, C.C.; Liu, Y.N.; Hu, Y.; Yang, Y.; Chen, Z. Macrophage inflammatory protein-2 as mediator of inflammation in acute liver injury. *World J. Gastroenterol.* **2017**, *23*, 3043–3052. [CrossRef] [PubMed]
33. Lynch, S.V.; Pedersen, O. The Human Intestinal Microbiome in Health and Disease. *N. Engl. J. Med.* **2016**, *375*, 2369–2379. [CrossRef] [PubMed]
34. Carmody, R.N.; Gerber, G.K.; Jr Luevano, J.M.; Gatti, D.M.; Somes, L.; Svenson, K.L.; Turnbaugh, P.J. Diet dominates host genotype in shaping the murine gut microbiota. *Cell Host Microbe* **2015**, *17*, 72–84. [CrossRef] [PubMed]
35. Llopis, M.; Cassard, A.M.; Wrzosek, L.; Boschat, L.; Bruneau, A.; Ferrere, G.; Puchois, V.; Martin, J.C.; Lepage, P.; Le Roy, T.; et al. Intestinal microbiota contributes to individual susceptibility to alcoholic liver disease. *Gut* **2016**, *65*, 830–839. [CrossRef] [PubMed]
36. Yan, A.W.; Fouts, D.E.; Brandl, J.; Starkel, P.; Torralba, M.; Schott, E.; Tsukamoto, H.; Nelson, K.E.; Brenner, D.A.; Schnabl, B. Enteric dysbiosis associated with a mouse model of alcoholic liver disease. *Hepatology* **2011**, *53*, 96–105. [CrossRef] [PubMed]
37. Lowe, P.P.; Gyongyosi, B.; Satishchandran, A.; Iracheta-Vellve, A.; Ambade, A.; Kodys, K.; Catalano, D.; Ward, D.V.; Szabo, G. Alcohol-related changes in the intestinal microbiome influence neutrophil infiltration, inflammation and steatosis in early alcoholic hepatitis in mice. *PLoS ONE* **2017**, *12*, e0174544.
38. Neyrinck, A.M.; Etxeberria, U.; Taminiau, B.; Daube, G.; Van Hul, M.; Everard, A.; Cani, P.D.; Bindels, L.B.; Delzenne, N.M. Rhubarb extract prevents hepatic inflammation induced by acute alcohol intake, an effect related to the modulation of the gut microbiota. *Mol. Nutr. Food Res.* **2017**, *61*, 1–12. [CrossRef] [PubMed]
39. Surana, N.K.; Kasper, D.L. The yin yang of bacterial polysaccharides: Lessons learned from B. fragilis PSA. *Immunol. Rev.* **2012**, *245*, 13–26. [CrossRef] [PubMed]
40. Chung, L.; Thiele, O.E.; Geis, A.L.; Chan, J.L.; Fu, K.; DeStefano, S.C.E.; Dejea, C.M.; Fathi, P.; Chen, J.; Finard, B.B.; et al. Bacteroides fragilis Toxin Coordinates a Pro-carcinogenic Inflammatory Cascade via Targeting of Colonic Epithelial Cells. *Cell Host Microbe* **2018**, *23*, 203–214.e5. [CrossRef] [PubMed]
41. Shin, N.R.; Whon, T.W.; Bae, J.W. Proteobacteria: Microbial signature of dysbiosis in gut microbiota. *Trends Biotechnol.* **2015**, *33*, 496–503. [CrossRef] [PubMed]
42. Derrien, M.; Vaughan, E.E.; Plugge, C.M.; de Vos, W.M. *Akkermansia muciniphila* gen. nov., sp. nov., a human intestinal mucin-degrading bacterium. *Int. J. Syst. Evol. Microbiol.* **2004**, *54*, 1469–1476. [CrossRef] [PubMed]
43. Li, J.; Lin, S.; Vanhoutte, P.M.; Woo, C.W.; Xu, A. Akkermansia Muciniphila Protects Against Atherosclerosis by Preventing Metabolic Endotoxemia-Induced Inflammation in Apoe$^{-/-}$ Mice. *Circulation* **2016**, *133*, 2434–2446. [CrossRef] [PubMed]
44. Grander, C.; Adolph, T.E.; Wieser, V.; Lowe, P.; Wrzosek, L.; Gyongyosi, B.; Ward, D.V.; Grabherr, F.; Gerner, R.R.; Pfister, A.; et al. Recovery of ethanol-induced *Akkermansia muciniphila* depletion ameliorates alcoholic liver disease. *Gut* **2018**, *67*, 891–901. [CrossRef] [PubMed]
45. Derrien, M.; Belzer, C.; de Vos, W.M. *Akkermansia muciniphila* and its role in regulating host functions. *Microb. Pathog.* **2017**, *106*, 171–181. [CrossRef] [PubMed]
46. Wu, W.; Lv, L.; Shi, D.; Ye, J.; Fang, D.; Guo, F.; Li, Y.; He, X.; Li, L. Protective Effect of *Akkermansia muciniphila* against Immune-Mediated Liver Injury in a Mouse Model. *Front. Microbiol.* **2017**, *8*, 1804. [CrossRef] [PubMed]

47. Ottman, N.; Geerlings, S.Y.; Aalvink, S.; de Vos, W.M.; Belzer, C. Action and function of *Akkermansia muciniphila* in microbiome ecology, health and disease. *Best Pract. Res. Clin. Gastroenterol.* **2017**, *31*, 637–642. [CrossRef] [PubMed]
48. Power, K.A.; Lu, J.T.; Monk, J.M.; Lepp, D.; Wu, W.; Zhang, C.; Liu, R.; Tsao, R.; Robinson, L.E.; Wood, G.A.; et al. Purified rutin and rutin-rich asparagus attenuates disease severity and tissue damage following dextran sodium sulfate-induced colitis. *Mol. Nutr. Food Res.* **2016**, *60*, 2396–2412. [CrossRef] [PubMed]
49. Mastrocola, R.; Ferrocino, I.; Liberto, E.; Chiazza, F.; Cento, A.S.; Collotta, D.; Querio, G.; Nigro, D.; Bitonto, V.; Cutrin, J.C.; et al. Fructose liquid and solid formulations differently affect gut integrity, microbiota composition and related liver toxicity: A comparative in vivo study. *J. Nutr. Biochem.* **2018**, *55*, 185–199. [CrossRef] [PubMed]
50. Stanislawski, M.A.; Lozupone, C.A.; Wagner, B.D.; Eggesbo, M.; Sontag, M.K.; Nusbacher, N.M.; Martinez, M.; Dabelea, D. Gut microbiota in adolescents and the association with fatty liver: The EPOCH study. *Pediatr. Res.* **2018**. [CrossRef] [PubMed]
51. Everard, A.; Belzer, C.; Geurts, L.; Ouwerkerk, J.P.; Druart, C.; Bindels, L.B.; Cani, P.D. Cross-talk between Akkermansia muciniphila and intestinal epithelium controls diet-induced obesity. *Proc. Natl. Acad. Sci. USA* **2013**, *110*, 9066–9071. [CrossRef] [PubMed]
52. Macpherson, A.J.; Heikenwalder, M.; Ganal-Vonarburg, S.C. The Liver at the Nexus of Host-Microbial Interactions. *Cell Host Microbe* **2016**, *20*, 561–571. [CrossRef] [PubMed]
53. Kaulmann, A.; Bohn, T. Carotenoids, inflammation, and oxidative stress—Implications of cellular signaling pathways and relation to chronic disease prevention. *Nutr. Res.* **2014**, *34*, 907–929. [CrossRef] [PubMed]
54. Speranza, L.; Pesce, M.; Patruno, A.; Franceschelli, S.; de Lutiis, M.A.; Grilli, A.; Felaco, M. Astaxanthin Treatment Reduced Oxidative Induced Pro-Inflammatory Cytokines Secretion in U937: SHP-1 as a Novel Biological Target. *Mar. Drugs* **2012**, *10*, 890–899. [CrossRef] [PubMed]

5

Dietary Carotenoids and Non-Alcoholic Fatty Liver Disease among US Adults, NHANES 2003–2014

Krista Christensen [1,*], Thomas Lawler [2] and Julie Mares [1]

1 Department of Ophthalmology and Visual Sciences, University of Wisconsin, 610 N. Walnut Street, 1069 WARF Building, Madison, WI 53726, USA; jmarespe@wisc.edu

2 Department of Nutritional Sciences, University of Wisconsin, 1415 Linden Drive, Madison, WI 53706, USA; tlawler2@wisc.edu

* Correspondence: krista.christensen@wisc.edu;

Abstract: Non-alcoholic fatty liver disease (NAFLD) is highly prevalent worldwide. Oxidative stress is thought to be a major mechanism, and previous epidemiological studies found higher serum levels of antioxidant carotenoids were associated with reduced risk for development and progression of NAFLD. The objective of this analysis is to examine cross-sectional associations between dietary and serum levels of carotenoids in relation to NAFLD among a nationally representative sample of US adults. We used data from the 2003–2014 National Health and Nutrition Examination Survey (NHANES). Dietary carotenoid intake was estimated from a 24-hour recall, while serum carotenoids were measured from 2003 to 2006. The NAFLD status was determined based upon US Fatty Liver Index (FLI) value ≥30. Regression models were used to estimate associations between carotenoids and NAFLD by controlling for covariates and adjusting for survey design variables. Overall, 33% of participants were classified as having NAFLD. Intake of all carotenoids, with the exception of lycopene, was lower among those with NAFLD. This association was significant for the highest quartiles of intake of α-carotene, β-carotene, β-cryptoxanthin, and lutein/zeaxanthin. For serum measures, the highest level of all carotenoids was associated with significantly reduced odds of NAFLD. In conclusion, higher intake and serum levels of most carotenoids were associated with lower odds of having NAFLD. Identification of such modifiable lifestyle factors provide an opportunity to limit or prevent the disease and its progression.

Keywords: nutrition; chronic disease; lutein; zeaxanthin; lycopene; beta-carotene; alpha-carotene; beta-cryptoxanthin

---

1. Introduction

Non-alcoholic fatty liver disease (NAFLD) is highly prevalent worldwide, and is the most common liver disease in the United States with an estimated prevalence of 30% among adults [1], and 3% to 12% among children [2]. NAFLD is conceptualized as the hepatic manifestation of the metabolic syndrome, and comprises a range of conditions across the clinical spectrum. The American Association for the Study of Liver Diseases defines NAFLD as presence of both *"evidence of hepatic steatosis (HS), either by imaging or histology"* and *"lack of secondary causes of hepatic fat accumulation such as significant alcohol consumption, long-term use of a steatogenic medication, or monogenic hereditary disorders"* [3]. Hepatic steatosis increases risk for progression to non-alcoholic steatohepatitis (NASH), which is characterized by activation of hepatic macrophages, infiltration of inflammatory immune cells, hepatocyte ballooning, and cell death. NASH, in turn, drastically increases risk for fibrosis, cirrhosis leading to liver failure, and hepatocellular carcinoma [3,4]. Since there is currently no accepted pharmaceutical or surgical treatment for NAFLD [5], lifestyle modifications such as dietary changes are typically recommended to prevent the development of NAFLD, and to mitigate severity once disease has developed.

NAFLD is thought to develop through a series of 'hits' or stressors to the liver ('multiple hit' hypothesis). Although the pathophysiology of NAFLD is complex, abdominal adiposity, aberrant lipid metabolism, insulin resistance, oxidative stress, and inflammation likely contribute to NAFLD by overlapping and mutually reinforcing pathways. The proximal cause of NAFLD is accumulation of fat in liver cells (hepatocytes) combined with oxidative stress and other insults to the liver. Hence, antioxidant activity by carotenoids may reduce risk, severity, or progression of this disease. A growing body of epidemiological research indicates that higher levels of carotenoids in serum are associated with reduced risk for NAFLD or for disease progression [6–11]. Previous studies found increased risk for NAFLD and NASH with lower levels of serum β-carotene, α-carotene, β-cryptoxanthin, and lycopene [7,10,12], and lower total serum carotenoids [6]. Higher levels of both specific and total serum carotenoids were prospectively associated with improvements in NAFLD as assessed by abdominal ultrasonography in a cohort of Chinese adults [11]. However, there is little evidence for association with dietary intake of carotenoids, and no identified trials of carotenoid interventions to treat NAFLD or slow its progression.

Despite the incomplete body of evidence from epidemiological studies, there are animal studies to support the association of carotenoid exposure and risk of NAFLD. Multiple rodent studies demonstrate that both lycopene [13–16] and lutein [17] can slow the rate of hepatic lipid accumulation in mice fed a high-fat diet. Proposed mechanisms for this effect include activation of SIRT1, which is a master regulator of mitochondrial biogenesis and lipid oxidation, and improvement in insulin sensitivity. Lycopene feeding also reduced markers of liver damage including ALT and AST [14,16], and attenuated circulating levels of pro-inflammatory cytokine TNF-α [14], implicated in NAFLD progression. The antioxidant capacity of carotenoids may directly prevent liver damage and progression of hepatic steatosis to NASH, by mitigating the injurious effects of oxidative stress in hepatocytes. Likewise, carotenoids may attenuate pro-inflammatory signaling through transcription factor NFKβ [18], and inhibit activation of macrophages to an M1 phenotype (characteristic of NAFLD progression) [19]. A recent review concluded that carotenoids may confer protection via multiple pathways, including decreased hepatic levels of cholesterol, glucose, MDA (malondialdehyde, marker of lipid peroxidation), TNF-α, and NFKβ binding activity [20].

In this analysis, we examine cross-sectional associations between dietary and serum carotenoids in relation to NAFLD-related outcomes among a nationally representative sample of US adults. We hypothesize that greater exposure to carotenoids in diet and serum will be associated with lower odds of NAFLD, as assessed when utilizing the US Fatty Liver Index (FLI).

2. Materials and Methods

2.1. Design

The National Health and Nutrition Examination Survey (NHANES) is a cross-sectional survey designed to provide a representative sample of the US non-institutionalized civilian population [21]. This work is not considered human subjects research since it relies on free, publicly available datasets only, and is, thus, not subject to IRB review.

For these analyses, we used information on dietary (2003–2014) and serum (2003–2006) carotenoids, and factors needed to construct the US FLI (race/ethnicity, age, gammaglutamyl transferase level, waist circumference, insulin level, and glucose level). Participants were excluded for the following reasons: missing information needed to calculate US FLI (e.g., non-participation in the fasting sample) or on carotenoid dietary intake, age less than 20 years, presence of hepatitis B or C antibody, missing or elevated alcohol intake (≥10 g or 1 drink/day for women or 20 g or 2 drinks/day for men), and self-reported liver disease.

2.2. Carotenoids in Diet and Supplements and in Serum

NHANES participants provide detailed dietary intake information for up to two 24-h periods. These recalls are used to estimate intakes of energy, nutrients, and other food components. The first dietary recall is collected in-person during the NHANES visit, while the second recall is collected by telephone 3 to 10 days later. For these analyses, total estimated dietary carotenoid intake (micrograms, μg) was averaged over the two recall periods (if only the first day was available, that value was used). For the NHANES cycles used, information was available on α-carotene, β-carotene, β-cryptoxanthin, lycopene, and lutein/zeaxanthin (combined). While the main focus of this analysis is on dietary intake, participants are also queried about supplement use for the same two 24-h periods with respect to carotenoids and supplement intake of lycopene and lutein/zeaxanthin were available for later NHANES cycles (2007 onward). For participants reporting supplement use, total intake of lycopene and of lutein/zeaxanthin was calculated as the sum of dietary and supplement intake for sensitivity analyses.

For two of the NHANES cycles in this analysis (2003/2004, 2005/2006), serum measurements of carotenoids were also available. In these two cycles, participants aged 6 years and older provided serum samples for measurement of six carotenoids (α-carotene, trans-β-carotene, cis β-carotene, β-cryptoxanthin, combined lutein/zeaxanthin, trans-lycopene, and total lycopene) using high performance liquid chromatography (HPLC). We evaluated serum levels of carotenoids in relation to NAFLD outcomes as a sub-analysis.

2.3. NAFLD-Related Outcomes

Outcome status is based upon the US Fatty Liver Index (FLI), as described in Ruhl et al. [22]. The FLI was developed using NHANES III data and evaluated against hepatic steatosis, as diagnosed by an abdominal ultrasound. A cutoff of 30 was used to define NAFLD as suggested by the authors.

2.4. Statistical Analysis

All data analysis was performed using SAS/STAT software (Version 9.4, SAS Institute Inc., Cary, NC, USA). Regression models were used to identify associations between carotenoid intake and NAFLD-related outcomes, controlling for potential confounders. The primary models included adjustment for survey design variables, and for survey cycle, sex, and age in years. To evaluate whether the effects of carotenoid intake might be attributable more generally to a healthy diet, we also looked at models additionally adjusted for the healthy eating index (HEI) 2015 score. This score was only available for 2005 onwards. As a sensitivity analysis, we evaluated regression models including primary adjustment variables, as well as poverty income ratio (PIR) and educational attainment. These additional factors may be related to both carotenoid intake and risk for NAFLD, but it is likely that their association with NAFLD is mediated through diet. Serum cotinine as a proxy for smoke exposure was evaluated, but was not associated with carotenoid intake nor with an NAFLD status. To evaluate potential non-linear effects, carotenoid exposures were treated as both continuous and categorical (quartiles) variables. Statistically significant was defined as p-value < 0.05 for categorical variables and for a linear trend.

Both logistic (binary outcome of NAFLD, SURVEYLOGISTIC procedure) and linear (continuous outcome of US FLI, SURVEYREG procedure) regression models were used to evaluate associations with carotenoid intake. All statistical analyses were adjusted for survey design and weighting variables. For the full dataset analysis (dietary intake of carotenoids), we created 12-year weights as one-sixth of the value of the fasting subsample MEC weight (WTSAF2YR * 1/6) since this represented the smallest subsample of the study population. For sensitivity analyses of total (diet and supplement) lycopene and lutein/zeaxanthin intake, eight-year weights were calculated as one fourth of the value (WTSAF2YR * 1/4). When including HEI 2015 score as an adjustment variable, we used 10-year weights calculated as one-fifth the value (WTSAF2YR * 1/5). For the sub-analysis of serum carotenoids, we created 4-year weights as one-half of the value (WTSAF2YR * 1/2), and for analysis of serum carotenoids including HEI 2015 score (2005–2006 serum data only), the original 2-year weights were used.

3. Results

Table 1 displays characteristics of the study population stratified by NAFLD status. About one-third (33%) were classified as having NAFLD based on a US FLI score. Not surprisingly, those with NAFLD tended to be older and were more often male, Mexican-American, or non-Hispanic white, and were more likely to be obese or have diabetes or hypertensive factors.

Intake of all carotenoids with the exception of lycopene, was lower among those with NAFLD. The dietary intakes of the specific carotenoids did show correlations in some cases. When accounting for survey weighting, Pearson correlations were highest between intakes of α and β-carotene ($\rho = 0.75$), α-carotene, and lutein/zeaxanthin ($\rho = 0.48$), and β-carotene and lutein/zeaxanthin ($\rho = 0.69$). Correlations between other carotenoids were lower but significant. When looking at the NHANES cycles where serum carotenoids were measured, all were highly correlated with each other ($p < 0.001$). An especially high correlation was noted between serum α and β-carotene levels ($\rho = 0.66$), while other correlations were weaker ($\rho = 0.19–0.45$) but still highly significant. Dietary intake levels for each carotenoid were significantly associated with corresponding serum levels ($p < 0.001$ for all) although Pearson correlation coefficients were modest ($\rho = 0.25–0.37$), which may reflect an error in assessment of carotenoid intake, or inter-individual variation in carotenoid absorption.

Table 2 shows odd ratios (ORs, 95% confidence intervals [CIs]) for the presence of NAFLD as a binary outcome. Analogous results from modeling the US FLI score as a continuous outcome are shown in Supplementary Table S1. In both tables, results are presented treating carotenoid intake as a categorical variable (quartiles) since there was evidence of non-linearity in some cases. However, we do include a p-value for the trend calculated from models including the carotenoid as a continuous exposure, for reference. In adjusted logistic models, the highest quartiles of intake of α-carotene, β-carotene, β-cryptoxanthin, and lutein/zeaxanthin were all associated with lower odds of NAFLD compared to the lowest quartile of intake. Associations were attenuated when including the HEI 2015 score in the model, but the direction of association was unchanged and remained significant for β-carotene and lutein/zeaxanthin. In sensitivity analyses including education and income, results were largely similar but somewhat attenuated. Similarly, significant associations in linear models for US FLI as a continuous outcome were seen for the highest quartiles of intake of each carotenoid with the exception of lycopene. In logistic regression models, results were attenuated when including the HEI 2015 score (or education and income) but unchanged with respect to the direction of association.

Table 1. Characteristics of NHANES participants, 2003–2014, by the NAFLD status.

Group	No NAFLD		NAFLD		*p*-Value * for Difference between Those With and Without NAFLD
	Weighted *n* (SD)	Weighted Percent (SE)	Weighted *n* (SD)	Weighted Percent (SE)	
Total	61,456,846 (2,218,754)	100 (0)	30,295,373 (1,301,957)	100 (0)	
Survey Cycle					0.02
2003–2004	10,566,907 (1,252,551)	17.2 (1.8)	4,397,048 (603,680)	14.5 (1.8)	
2005–2006	9,983,650 (701,413)	16.2 (1.1)	4,560,556 (428,466)	15.1 (1.3)	
2007–2008	10,630,944 (843,068)	17.3 (1.3)	5,188,078 (602,156)	17.1 (1.8)	
2009–2010	9,483,325 (665,022)	15.4 (1.1)	5,996,470 (478,479)	19.8 (1.5)	
2011–2012	10,439,332 (1,024,219)	17.0 (1.5)	4,980,308 (513,756)	16.4 (1.6)	
2013–2014	10,352,685 (812,379)	16.8 (1.2)	5,172,910 (539,998)	17.1 (1.6)	
Age Group (years)					<0.0001
20–39	20,935,959 (928,501)	35.8 (1.2)	6,195,884 (420,329)	21.1 (1.2)	
40–59	20,750,665 (1,067,685)	35.5 (1.2)	11,253,296 (747,129)	38.4 (1.6)	
60–79	13,098,637 (712,268)	22.4 (0.8)	10,320,193 (568,536)	35.2 (1.5)	
≥80	3,682,338 (262,507)	6.3 (0.4)	1,547,004 (175,185)	5.3 (0.6)	
Sex					<0.0001
Male	26,036,711 (1,090,038)	42.4 (0.9)	16,577,926 (822,807)	54.7 (1.2)	
Female	35,420,134 (1,373,568)	57.6 (0.9)	13,717,446 (675,055)	45.3 (1.2)	
Race/Ethnicity					<0.0001
Mexican American	4,040,549 (353,152)	6.6 (0.7)	3,214,449 (336,258)	10.6 (1.3)	
Other Hispanic	2,502,869 (294,586)	4.1 (0.5)	1,169,495 (146,235)	3.9 (0.5)	
Non-Hispanic White	42,084,359 (2,357,817)	68.5 (1.6)	22,580,348 (1,364,103)	74.5 (1.8)	
Non-Hispanic Black	8,406,747 (589,390)	13.7 (1.1)	1,986,698 (189,877)	6.6 (0.7)	
Other/Multiracial	4,422,319 (386,390)	7.2 (0.6)	1,344,381 (187,613)	4.4 (0.6)	
BMI Category					<0.0001
Underweight (<18.5)	1,267,523 (190,732)	2.1 (0.3)	11,483 (11,483)	0 (0)	
Normal (18.5–24.9)	23,267,000 (1,199,452)	37.9 (1.1)	1,067,429 (166,431)	3.5 (0.5)	
Overweight (25–29.9)	24,039,650 (975,583)	39.1 (1)	6,865,896 (515,913)	22.7 (1.3)	
Obese (≥30)	12,882,671 (625,090)	21.0 (0.8)	22,350,563 (1,000,989)	73.8 (1.4)	

Table 1. *Cont.*

Group	No NAFLD		NAFLD		p-Value * for Difference between Those With and Without NAFLD
	Weighted *n* (SD)	Weighted Percent (SE)	Weighted *n* (SD)	Weighted Percent (SE)	
Smoking Status					<0.0001
Never	39,936,202 (1,411,228)	65 (1)	17,112,945 (831,979)	56.5 (1.5)	
Current	8,772,599 (631,562)	14.3 (0.8)	3,937,101 (329,377)	13 (1)	
Former	12,734,901 (761,119)	20.7 (0.9)	9,242,180 (599,355)	30.5 (1.2)	
Missing	13,143 (7800)	0 (0)	3146 (3146)	0 (0)	
Education Level					<0.0001
Less than HS	996,9649 (566,262)	16.2 (0.9)	6,847,959 (414,383)	22.6 (1.3)	
HS or some college	31,596,068 (1,513,799)	51.4 (1.3)	17,238,418 (1,037,220)	56.9 (1.7)	
College or more	19875667 (1,131,428)	32.3 (1.4)	6,208,995 (464,059)	20.5 (1.4)	
Missing	15,459 (9780)	0 (0)	0 (0)	0 (0)	
Diabetes (doctor's diagnosis)					<0.0001
No	57,768,923 (2,130,004)	94 (0.5)	24,365,926 (1,187,983)	80.4 (1.3)	
Yes	3687,922 (301,760)	6 (0.5)	5,929,446 (413,180)	19.6 (1.3)	
Diabetes (plasma fasting glucose ≥127 mg/dL)					<0.0001
No	58,992,373 (2,196,856)	96 (0.4)	23,910,800 (1,125,079)	78.9 (1.2)	
Yes	2,464,472 (221,631)	4 (0.4)	6,384,573 (417,802)	21.1 (1.2)	
Diabetes (either criteria)					<0.0001
No	56,999,582 (2,117,147)	92.7 (0.5)	22,113,112 (1,076,534)	73 (1.3)	
Yes	4,457,263 (331,259)	7.3 (0.5)	8,182,260 (487,535)	27 (1.3)	
High blood pressure at exam (systolic ≥130 and/or diastolic ≥85 mm Hg)					<0.0001
No	44,620,732 (1,833,006)	74.5 (0.9)	17,861,138 (883,010)	61.1 (1.4)	
Yes	15,263,826 (689,875)	25.5 (0.9)	11,373,199 (622,176)	38.9 (1.4)	

Table 1. *Cont.*

Group	No NAFLD		NAFLD		*p*-Value * for Difference between Those With and Without NAFLD
	Weighted *n* (SD)	Weighted Percent (SE)	Weighted *n* (SD)	Weighted Percent (SE)	
	Mean (SE)		**Mean (SE)**		
Age (years)	48.28 (0.4)		53.77 (0.47)		<0.0001
Family Income (poverty income ratio, PIR)	3.02 (0.04)		2.83 (0.06)		0.001
Body Mass Index (kg/m^2)	26.59 (0.1)		34.66 (0.23)		<0.0001
Waist Circumference (cm)	92.81 (0.25)		114.7 (0.47)		<0.0001
Dietary Measures					
Total Energy (kcal/day)	2018.42 (17.58)		2070.52 (23.51)		0.05
Dietary α-carotene (mcg)	489.85 (51.53)		387.73 (25.77)		0.16
Dietary β-carotene (mcg)	2547.38 (170.97)		1933.4 (70.65)		0.0003
Dietary β-cryptoxanthin (mcg)	110.22 (4.6)		93.48 (5.15)		0.05
Dietary lycopene (mcg)	5372.32 (190.38)		5624.4 (228.24)		0.37
Dietary lutein/zeaxanthin (mcg)	1748.17 (109.42)		1275.8 (49.83)		<0.0001
Laboratory Measures					
Insulin (pmol/L)	47.3 (0.62)		137.44 (3.38)		<0.0001
Glucose, plasma (mg/dL)	98.98 (0.43)		119.59 (1.17)		<0.0001
Cholesterol (mg/dL)	196.21 (1)		194.76 (1.33)		0.35
Triglycerides (mg/dL)	107.73 (2.15)		175.63 (4.18)		<0.0001
LDL-cholesterol (mg/dL)	116.69 (0.78)		115.08 (1.13)		0.24
Direct HDL-Cholesterol (mg/dL)	56.4 (0.38)		45.29 (0.34)		<0.0001
Gamma glutamyl transferase (U/L)	18.58 (0.26)		35.82 (0.85)		<0.0001
US Fatty Liver Index	12.39 (0.17)		52.8 (0.52)		<0.0001
Serum Measures (2003–2006 only)					
Serum α-carotene (μg/dL)	5.03 (0.28)		2.96 (0.14)		<0.0001
Serum β-carotene (μg/dL)	23.25 (1.14)		12.96 (0.6)		<0.0001
Serum β-cryptoxanthin (μg/dL)	10.32 (0.39)		7.6 (0.29)		<0.0001
Serum lycopene (μg/dL)	43.8 (0.72)		40.37 (1.07)		0.02

Table 2. Odds ratios * (95% confidence interval) for association between the quartile of carotenoid intake, relative to Quartile 1, and presence of NAFLD. The median (range) for each quartile of carotenoid intake is also displayed (μg/day).

	Quartile 1	**Quartile 2**	**Quartile 3**	**Quartile 4**	***p*-Value for Trend**
α-carotene					
Median (Range)	10.0 (0–27)	49.8 (27–95.5)	217.4 (96–477)	1007.4 (477.5–72,037)	
Model 1	Referent	0.99 (0.84, 1.16)	0.95 (0.79, 1.15)	**0.75 (0.63, 0.89)**	0.11
Model 2	Referent	**1.23 (1.04, 1.46)**	1.19 (0.98, 1.44)	0.99 (0.81, 1.21)	0.37
β-carotene					
Median (Range)	248.8 (0–435)	682.6 (435.5–1092.5)	1738.8 (1094–2726.5)	4691.2 (2728–246,122)	
Model 1	Referent	0.99 (0.82, 1.20)	**0.82 (0.70, 0.97)**	**0.63 (0.52, 0.76)**	**<0.001**
Model 2	Referent	1.04 (0.84, 1.28)	0.92 (0.76, 1.12)	**0.75 (0.60, 0.94)**	**0.02**
β-cryptoxanthin					
Median (Range)	5.7 (0–14.5)	26.3 (15–47)	76.6 (47.5–124)	229.5 (124.5–6088.5)	
Model 1	Referent	0.86 (0.72, 1.03)	0.82 (0.64, 1.04)	**0.64 (0.52, 0.80)**	**0.04**
Model 2	Referent	0.91 (0.74, 1.11)	0.97 (0.73, 1.28)	0.84 (0.65, 1.09)	0.50
Lycopene (Diet)					
Median (Range)	4.1 (0–564.5)	1273.5 (566.5–2233)	3792.1 (2234.5–6417.5)	12110 (6419–108,852)	
Model 1	Referent	0.94 (0.78, 1.14)	0.89 (0.74, 1.09)	1.12 (0.91, 1.37)	0.29
Model 2	Referent	0.99 (0.80, 1.23)	0.93 (0.75, 1.16)	1.07 (0.84, 1.35)	0.97
Lutein/Zeaxanthin (Diet)					
Median (Range)	277.0 (0–430.5)	600.2 (431–786.5)	1050.7 (787–1506)	2570.3 (1506.5–146,912)	
Model 1	Referent	0.94 (0.75, 1.17)	0.88 (0.73, 1.06)	**0.63 (0.51, 0.77)**	**<0.001**
Model 2	Referent	1.02 (0.81, 1.28)	1.02 (0.83, 1.26)	**0.78 (0.63, 0.96)**	**<0.001**
Total Lycopene (Diet and Supplement)					
Median (Range)	35.9 (0–590.5)	1313.8 (591–2276)	3838.2 (2280–6451.5)	12,203 (6455–108,852)	
Model 1	Referent	0.97 (0.81, 1.17)	0.92 (0.76, 1.1)	1.12 (0.92, 1.37)	0.42
Model 2	Referent	1.04 (0.86, 1.27)	0.96 (0.79, 1.18)	1.08 (0.86, 1.35)	0.72
Total Lutein/Zeaxanthin (Diet and Supplement)					
Median (Range)	281.6 (0–444.5)	627.6 (445–816.5)	1096.9 (817–1556)	2751.3 (1556.5–161,912)	
Model 1	Referent	0.92 (0.75, 1.14)	0.85 (0.71, 1.02)	**0.59 (0.48, 0.73)**	**<0.001**
Model 2	Referent	1.02 (0.82, 1.28)	1.01 (0.81, 1.25)	**0.73 (0.59, 0.91)**	**0.002**

* Model 1 is adjusted for age, sex, and the survey cycle year. Model 2 is adjusted for age, sex, and survey year, along with HEI 2015 score. All analyses are adjusted for survey design variables. Bold text indicates statistically significant associations.

Table 3 displays results from logistic regression modeling of serum carotenoid exposures and the NAFLD status as a binary outcome, while analogous results for US FLI as a continuous outcome are shown in Supplementary Table S2. As shown above for dietary intakes, serum carotenoids were treated as categorical exposures, with p-value for the trend calculated from models including serum carotenoids as a continuous variable. For serum carotenoid levels, a dose-response pattern was more apparent (compared with dietary intake exposures), with most of the *p*-values for the trend being statistically significant. In the fully adjusted model, the highest quartile was associated with significantly reduced risk for NAFLD among all carotenoids except lycopene. Statistically significant inverse associations were observed for Quartiles 2–4 of serum β-carotene, and Quartiles 3 and 4 of serum α-carotene, β-cryptoxanthin, and lutein/zeaxanthin. In general, estimates were largely unaffected by adjusting the HEI 2015 score, or for income and education. Similar results were seen in fully adjusted linear models for US FLI as a continuous outcome, but the highest quartile of serum lycopene was associated with lower US FLI in the fully adjusted model (see Supplementary Table S2).

Table 3. Logistic regression results (odds ratio (95% confidence interval)) for association between the quartile of serum carotenoids, relative to Quartile 1, and presence of NAFLD. The median (range) for each quartile of serum concentration is also displayed (μg/dL).

	Quartile 1	Quartile 2	Quartile 3	Quartile 4	*p*-Value for Trend
α-carotene					
Median (Range)	1.0 (0.2–1.5)	2.1 (1.6–3.0)	4.0 (3.0–5.4)	8.6 (5.4–96.5)	
Model 1	Referent	0.81 (0.62, 1.06)	**0.48 (0.33, 0.69)**	**0.33 (0.22, 0.5)**	**<0.001**
Model 2	Referent	0.7 (0.43, 1.13)	**0.35 (0.17, 0.71)**	**0.3 (0.15, 0.6)**	**<0.001**
β-carotene					
Median (Range)	6.0 (0.6–8.3)	10.5 (8.3–14.1)	18.2 (14.1–25.1)	36.1 (25.1–292.9)	
Model 1	Referent	**0.40 (0.28, 0.57)**	**0.31 (0.20, 0.46)**	**0.14 (0.09, 0.21)**	**<0.001**
Model 2	Referent	**0.28 (0.18, 0.45)**	**0.26 (0.14, 0.48)**	**0.13 (0.07, 0.23)**	**<0.001**
β-cryptoxanthin					
Median (Range)	3.5 (0.6–4.9)	6.4 (4.9–8.2)	10.3 (8.3–13.8)	19.4 (13.8–93.1)	
Model 1	Referent	0.73 (0.52, 1.03)	**0.49 (0.35, 0.68)**	**0.37 (0.26, 0.52)**	**<0.001**
Model 2	Referent	0.75 (0.44, 1.28)	**0.53 (0.31, 0.91)**	**0.45 (0.22, 0.92)**	**0.02**
Lycopene					
Median (Range)	19.2 (0.7–26.2)	32.6 (26.2–37.9)	43.5 (37.9–51.1)	64.0 (51.2–148.0)	
Model 1	Referent	0.91 (0.62, 1.32)	0.8 (0.53, 1.21)	**0.63 (0.41, 0.96)**	**0.03**
Model 2	Referent	0.99 (0.66, 1.49)	0.75 (0.4, 1.41)	0.68 (0.39, 1.21)	0.17
Lutein/Zeaxanthin					
Median (Range)	8.6 (2.4–10.9)	13.0 (10.6–15.2)	17.7 (15.2–27.0)	26.0 (20.7–113.1)	
Model 1	Referent	0.72 (0.51, 1.01)	**0.54 (0.36, 0.79)**	**0.33 (0.24, 0.47)**	**<0.001**
Model 2	Referent	0.78 (0.44, 1.38)	**0.53 (0.29, 0.97)**	**0.31 (0.2, 0.5)**	**<0.01**

Model 1 is adjusted for age, sex, and the survey cycle year. Model 2 is adjusted for age, sex, and survey year, along with the HEI 2015 score. All analyses are adjusted for survey design variables. Bold text indicates statistically significant associations.

4. Discussion

In this nationally representative sample of the US adult population, higher intake of certain carotenoids, and higher concentrations of carotenoids in the serum were associated with lower odds of having NAFLD, and with a better score of the US Fatty Liver Index. This is very promising given that there are no currently accepted therapeutic interventions for NAFLD. The dietary modification to increase carotenoid intake represents a possible route for prevention and amelioration of a common chronic health condition.

These findings build on a body of evidence suggesting relationships between carotenoid status to lipid metabolism and obesity, and are consistent with other epidemiological studies that demonstrate a prospective association between serum carotenoid levels and NAFLD [6,7,11], or between serum carotenoids and serum ALT [8,9]. These previous studies included a variety of designs. In a cross-sectional prevalence study (similar to the design of the NHANES analysis reported here), Cao et al. demonstrated that individuals with the highest serum levels of α and β-carotene, β-cryptoxanthin, lycopene, and lutein/zeaxanthin, had significantly reduced risk (ORs 0.32–0.62) for NAFLD, as diagnosed using abdominal ultrasonography [6]. A prospective study from the same group revealed that serum carotenoids were approximately 9% to 30% higher in individuals whose NAFLD improved compared to those who experienced disease progression [11]. Lastly, a case-control study demonstrated that serum lutein, zeaxanthin, lycopene, and α and β-carotene levels were 30% to 60% lower in NASH cases compared to controls [7]. Based on our knowledge, the present study is the first to report a statistically significant inverse association between dietary carotenoid intake and both risk of NAFLD and score on the US FLI, which is consistent with reduced risk for NAFLD. Our results are supported by animal studies in which the administration of carotenoids (including lycopene and lutein) attenuated the hepatic accumulation of lipids on a high-fat diet, as well as increased expression of SIRT1, which is a key regulator of fatty acid oxidation [15,17]. Higher carotenoid intake may reduce risk for NAFLD, and, in particular, the progression of simple hepatic steatosis to NASH, through several different pathways, including the attenuation of oxidative stress in the liver, with downstream effects on secretion of pro-inflammatory cytokines by hepatic macrophages, immune infiltration, and insulin sensitivity [20].

Many of the carotenoid measures were correlated with each other, which can make it difficult to distinguish individual effects (for example, correlations between intakes of α and β-carotene, and each of these with lutein/zeaxanthin, were between 0.78 to 0.94). For the logistic model (NAFLD as a binary outcome), when comparing the fully adjusted model with one carotenoid included at a time versus all included in the model, effect estimates were generally similar but attenuated (and confidence intervals increased in width). We investigated the possibility that beneficial associations of higher carotenoid intake are due to benefits of eating foods high in carotenoids (e.g., fruits and vegetables). Inclusion of the healthy eating index 2015 score did attenuate—but did not eliminate—associations with dietary carotenoids. Conversely, associations for serum carotenoids were largely unaffected by adjusting the healthy eating index score. It is likely that some of the protective association is due to healthier eating patterns. In addition, healthy diet patterns may enhance absorption of carotenoids from the diet. However, some effect may be due to carotenoid mechanisms specifically. This would be consistent with the observation that inverse associations were generally stronger and more consistent for serum carotenoids compared with dietary intake, which may reflect heterogeneity in the absorption of carotenoids into the bloodstream and greater measurement error or misclassification in the self-reported dietary data [23].

Limitations of this analysis included the use of self-reported dietary data, which may be due to a greater measurement error. The NAFLD status was inferred based upon a previously validated index, but is not a perfect proxy for NAFLD diagnosis based upon liver biopsy or other more invasive methods. However, evaluation of the FLI in the NHANES has shown good sensitivity, with the area under the receiver operator curve reported to be 78% [22], which suggests less potential for the outcome misclassification error. Furthermore, use of this index with the NHANES population made it impossible to adjust for potentially important covariates including body composition and markers of insulin sensitivity. Since the FLI is a surrogate marker for NAFLD based on markers of metabolic health, it is not clear whether carotenoid exposure is correlated with NAFLD independently of these markers. Another limitation is that the dietary analysis does not include an estimation of intake for certain carotenoids—such as astaxanthin and fucoxanthin—which may also have associations with NAFLD. Strengths include the use of multiple years of data from a large and nationally representative sample, consideration of multiple potential confounders, and examination of multiple carotenoids singly and in combination.

5. Conclusions

We found that higher intake and serum levels of certain carotenoids were cross-sectionally associated with lower odds of NAFLD. These findings are promising given the limited therapeutic options for treating NAFLD, in that identification of modifiable lifestyle factors provide an opportunity to limit or prevent the disease and its progression.

Supplementary Materials:
Table S1: Beta coefficients (standard error), *p*-values, for association between quartile of carotenoid intake, relative to quartile 1, and the US Fatty Liver Index. The median (range) for each quartile of carotenoid intake is also displayed (μg/day). Table S2: Beta coefficients (standard error), *p*-values, for association between quartile of serum carotenoids, relative to quartile 1, and the US Fatty Liver Index. The median (range) for each quartile of serum concentration is also displayed (μg/dL).

Author Contributions: Conceptualization, K.C. Formal analysis, K.C. and T.L. Funding acquisition, J.M. Investigation, K.C. Methodology, K.C. and J.M. Resources, J.M. Writing—original draft, K.C. and T.L. Writing—review & editing, J.M.

References

1. Le, M.H.; Devaki, P.; Ha, N.B.; Jun, D.W.; Te, H.S.; Cheung, R.C.; Nguyen, M.H. Prevalence of non-alcoholic fatty liver disease and risk factors for advanced fibrosis and mortality in the United States. *PLoS ONE* **2017**, *12*, e0173499. [CrossRef] [PubMed]
2. Bush, H.; Golabi, P.; Younossi, Z.M. Pediatric Non-Alcoholic Fatty Liver Disease. *Children* **2017**, *4*, 48. [CrossRef] [PubMed]
3. Chalasani, N.; Younossi, Z.; Lavine, J.E.; Charlton, M.; Cusi, K.; Rinella, M.; Harrison, S.A.; Brunt, E.M.; Sanyal, A.J. The diagnosis and management of nonalcoholic fatty liver disease: Practice guidance from the American Association for the Study of Liver Diseases. *Hepatology* **2018**, *67*, 328–357. [CrossRef]
4. Brunt, E.M.; Wong, V.W.; Nobili, V.; Day, C.P.; Sookoian, S.; Maher, J.J.; Bugianesi, E.; Sirlin, C.B.; Neuschwander-Tetri, B.A.; Rinella, M.E. Nonalcoholic fatty liver disease. *Nat. Rev. Dis. Primers* **2015**, *1*, 15080. [CrossRef] [PubMed]
5. Rinella, M.E.; Loomba, R.; Caldwell, S.H.; Kowdley, K.; Charlton, M.; Tetri, B.; Harrison, S.A. Controversies in the Diagnosis and Management of NAFLD and NASH. *Gastroenterol. Hepatol.* **2014**, *10*, 219–227.
6. Cao, Y.; Wang, C.; Liu, J.; Liu, Z.M.; Ling, W.H.; Chen, Y.M. Greater serum carotenoid levels associated with lower prevalence of nonalcoholic fatty liver disease in Chinese adults. *Sci. Rep.* **2015**, *5*, 12951. [CrossRef]
7. Erhardt, A.; Stahl, W.; Sies, H.; Lirussi, F.; Donner, A.; Haussinger, D. Plasma levels of vitamin E and carotenoids are decreased in patients with Nonalcoholic Steatohepatitis (NASH). *Eur. J. Med. Res.* **2011**, *16*, 76–78. [CrossRef]
8. Ruhl, C.E.; Everhart, J.E. Relation of elevated serum alanine aminotransferase activity with iron and antioxidant levels in the United States. *Gastroenterology* **2003**, *124*, 1821–1829. [CrossRef]
9. Sugiura, M.; Nakamura, M.; Ogawa, K.; Ikoma, Y.; Yano, M. High serum carotenoids are associated with lower risk for developing elevated serum alanine aminotransferase among Japanese subjects: The Mikkabi cohort study. *Br. J. Nutr.* **2016**, *115*, 1462–1469. [CrossRef]
10. Villaca Chaves, G.; Pereira, S.E.; Saboya, C.J.; Ramalho, A. Non-alcoholic fatty liver disease and its relationship with the nutritional status of vitamin A in individuals with class III obesity. *Obes. Surg.* **2008**, *18*, 378–385. [CrossRef]
11. Xiao, M.L.; Chen, G.D.; Zeng, F.F.; Qiu, R.; Shi, W.Q.; Lin, J.S.; Cao, Y.; Li, H.B.; Ling, W.H.; Chen, Y.M. Higher serum carotenoids associated with improvement of non-alcoholic fatty liver disease in adults: A prospective study. *Eur. J. Nutr.* **2018**. [CrossRef]
12. Park, S.K.; Lee, H.J.; Lee, D.H.; Lee, S.K.; Chun, B.Y.; Kim, S.A.; Lee, H.S.; Son, H.K.; Kim, S.H. Associations of non alcoholic fatty liver with the metabolic syndrome and serum carotenoids. *J. Prev. Med. Public Health* **2008**, *41*, 39–44. [CrossRef] [PubMed]
13. Ahn, J.; Lee, H.; Jung, C.H.; Ha, T. Lycopene inhibits hepatic steatosis via microRNA-21-induced downregulation of fatty acid-binding protein 7 in mice fed a high-fat diet. *Mol. Nutr. Food Res.* **2012**, *56*, 1665–1674. [CrossRef]
14. Bahcecioglu, I.H.; Kuzu, N.; Metin, K.; Ozercan, I.H.; Ustundag, B.; Sahin, K.; Kucuk, O. Lycopene prevents development of steatohepatitis in experimental nonalcoholic steatohepatitis model induced by high-fat diet. *Vet. Med. Int.* **2010**. [CrossRef]

15. Chung, J.; Koo, K.; Lian, F.; Hu, K.Q.; Ernst, H.; Wang, X.D. Apo-10′-lycopenoic acid, a lycopene metabolite, increases sirtuin 1 mRNA and protein levels and decreases hepatic fat accumulation in ob/ob mice. *J. Nutr.* **2012**, *142*, 405–410. [CrossRef]
16. Jiang, W.; Guo, M.H.; Hai, X. Hepatoprotective and antioxidant effects of lycopene on non-alcoholic fatty liver disease in rat. *World J. Gastroenterol.* **2016**, *22*, 10180–10188. [CrossRef]
17. Qiu, X.; Gao, D.H.; Xiang, X.; Xiong, Y.F.; Zhu, T.S.; Liu, L.G.; Sun, X.F.; Hao, L.P. Ameliorative effects of lutein on non-alcoholic fatty liver disease in rats. *World J. Gastroenterol.* **2015**, *21*, 8061–8072. [CrossRef]
18. Kim, J.H.; Na, H.J.; Kim, C.K.; Kim, J.Y.; Ha, K.S.; Lee, H.; Chung, H.T.; Kwon, H.J.; Kwon, Y.G.; Kim, Y.M. The non-provitamin A carotenoid, lutein, inhibits NF-kappaB-dependent gene expression through redox-based regulation of the phosphatidylinositol 3-kinase/PTEN/Akt and NF-kappaB-inducing kinase pathways: Role of H(2)O(2) in NF-kappaB activation. *Free Radic. Biol. Med.* **2008**, *45*, 885–896. [CrossRef] [PubMed]
19. Ni, Y.; Zhuge, F.; Nagashimada, M.; Ota, T. Novel Action of Carotenoids on Non-Alcoholic Fatty Liver Disease: Macrophage Polarization and Liver Homeostasis. *Nutrients* **2016**, *8*, 391. [CrossRef]
20. Murillo, A.G.; DiMarco, D.M.; Fernandez, M.L. The Potential of Non-Provitamin A Carotenoids for the Prevention and Treatment of Non-Alcoholic Fatty Liver Disease. *Biology* **2016**, *5*, 42. [CrossRef] [PubMed]
21. Centers for Disease Control and Prevention (CDC); National Center for Health Statistics (NCHS). National Health and Nutrition Examination Survey. NHANES Questionnaires, Datasets, and Related Documentation. Available online: https://wwwn.cdc.gov/nchs/nhanes/Default.aspx (accessed on 30 May 2018).
22. Ruhl, C.E.; Everhart, J.E. Fatty liver indices in the multiethnic United States National Health and Nutrition Examination Survey. *Aliment. Pharmacol. Ther.* **2015**, *41*, 65–76. [CrossRef] [PubMed]
23. Borel, P. Genetic variations involved in interindividual variability in carotenoid status. *Mol. Nutr. Food Res.* **2012**, *56*, 228–240. [CrossRef] [PubMed]

6

Carotenoid Content in Human Colostrum is Associated to Preterm/Full-Term Birth Condition

Ana A. O. Xavier [1], Elena Díaz-Salido [2], Isabel Arenilla-Vélez [2], Josefa Aguayo-Maldonado [2], Juan Garrido-Fernández [1], Javier Fontecha [3], Alicia Sánchez-García [4] and Antonio Pérez-Gálvez [1,*]

1 Department of Food Phytochemistry, Instituto de la Grasa (CSIC), Campus Universitario, Building 46, 41013 Sevilla, Spain; anaaugustax@gmail.com (A.A.O.X.); jgarrido@ig.csic.es (J.G.-F.)
2 Unidad de Neonatología, Hospital Virgen del Rocío, 41013 Sevilla, Spain; elenam.diaz.sspa@juntadeandalucia.es (E.D.-S.); Isaareni@yahoo.es (I.A.-V.); pepaaguayo@gmail.com (J.A.-M.)
3 Institute of Food Science Research (CSIC-UAM), 28049 Madrid, Spain; j.fontecha@csic.es
4 Laboratorio de Espectrometría de Masas, Instituto de la Grasa (CSIC), 41013 Sevilla, Spain; asangar@ig.csic.es
* Correspondence: aperez@ig.csic.es;

Abstract: Factors such as lactation stage and premature and small-for-gestational conditions could lead to great inter-individual variability in the carotenoid content of human milk. The aim was to analyze the carotenoid content in colostrum and mature milk of preterm (PT) and full-term (FT) mothers to establish whether they are significantly different and, if so, the stage of lactation when the differences are established. Samples of blood, colostrum, and mature milk were collected from Spanish donating mothers who gave birth to PT or FT infants. Carotenoids from serum and milk samples were analyzed by HPLC-atmospheric pressure chemical ionization (APCI)-MS. Quantitatively, colostrum from PT mothers presented lower total carotenoid content when compared to that from FT mothers. The only exception was lutein, where levels were not different. The transition from colostrum to mature milk makes observed differences in the carotenoid content disappear, since there were no variances between PT and FT groups for both individual and total carotenoid content. The premature birth condition affects the quantitative carotenoid composition of the colostrum but has no effect on the lutein content. This fact could be related to the significant role of this xanthophyll in the development of infant retina and feasibly to cognitive function.

Keywords: breastfeeding; new-born; full-term mothers; preterm mothers; xanthophylls; carotenes; lutein; colostrum; mature milk

1. Introduction

Breastfeeding provides health advantages for the immediate growth and development of the new-born, benefits that will extend into adulthood [1], and decreases the risk of child morbidity and mortality [2,3]. International policy agencies recommend exclusive breastfeeding for six months, followed by continued breastfeeding with appropriate complementary foods for up to two years or beyond [4]. Breast milk contains the macro and micronutrients necessary to fulfil nutritional requirements of the infant, as well as immune and nonimmune properties and growth factors [5,6]. Many of these constituents in the milk are derived from maternal blood, which is enriched through diet. This is the case of carotenoid pigments that are exclusively synthesized de novo by photosynthetic organisms, bacteria, yeasts, and some fungi, and incorporated into human tissues and blood through food sources, fruits, vegetables, algae, eggs, and fish [7]. The human milk carotenoids with provitamin

A activity contribute to the vitamin A needs of the infant, a key issue in those developing countries where the dietary supply of vitamin A sources is often limited [8]. Independently of the provitamin A activity, carotenoids exert important functions in immunity, participate in the antioxidant defense system, and are related to a reduced risk of developing chronic diseases [9,10]. The specific accumulation of lutein and zeaxanthin in the fovea of the retina is of remarkable interest, given that this tissue continues to develop during infancy [11]. These carotenoids, known as macular pigments, prevent retinal damage through their blue light filtration and antioxidant properties [12–14], and contribute to the proper structural development of the retina [15]. Furthermore, it has been shown that enriching the macular pigment density by lutein supplementation positively impacts on contrast sensitivity and glare disability [16]. Recent research correlates macular pigment content with cognitive function through different evidence, as it has been shown that the increase in visual performance reached with lutein supplementation is associated with better cognition [17,18], in a similar fashion as the levels of macular lutein and zeaxanthin are related to brain lutein and zeaxanthin content [19]. Also, it would be important to point out that these levels were significantly related to pre-mortem measures of cognitive function [20,21].

These statements may apply in the prenatal and postnatal developing infant. Vishwanathan et al. [22] have shown that lutein is the predominant carotenoid in the infant brain, with much lower levels of zeaxanthin, β-cryptoxanthin, and β-carotene. This accumulation is the starting point to support that carotenoids contribute to early neurodevelopment [23,24]. It could be assumed that the accumulation of carotenoids in the infant brain behave in a similar fashion to the macular pigments in the infant retina, where the carotenoids tend to accumulate in the final months of gestation [25,26]. Indeed, the content of macular pigments is variable in the developing retina [27] and such variability would extend to their brain content if both quantities are correlated as noted above.

The macular and brain carotenoid levels after delivery are a consequence of the infant intake of carotenoids from colostrum and mature milk or infant formula, because these are the only dietary sources containing carotenoids that the new-born receives [23]. Also, it is well established that there is a high-amount of inter-individual and intra-individual variability in milk carotenoid content, which it is associated to maternal dietary habits [28,29], lactation stage [30–33], and health status of the mother, including alcohol intake and smoking [34,35]. With this knowledge, we are beginning to understand the factors contributing to the efficiency of the carotenoid accumulation in infant tissues during the initial months of age. In addition, some inputs are now identified regarding the similarities and differences associated with the carotenoid transfer from maternal blood with the transport of bulk lipids during lactation. Even the existence of transport mechanism of xanthophylls [36] and an active acylation pathway in the mammary glands [37] have been observed. Other features influencing the carotenoid status of the infant at birth, which are now under analysis, are the premature and small-for-gestational conditions. The highest utero accretion of energy and nutrients takes place during the last weeks of pregnancy and prematurity impairs the accumulation of carotenoids into the tissues of the child as shown by Vishwanathan et al. [22], who reported lower carotenoid content in brain of preterm (PT) infants compared to those born at full-term (FT) condition.

The aim of this work was to analyze the carotenoid content in the colostrum and mature milk of preterm and full-term mothers to determine whether they are significantly different and, if so, the stage of lactation when the differences are established and whether they are transitory or not. Prematurity is not a condition only affecting the developmental and nutritional stages of the infant, but also the maturity of the mammary gland and its ability to secrete milk with the appropriate composition for the situation of the new-born. An incomplete gestational period affects the deposition of nutrients in the mammary gland—as it has been described for the accumulation of fatty acids [38]—and the deficiencies may happen at birth or appear during the lactation transition to mature milk [39]. Thus, the incomplete maturity of the mammary gland could be a significant factor that may affect the potential of the breastfeeding to compensate for the nutritional deficits of the PT child. Neither the carotenoid content of the colostrum nor the dynamics of carotenoid content changes occurring in mothers who gave birth prematurely and the comparison with mothers whose children were born at full-term, have been analyzed so far.

2. Materials and Methods

2.1. Subjects

The study population comprised 144 healthy women, which were recruited within a 12 month period between 2015 and 2016 and classified into two groups: mothers (n = 72) who gave birth to full-term neonates (37–40 weeks) and mothers (n = 72) who gave birth to preterm neonates (28–35 weeks). Eligible participants in this study were non-smoking mothers with no chronic diseases. Mothers following any special diets, vegetarians, or those taking supplements were not included. Exclusion criteria applied were pathologies and/or infections during the gestation, developmental anomalies in the fetus, or death of the child. They provided informed consent to participate in the research program and none of the initially enrolled mothers dropped out of the study.

Our previous study [37] indicated that 70 volunteers per group would be necessary to detect significant differences of the individual carotenoid profile between preterm and full-term delivery conditions and between lactation stages at a significance level of $p = 0.05$.

2.2. Measures

2.2.1. Milk and Blood Sample Collection

The samples were collected at the Unidad de Neonatología of the Hospital Universitario Virgen del Rocío (Seville, Spain). Preterm and full-term mothers donated colostrum at 3–5 days postpartum and the same mothers donated mature milk at 30 days postpartum. Milk samples were obtained by collection of the total milk volume of one breast during one milk expression session into a polypropylene bottle. Fasting blood samples (10 mL) were collected at the same time of milk samples. Blood was centrifuged after clotting for 10 min at 2000× g at 4 °C to obtain serum. The samples were transported directly to the laboratory and stored at −80 °C until analysis.

2.2.2. Extraction of the Carotenoid Fraction

The experimental conditions previously described by Ríos et al. [37] were used for extraction of carotenoids from human milk samples. Human milk (3 mL) was mixed with 3 mL of KOH:methanol (20% w/v), and the mixture was incubated for 1 h. After hydrolysis, 6 mL of methanol were added, and the mixture was vortex-mixed for 2 min and cooled at −20 °C for 20 min. Subsequently, the cooled mixture was centrifuged at 10,000× g and 4 °C for 5 min, discarding the upper layer. Diethyl ether (5 mL) and hexane (2 mL) were added to the pellet and vortex-mixed for 2 min. Then, 5 mL of NaCl 10% (w/v) was added, and the sample was vortex-mixed again for 2 min. After centrifugation (10,000× g at 4 °C for 5 min), the organic layer was washed with water until neutral pH was reached. The organic extract was evaporated to dryness in a rotatory evaporator at 25 °C, and the residue was dissolved in 1 mL of methanol:methyl tert-butyl ether (8:2). This solution was filtered through a 0.22-µm filter and stored at −20 °C until analysis. Carotenoid extraction from serum samples was carried out according to the method described by Pérez-Gálvez et al. [40]. Serum (0.1 mL) was extracted with 6 mL hexane:dichloromethane (5:1). The mixture was vortex-mixed for 1 min and centrifuged at 2000× g at 20 °C for 10 min. A portion of the upper phase (5 mL) was withdrawn and the solvent evaporated under N_2. The extract was dissolved in 100 µL of acetone and stored at −20 °C until analysis by HPLC-MS, which was performed within 1 week.

2.2.3. Identification and Quantification of Carotenoids in the Carotenoid Extracts

The carotenoids from human milk and serum samples were separated using a Dionex Ultimate 3000RS U-HPLC (Thermo Fisher Scientific, Waltham, MA, USA) using the method developed by

Breithaupt et al. [41] with slight modifications [37]. High-resolution mass spectrometry measurements were completed on the basis of mass accuracy and in combination with the isotopic pattern in the SigmaFit algorithm [37]. The characteristics of experimental mass spectrum and the MS^2 data were compared with the data available in the literature for carotenoid identification in human milk and serum samples [42–48]. For carotenoid quantification, stock solutions of β-carotene, β-cryptoxanthin, lutein, and lycopene were prepared at a concentration of 25 mg/L. Once the exact concentration was determined (2% maximum total error), working stock solutions for external calibration curves were prepared at 5 concentration levels ranging from 0.15 to 10.0 mg/L. The content of xanthophylls and carotenes was determined in the unsaponified extract. Zeaxanthin was quantified with the calibration curve of lutein, while xanthophyll esters were quantified as their corresponding free xanthophyll [47,48].

2.2.4. Determination of the Lipid Content

The lipid content of human milk samples was determined according to the solvent extraction procedure and then by gravimetry [49].

2.3. Ethics Approval

All subjects gave their informed consent for inclusion before they participated in the study, which was conducted in accordance with the Declaration of Helsinki. The study protocol was approved by the Ethics Committee of the Hospital Universitario Virgen del Rocío and the Bioethics Subcommittee of the Spanish National Research Council (AGL2013-42757R).

2.4. Statistical Analysis

Data are reported as the median, including 25th and 75th percentiles. Due to the non-normality of content of individual carotenoids (Kolmogorov–Smirnov test), the data were analyzed using a non-parametric statistical procedure in the SPSS software (IBM® SPSS® Statistics version 24, IBM, New York, NY, USA). The Mann–Whitney test was applied to analyze the differences in carotenoid content of colostrum and mature milk of PT and FT mothers, and to compare the carotenoid content of colostrum and mature milk within each group of lactating mothers. The same test was applied for carotenoid content in serum samples of both groups and at both collection stages (colostrum and mature milk). The significance was set at $p < 0.05$.

3. Results

The carotenoid composition of the colostrum and mature milk samples from PT and FT mothers is shown in Table 1. Colostrum samples from both groups were qualitatively equal regarding the carotenoid profile, but significant differences were observed when the groups were compared quantitatively. Specifically, the colostrum of FT mothers showed higher carotenoid content, both for individual carotenoids and for the total amount (median of total carotenoid content of 4961.1 nM in the colostrum of full-term mothers vs. 2641.1 nM in the colostrum from preterm mothers, $p < 0.05$), except for the lutein content that was not different between groups (486.31 nM vs. 432.83 nM, $p = 0.238$). Figure 1 shows the percentage distribution of the carotenoids in colostrum and mature milk of both groups of mothers. Xanthophylls, which are carotenoids containing oxygenated functions in their structure, and carotenes, which are strictly hydrocarbons, were similarly accumulated in colostrum samples of PT and FT mothers, as the ratio between both groups of pigments was close to 1 (0.97 and 0.90 for the preterm and the full-term group, respectively). The ranking of individual carotenoids in the colostrum samples was recurrent for both groups, with zeaxanthin presenting the lowest content value followed by the pool of xanthophyll esters (sum of lutein, zeaxanthin, and β-cryptoxanthin esters), the free xanthophylls lutein and β-cryptoxanthin, and finally by the carotenes α- and β-carotene and lycopene. The total fat content of colostrum was not related with the PT or FT condition, with values in the range of 35–45 mg/mL showing no significant differences. Regarding the carotenoid content of the mature milk, both individual and total amounts of carotenoids from PT mothers did not differ from that of FT mothers, either qualitatively or quantitatively. Thus, the total carotenoid content was not statistically different (median 768.0 nM vs. 693.54 nM, $p = 0.278$). The ratio of xanthophylls/carotenes in the mature milk samples was higher than 1 (1.61 and 1.70 for the FT and the PT groups, respectively), unlike the distribution pattern of carotenoids found in the colostrum samples. Zeaxanthin was the minor carotenoid present in the mature milk samples, likewise in the colostrum samples, but the xanthophyll esters were undetectable in both groups. Then, α- and β-carotene and lycopene followed, and finally β-cryptoxanthin and lutein. Again, the total milk fat content was similar in both groups, similar to the values reached in colostrum samples (30–40 mg/mL) and unrelated with the PT or FT condition, with no significant differences between groups.

Table 1. Carotenoid content in colostrum and mature milk of preterm (PT, $n = 70$) and full-term (FT, $n = 70$) mothers. Data are expressed in nM concentration.

	PT Mothers [1]			FT Mothers [1]		
	25th Percentile	Median	75th Percentile	25th Percentile	Median	75th Percentile
			Colostrum [2]			
Zeaxanthin (X) [3]	35.9	63.2	112.6	73.7	106.4	141.4
Lutein (X)	231.6	432.8 [a]	667.9	322.9	486.3 [a]	745.8
β-Cryptoxanthin (X)	231.4	406.7	853.0	429.6	754.6	1486
Lycopene (C) [4]	388.1	669.9	931.6	483.0	1065	1846
α+β-Carotene (C)	331.0	594.6	1364	602.3	1103	2238
Xanthophyll esters (X)	144.5	334.6 [b]	733.4	251.5	598.7 [b]	1211
Total	1810	2641	4498	2854	4961	7209
			Mature milk [5]			
Zeaxanthin	36.7	46.6	65.9	38.4	59.9	91.9
Lutein	170.0	217.3	283.0	150.3	195.9	270.8
β-Cryptoxanthin	53.0	135.1	224.6	87.4	190.6	353.9
Lycopene	89.4	125.8	173.6	118.8	192.7	221.2
α+β-Carotene	50.0	106.4	202.2	59.4	84.8	315.0
Xanthophyll esters	0	0	0	0	0	0
Total	508.7	693.5	934.0	512.3	768.0	1174

[1]: Data are significantly different when colostrum and mature milk values are compared within each group of lactating mothers, except for zeaxanthin of the preterm group. [2]: Data of colostrum samples were significantly different between both groups of lactating mothers except for values marked with superscript letters ($p < 0.05$). [3]: X means xanthophyll. [4]: C means carotene. [5]: No significant differences were observed for data of both groups of lactating mothers.

Evolution of the carotenoid content from colostrum to mature milk followed a similar sharp decline but it was lower for the carotenoid content in mature milk of PT mothers (74% of the total carotenoid content) than for the FT mothers (85% of the total carotenoid content). Significant differences were observed when individual and total carotenoid contents of colostrum and mature milk samples were compared within each group of lactating mothers, except for zeaxanthin content of the group of PT mothers.

No significant differences were observed in both groups both for individual and total carotenoid content, as shown in Table 2 and Figure 1, in the serum from lactating mothers, either at the initial lactation stage (3–5 days after delivery) or once the milk reached the mature state (30 days after delivery). Within each group and during the progress of lactation, individual and total carotenoid content did not differ also, as shown in Table 2 and Figure 1. Xanthophylls and carotenes were similarly distributed in both groups of lactating mothers and this ratio was the same at both stages of lactation. Zeaxanthin was the minor carotenoid found in the serum, and the close similarity in the data of the rest of carotenoids makes it tough to establish a clear ranking.

Table 2. Carotenoid content in serum of preterm (PT, $n = 70$) and full-term (FT, $n = 70$) mothers at two lactation stages. Data are expressed in nM concentration.

	PT Mothers			FT Mothers		
	25th Percentile	Median	75th Percentile	25th percentile	Median	75th Percentile
Serum samples collected at 3–5 day postpartum [1]						
Zeaxanthin	108.2	142.9	171.8	94.4	122.1	152.4
Lutein	658.3	744.8	911.9	552.4	656.0	834.7
β-Cryptoxanthin	419.8	814.1	964.7	617.8	737.3	1084
Lycopene	481.7	712.9	980.2	450.3	673.5	887.3
α+β-Carotene	519.6	816.8	1089	494.6	671.2	1547
Xanthophyll esters	0	0	0	0	0	0
Total	2984	3288	3751	2869	3222	3811
Serum samples collected at 15–30 day postpartum [1]						
Zeaxanthin	105.3	136.1	187.4	96.0	135.5	158.6
Lutein	622.6	768.4	1010	579.0	673.9	809.1
β-Cryptoxanthin	329.9	729.3	1152	669.2	822.4	925.2
Lycopene	555.3	824.0	1007	473.9	730.4	905.7
α+β-Carotene	583.3	967.4	1594	549.2	743.8	1087
Xanthophyll esters	0	0	0	0	0	0
Total	3279	3636	3898	2938	3295	3711

[1]: No significant differences were observed for data of both groups of lactating mothers or at each collection time within a group.

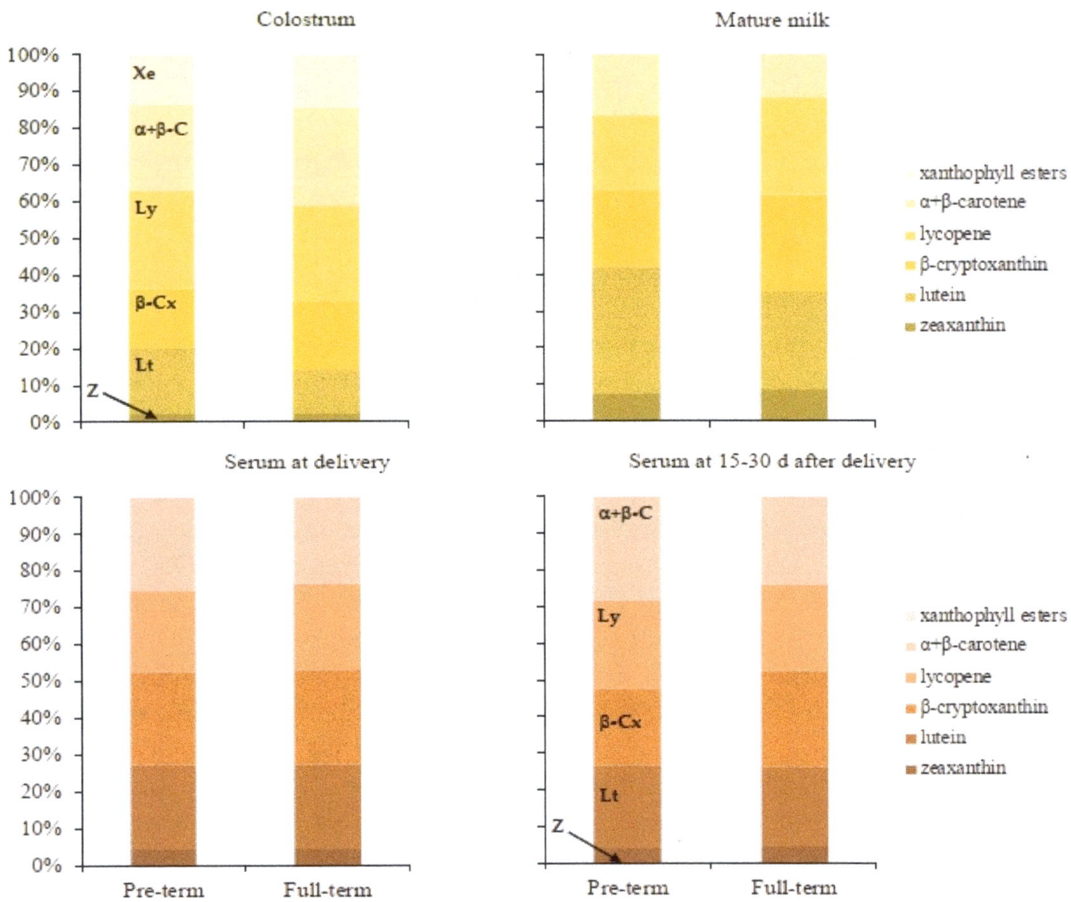

Figure 1. Percentage distribution of the individual carotenoids and xanthophyll esters in colostrum and mature milk samples, and in serum collected at delivery or at 15–30 days after delivery, from preterm and full-term mothers. Xe: xanthophyll esters; α+β-C: α+β-carotene; Ly: lycopene; β-Cx: β-cryptoxanthin; Lt: lutein; Z: zeaxanthin.

4. Discussion

Individual and total content of the major carotenoids in human milk samples have been determined in previous studies [28,29,32,33,36], and our data are in the same order of magnitude and follow similar changes and trends regarding the transition from colostrum to mature milk and the distribution pattern of individual carotenoids. We also noted the high variability of data observed before. Giuliano et al. [28] showed that although the carotenoid content might fluctuate daily and even during feeding, the large variability in carotenoid content is due to inter-individual differences in dietary intake of food sources of carotenoids, the carotenoid bioavailability, and the bioconversion of pro-vitamin A carotenoids to retinoid. Indeed, the bioconversion to retinoid in addition to the nutritional status of the mother may explain the extreme inter-individual differences in the case of α- and β-carotene.

Studies focused on carotenoid content in human colostrum are less frequent in the literature [30,36,37,50], and the characterization of the full carotenoid profile in some of them is incomplete, in comparison with the extensive surveys done with mature human milk samples. Colostrum is a secretion of the mammary gland only available during the few days immediately after delivery, and its composition does not represent the stabilized nutrient contents of mature milk. These are reasonable causes to explain the less intensive attention paid to carotenoids in human colostrum. Most longitudinal studies do not include colostrum collection in the sampling, while some others do. In the latter cases, data should be considered carefully as the carotenoid content in colostrum is significantly higher than in mature milk and even the distribution of carotenoids (xanthophylls, carotenes, and presence of xanthophyll esters) may be different as well [37]. It is well established that carotenoid levels decrease significantly from the colostrum to the mature milk samples as observed in preceding longitudinal and comparative studies [32]. We found a drop of carotenoid levels similar (4-fold for PT mothers and 6-fold for FT mothers) to those reported by Sommerburg et al. [51], Macias and Schweigert [52], and Schweigert et al. [36].

The total carotenoid content observed for mature milk in this study are in the highest range of data reported for North American mothers [28], close to the mean values reported for Irish mothers [53], and higher than those found in a study on milk of German mothers [36]. Finally, the data presented in this study are higher when compared with the largest multinational study of breast milk carotenoids published by Canfield et al. [29]. The main reasons for the differences and similarities are dietary habits including individual preferences, seasonal/regional changes in fruit and vegetable availability, and cooking methods. Qualitatively, the carotenoids were distributed in colostrum samples in a different fashion in comparison to mature milk, with an almost equal presence of carotenes and xanthophylls, while this equilibrium is significantly displaced to the preferential accumulation of xanthophylls during the progress of lactation in agreement with previous reports [32,36]. Mature milk showed a distribution pattern with the prevalence of the xanthophylls lutein and β-cryptoxanthin, followed by the apolar carotenes lycopene and α+β-carotene. Zeaxanthin was a minor carotenoid. This displacement is not correlated with the carotenoid distribution in plasma samples, which was the same at both collection stages, with similar distribution of carotenes and xanthophylls, as shown in Figure 1. This constancy of carotenoid distribution and quantitative content in plasma could indicate that the volunteers had similar food sources of carotenoids throughout the study and that they did not introduce significant changes in their dietary habits after delivery. Circulating carotenoid content is positively associated with the daily intake of fruits and vegetables. It has been shown that qualitative carotenoid composition of serum correlates with short-term carotenoid intake [54,55] and particularly, β-cryptoxanthin and lutein are robust biomarkers of fruit and vegetable consumption [56]. Therefore, the shift of carotenoid distribution towards a higher xanthophyll presence in mature milk would not likely be due to a change in dietary habits. It seems that during the transition of the carotenoid content from colostrum to mature milk, xanthophylls are preferentially accumulated in the mammary epithelium. Transport mechanisms operative at the intestinal epithelium that are involved in the uptake of carotenoids from the lumen, may be active at the mammary epithelium. In fact, it has been demonstrated that SR-BI, CD36, and NPC1L1 facilitate the uptake of carotenoids in the small intestine [57–59], and these proteins are also expressed in the mammary glands [60,61]. Even the expression of some of these proteins has been shown to increase in the mammary tissue of lactating animals. This is the case of CD36 in lactating cows [62] which increases its expression levels after delivery, reaching a maximum at 6 weeks postpartum. Whether such an increase in the expression levels of any of these proteins take place coordinately after delivery in the human mammary gland, and whether they are specific for some protein kind remains to be elucidated, though this would help to explain differences in the xanthophyll to carotene proportion in colostrum and mature milk.

Regarding the influence of the gestational age on the carotenoid content, we observed that significant differences appeared only in colostrum samples. The group of PT mothers produced colostrum with lower carotenoid levels, except for lutein that reached a similar content to the one observed in the group of FT mothers. The carotenoid distribution in colostrum was similar in both groups (equal xanthophyll:carotene ratio), so that the differences were only quantitative. Jewell et al. [53] reported differences in lutein and zeaxanthin content in colostrum between PT and FT mothers, but the statistical power was limited in their study and differences were not significant. The differences observed here should not be attributed to diverse dietary habits of the mothers of the PT group, since the plasma carotenoid contents were not different from those observed in the mothers of the FT group. Several changes take place in the mammary glands during pregnancy to prepare for lactation, including gland maturation and alveologenesis [63], with the start of several signaling pathways that develop the structural and functional changes required to generate and deliver milk. The maternal metabolism is remodeled to flow nutrients to the placenta and the mammary glands for support fetal and infant growth. In this scenario, the premature delivery breaks the regular process of utero accretion and transfer of nutrients to the developing fetus, as well as the accumulation of nutrients and phytochemicals in the mammary glands from the mother stores. It has been shown that carotenoid content in PT infants' tissues is abnormally low or undetectable [26]. Our data show the differences in the carotenoid contents are also extended to the colostrum secretion in the case of premature delivery, with a trend to lower carotenoid content. However, it does not affect the lutein content in colostrum of PT mothers, which reached the same value as in the group of FT mothers. This fact could be related with the significance of lutein to the health of the new born. Lutein content is associated with proper condition of the infant retina [64] and its accumulation in the brain points to a role in cognitive function [21]. Such impact at the initial stage of life implies a mechanism assuring the lutein supply from human milk. Thus, it would not be impaired by factors like the premature condition. Again, the presence of a facilitated transport mechanism, principally active for lutein accumulation, is a reasonable hypothesis to explain this result. As it has been noted above, the measurement of the levels of those proteins involved in carotenoid transport in mammary glands would provide evidence to support this hypothesis. The subsequent regularization process of the carotenoid content from colostrum to mature milk is not affected by the premature condition since the mature milk of both groups of mothers showed carotenoid levels without significant differences both qualitatively and quantitatively.

To our knowledge, this is the first study to examine and compare the qualitative and quantitative carotenoid profile in colostrum and mature milk samples from lactating mothers that gave birth either prematurely or at full-term. The homogeneous sample, regarding the dietary habits, controlled one of the main factors that determine carotenoid levels in human tissues, including colostrum and milk samples. The qualitative findings replicated those reported in previous studies, but through the inclusion of an adequate number of volunteers, we had statistical power to find the differences in carotenoid content of the colostrum samples. Thus, our data give support to the hypothesis of the targeted accumulation of lutein and that this process is not limited by the premature condition at birth. Indeed, this condition reduced the amount of the rest of carotenoids in colostrum but the subsequent transition stage to mature milk made differences disappear. However, we are not able to predict whether our findings will reproduce in other populations with different dietary habits.

5. Conclusions

In our study, we have determined the qualitative and quantitative features of the carotenoid composition of colostrum and mature milk of mothers who gave birth to babies born between 28 and 35 weeks of gestation and to infants at full-term. Our results have shown that the qualitative profile does not vary between groups, but there is a shift from a balanced composition in carotenes and xanthophylls in colostrum to a higher presence of the latter in mature milk. Quantitatively, we found significant differences between the groups in the colostrum samples, with lower content in the preterm group, except for lutein, which behaves in a different fashion. The transition from colostrum to mature milk results in no difference in the carotenoid content between the two groups. These results lead to the conclusion that the premature condition affects the quantitative carotenoid composition of the colostrum, but that condition does not impair the lutein content, which is related to the significant role of the xanthophyll in development of the infant retina and brain. Our study points to the need of research regarding the presence of protein-type transporters in mammary epithelium as one key issue for the existing dynamics on carotenoid content in human milk.

Author Contributions: E.D.-S., I.A.-V., and J.A.-M. carried out all human studies and sample collection. J.G.-F., A.A.O.X., and A.S.-G. conducted research. J.A.-M., J.G.-F., and A.P.-G. analyzed data. A.A.O.X., J.G.-F., J.F., and A.P.-G. wrote the paper. All authors read and approved the final manuscript.

Acknowledgments: Source of financial support: Ministry of Economy and Competitiveness of the Spanish Government, grants AGL2013-42757-R and AGL2017-87884-R. A.A.O.X. is a fellow of the Science without Borders Program of the Brazilian National Council for Scientific and Technological Development, fellowship 238163/2012-1.

Abbreviations

PT	preterm
FT	full-term
HPLC	high-performance liquid chromatography
APCI	atmospheric pressure chemical ionization
UHR	ultra-high resolution
TOF	time of flight

References

1. Leon-Cava, N.; Lutter, C.; Ross, J.; Martin, L. *Quantifying the Benefits of Breastfeeding: A Summary of the Evidence*; Pan American Health Organization: Washington, DC, USA, 2002; pp. 1–168, ISBN 9275123977.
2. Betran, A.P.; de Onis, M.; Lauer, J.A.; Villar, J. Ecological study of effect of breast feeding on infant mortality in Latin America. *BMJ* **2001**, *323*, 303–306. [CrossRef] [PubMed]
3. WHO Collaborative Study Team on the Role of Breastfeeding on the Prevention of Infant Mortality. Effect of breastfeeding on infant and child mortality due to infectious diseases in less developed countries: A pooled analysis. *Lancet* **2000**, *355*, 451–455. [CrossRef]
4. *WHO Global Strategy for Infant and Young Child Feeding*; World Health Organization: Geneva, Switzerland, 2003; pp. 1–30, ISBN 9241562218.
5. Picciano, M.F. Nutrient composition of human milk. *Pediatr. Clin. North Am.* **2001**, *48*, 53–67. [CrossRef]
6. Ballard, O.; Morrow, A.L. Human milk composition: Nutrients and bioactive factors. *Pediatr. Clin. North Am.* **2013**, *60*, 49–74. [CrossRef] [PubMed]
7. Liaaen-Jensen, S. Basic carotenoid chemistry. In *Carotenoids in Health and Disease*; Krinsky, N.I., Mayne, S.T., Sies, H., Eds.; Marcel Dekker: New York, NY, USA, 2004; pp. 1–30, ISBN 0203026640.
8. Stoltzfus, R.J.; Hakima, M.; Miller, K.W.; Rasmussen, K.M.; Dawiesah, S.I.; Habicht, J.P.; Dibley, M.J. High dose vitamin A supplementation of breast-feeding Indonesian mothers: Effects on the vitamin A status of mother and infant. *J. Nutr.* **1993**, *123*, 666–675. [CrossRef] [PubMed]
9. Bendich, A. Non-provitamin A activity of carotenoids: Immunoenhancement. *Trends Food Sci. Tech.* **1991**, *2*, 127–130. [CrossRef]

10. Stahl, W.; Sies, H. Bioactivity and protective effects of natural carotenoids. *Biochim. Biophys. Acta* **2005**, *1740*, 101–107. [CrossRef] [PubMed]
11. Provis, J.; Diaz, C.; Dreher, B. Ontogeny of the primate fovea: A central issue in retinal development. *Prog. Neurobiol.* **1998**, *54*, 549–581. [CrossRef]
12. Landrum, J.; Bone, R. Lutein, zeaxanthin, and the macular pigment. *Arch. Biochem. Biophys.* **2001**, *385*, 28–40. [CrossRef] [PubMed]
13. Pintea, A.; Socaciu, C.; Rugina, D.O.; Pop, R.; Bunea, A. Xanthophylls protect against induced oxidation in cultured human retinal pigment epithelial cells. *J. Food Compost. Anal.* **2011**, *26*, 830–836. [CrossRef]
14. Junghans, A.; Sies, H.; Stahl, W. Macular pigments lutein and zeaxanthin as blue light filters studied in liposomes. *Arch. Biochem. Biophys.* **2001**, *391*, 160–164. [CrossRef] [PubMed]
15. Leung, I.; Sandstrom, M.M.; Zucker, C.; Neuringer, M.; Snodderly, D. Nutritional manipulation of primate retinas, II: Effects of age, n-3 fatty acids, lutein, and zeaxanthin on retinal pigment epithelium. *Invest. Ophthalmol. Vis. Sci.* **2004**, *45*, 3244–3256. [CrossRef] [PubMed]
16. Loughman, J.; Nolan, J.M.; Howard, A.N.; Connolly, E.; Meagher, K.; Beatty, S. The impact of macular pigment augmentation on visual performance using different carotenoid formulations. *Invest. Ophthalmol. Vis. Sci.* **2012**, *53*, 7871–7880. [CrossRef] [PubMed]
17. Kelly, D.; Coen, R.F.; Akuffo, K.O.; Beatty, S.; Dennison, J.; Moran, R.; Stack, J.; Howard, A.N.; Mulcahy, R.; Nolan, J.M. Cognitive function and its relationship with macular pigment optical density and serum concentrations of its constituent carotenoids. *J. Alzheimers. Dis.* **2015**, *48*, 261–277. [CrossRef] [PubMed]
18. Vishwanathan, R.; Iannaccone, A.; Scott, T.M.; Kritchevsky, S.B.; Jennings, B.J.; Carboni, G.; Forma, G.; Satterfield, S.; Harris, T.; Johnson, K.C.; et al. Macular pigment optical density is related to cognitive function in older people. *Age Ageing* **2014**, *43*, 271–275. [CrossRef] [PubMed]
19. Vishwanathan, R.; Neuringer, M.; Snodderly, D.M.; Schalch, W.; Johnson, E.J. Macular lutein and zeaxanthin are related to brain lutein and zeaxanthin in primates. *Nutr. Neurosci.* **2013**, *16*, 21–29. [CrossRef] [PubMed]
20. Craft, N.E.; Haitema, T.B.; Garnett, K.M.; Fitch, K.A.; Dorey, C.K. Carotenoid, tocopherol, and retinol concentrations in elderly human brain. *J. Nutr. Health Aging* **2004**, *8*, 156–162. [PubMed]
21. Johnson, E.J.; Vishwanathan, R.; Johnson, M.A.; Hausman, D.B.; Davey, A.; Scott, T.M.; Green, R.C.; Miller, S.; Gearing, M.; Woodard, J.; et al. Relationship between serum and brain carotenoids, α-tocopherol, and retinol concentrations and cognitive performance in the oldest old from the Georgia Centenarian Study. *J. Aging Res.* **2013**, *2013*, 951786. [CrossRef] [PubMed]
22. Vishwanathan, R.; Kuchan, M.; Sen, S.; Johnson, E.J. Lutein and preterm infants with decreased concentration of brain carotenoids. *J. Pediatr. Gastroenterol. Nutr.* **2014**, *59*, 659–665. [CrossRef] [PubMed]
23. Hammond, B.R. Jr. Possible role for dietary lutein and zeaxanthin in visual development. *Nutr. Rev.* **2008**, *66*, 695–702. [CrossRef] [PubMed]
24. Johnson, E.J. Role of lutein and zeaxanthin in visual and cognitive function throughout the lifespan. *Nutr. Rev.* **2014**, *72*, 605–612. [CrossRef] [PubMed]
25. Henriksen, B.S.; Chan, G.; Hoffman, R.O.; Sharifzadeh, M.; Ermakov, I.V.; Gellermann, W.; Bernstein, P.S. Interrelationships between maternal carotenoid status and newborn infant macular pigment optical density and carotenoid status. *Invest. Ophthalmol. Vis. Sci.* **2013**, *54*, 5568–5578. [CrossRef] [PubMed]
26. Bernstein, P.S.; Sharifzadeh, M.; Liu, A.; Ermakiv, I.; Nelson, K.; Sheng, X.; Panish, C.; Carlstrom, B.; Hoffman, R.O.; Gellermann, W. Blue-light reflectance imaging of macular pigment in infants and children. *Invest. Ophthalmol. Vis. Sci.* **2013**, *54*, 4034–4040. [CrossRef] [PubMed]
27. Bone, R.A.; Landrum, J.T.; Friedes, L.M.; Gomez, C.M.; Kilburn, M.D.; Menendez, E.; Vidal, I.; Wang, W. Distribution of lutein and zeaxanthin stereoisomers in the human retina. *Exp. Eye Res.* **1997**, *64*, 211–218. [CrossRef] [PubMed]
28. Giuliano, A.R.; Neilson, E.M.; Yap, H.; Baier, M.; Canfield, L.M. Carotenoids of mature human milk: Inter/intraindividual variability. *J. Nutr. Biochem.* **1994**, *5*, 551–556. [CrossRef]
29. Canfield, L.M.; Clandinin, M.T.; Davies, D.P.; Fernandez, M.C.; Jackson, J.; Hawkes, J.; Goldman, W.J.; Pramuk, K.; Reyes, H.; Sablan, B.; et al. Multinational study of major breast milk carotenoids of healthy mothers. *Eur. J. Nutr.* **2003**, *42*, 133–141. [PubMed]
30. Patton, S.; Canfield, L.M.; Huston, G.E.; Ferris, A.M.; Jensen, R.G. Carotenoids of human colostrum. *Lipids* **1990**, *25*, 159–165. [CrossRef] [PubMed]

31. Khachik, F.; Spangler, C.J.; Smith, J.C.; Canfield, L.M.; Pfander, H.; Speck, A. Identification, quantification, and relative concentrations of carotenoids, and their metabolites in human milk and serum. *Anal. Chem.* **1997**, *69*, 1873–1881. [CrossRef] [PubMed]
32. Gossage, C.P.; Deyhim, M.; Yamini, S.; Douglas, L.W.; Moser-Veillon, P.B. Carotenoid composition of human milk during the first month postpartum and the response to β-carotene supplementation. *Am. J. Clin. Nutr.* **2002**, *76*, 193–197. [CrossRef] [PubMed]
33. Lipkie, T.E.; Morrow, A.L.; Jouni, Z.E.; McMahon, R.J.; Ferruzzi, M.G. Longitudinal survey of carotenoids in human milk from urban cohorts in China, Mexico, and the USA. *PLoS ONE* **2015**, *10*. [CrossRef] [PubMed]
34. Galan, P.; Viteri, F.E.; Bertrais, S.; Czernichow, S.; Faure, H.; Arnaud, J.; Ruffieux, D.; Chenal, S.; Arnault, N.; Favier, A.; et al. Serum concentrations of beta-carotene, vitamins C and E, zinc and selenium are influenced by sex, age, diet, smoking status, alcohol consumption and corpulence in a general French adult population. *Eur. J. Clin. Nutr.* **2005**, *59*, 1181–1190. [CrossRef] [PubMed]
35. Forman, M.R.; Beecher, G.R.; Lanza, E.; Reichman, M.E.; Graubard, B.I.; Campbell, W.S.; Marr, T.; Yong, L.C.; Judd, J.T.; Taylor, P.R. Effect of alcohol consumption on plasma carotenoid concentrations in premenopausal women, a controlled dietary study. *Am. J. Clin. Nutr.* **1995**, *62*, 131–135. [CrossRef] [PubMed]
36. Schweigert, F.J.; Bathe, K.; Chen, F.; Büscher, U.; Dudenhausen, J.W. Effect of the stage of lactation in humans on carotenoid levels in milk, blood plasma and plasma lipoprotein fractions. *Eur. J. Nutr.* **2004**, *43*, 39–44. [CrossRef] [PubMed]
37. Ríos, J.J.; Xavier, A.A.O.; Díaz-Salido, E.; Arenilla-Vélez, I.; Jarén-Galán, M.; Garrido-Fernández, J.; Aguayo-Maldonado, J.; Pérez-Gálvez, A. Xanthophyll esters are found in human colostrum. *Mol. Nutr. Food Res.* **2017**, *61*. [CrossRef] [PubMed]
38. Bokor, S.; Koletzko, B.; Decsi, T. Systematic review of fatty acid composition of human milk from mothers of preterm compared to full-term infants. *Ann. Nutr. Metab.* **2007**, *51*, 550–556. [CrossRef] [PubMed]
39. Bobiński, R.; Mikulska, M.; Mojska, H.; Simon, M. Comparison of the fatty acid composition of transitional and mature milk of mothers who delivered healthy full-term babies, preterm babies and full-term small for gestational age infants. *Eur. J. Clin. Nutr.* **2013**, *67*, 966–971. [CrossRef] [PubMed]
40. Pérez-Gálvez, A.; Martin, H.D.; Sies, H.; Stahl, W. Incorporation of carotenoids from paprika oleoresin into human chylomicrons. *Br. J. Nutr.* **2003**, *89*, 787–793. [CrossRef] [PubMed]
41. Breithaupt, D.E.; Wirt, U.; Bamedi, A. Differentiation between lutein monoester regioisomers and detection of lutein diesters from marigold flowers (*Tagetes erecta* L.) and several fruits by liquid chromatography-mass spectrometry. *J. Agric. Food Chem.* **2002**, *50*, 66–70. [CrossRef] [PubMed]
42. Liaaen-Jensen, S. Combined approach, identification and structure elucidation of carotenoids. In *Carotenoids, Volume 1B, Spectroscopy*; Britton, G., Liaaen-Jensen, S., Pfander, H., Eds.; Birkhäuser Verlag: Basel, Switzerland, 1995; pp. 343–354, ISBN 0817629092.
43. Enzell, C.R.; Back, S. Mass spectrometry. In *Carotenoids, Volume 1B, Spectroscopy*; Britton, G., Liaaen-Jensen, S., Pfander, H., Eds.; Birkhäuser Verlag: Basel, Switzerland, 1995; pp. 261–320, ISBN 0817629092.
44. Britton, G.; Liaaen-Jensen, S.; Pfander, H. *Carotenoids Handbook*; Birkhäuser Verlag: Basel, Switzerland, 2004; ISBN 3034878362.
45. Rodriguez-Amaya, D.B. *Food Carotenoids, Chemistry, Biology, and Technology*; Wiley Blackwell: Singapore, 2016.
46. Rivera, S.M.; Christou, P.; Canela-Garayoa, R. Identification of carotenoids using mass spectrometry. *Mass Spectrom. Rev.* **2014**, *33*, 353–372. [CrossRef] [PubMed]
47. De Rosso, V.V.; Mercadante, A.Z. Identification and quantification of carotenoids, by HPLC-PDA-MS/MS, from Amazonian fruits. *J. Agric. Food Chem.* **2007**, *55*, 5062–5072. [CrossRef] [PubMed]
48. Weller, P.; Breithaupt, D.E. Identification and quantification of zeaxanthin esters in plants using liquid chromatography-mass spectrometry. *J. Agric. Food Chem.* **2003**, *51*, 7044–7049. [CrossRef] [PubMed]
49. Jensen, R.G.; Lammi-Keefe, C.J.; Koletzko, B. Representative sampling of human milk and the extraction of fat for analysis of environmental lipophilic contaminants. *Toxicol. Environ. Chem.* **1997**, *62*, 229–247. [CrossRef]
50. Gebre-Medhin, M.; Vahlquist, A.; Hofvander, Y.; Uppsall, L.; Vahlquist, B. Breast milk composition in Ethiopean and Swedish mothers. I. Vitamin A and beta-carotene. *Am. J. Clin. Nutr.* **1976**, *29*, 441–451. [CrossRef] [PubMed]
51. Sommerburg, O.; Meissner, K.; Nelle, M.; Lenhartz, H.; Leichsenring, M. Carotenoid supply in breast-fed neonates. *Eur. J. Pediatr.* **2000**, *159*, 86–90. [CrossRef] [PubMed]

52. Macias, C.; Schweigert, F.J. Changes in the concentration of carotenoids, vitamin A, alpha-tocopherol and total lipids in human milk throughout early lactation. *Ann. Nutr. Metab.* **2001**, *45*, 82–85. [CrossRef] [PubMed]
53. Jewell, V.C.; Northrop-Clewes, C.A.; Tubman, R.; Thurnham, D.I. Nutritional factors and visual function in premature infants. *Proc. Nutr. Soc.* **2001**, *60*, 171–178. [CrossRef] [PubMed]
54. Olmedilla, B.; Granado, F.; Southon, S.; Wright, A.J.A.; Blanco, I.; Gil-Martínez, E.; van den Berg, H.; Corridan, B.; Roussel, A.M.; Chopra, M.; et al. Serum concentrations of carotenoids and vitamins A, E, and C in control subjects from five European countries. *Br. J. Nutr.* **2001**, *85*, 227–238. [CrossRef] [PubMed]
55. Thurnham, D.I.; Northrop-Clewes, C.A.; Chopra, M. Biomarkers of vegetable and fruit intakes. *Am. J. Clin. Nutr.* **1998**, *68*, 756–757. [CrossRef] [PubMed]
56. Couillard, C.; Lemieux, S.; Vohl, M.C.; Couture, P.; Lamarche, B. Carotenoids as biomarkers of fruit and vegetable intake in men and women. *Br. J. Nutr.* **2016**, *116*, 1206–1215. [CrossRef] [PubMed]
57. Borel, P.; Lietz, G.; Goncalves, A.; Edelenyi, F.S.; Lecompte, S.; Curtis, P.; Goumidi, L.; Caslake, M.J.; Miles, E.A.; Packard, C.; et al. CD36 and SR-BI are involved in cellular uptake of provitamin A carotenoids by Caco-2 and HEK cells, and some of their genetic variants are associated with plasma concentrations of these micronutrients in humans. *J. Nutr.* **2013**, *143*, 448–456. [CrossRef] [PubMed]
58. Moussa, M.; Gouranton, E.; Gleize, B.; Yazidi, C.E.; Niot, I.; Besnard, P.; Borel, P.; Landrier, J.F. CD36 is involved in lycopene and lutein uptake by adipocytes and adipose tissue cultures. *Mol. Nutr. Food Res.* **2011**, *55*, 578–584. [CrossRef] [PubMed]
59. Sato, Y.; Suzuki, R.; Kobayashi, M.; Itagaki, S.; Hirano, T.; Noda, T.; Mizuno, S.; Sugawara, M.; Iseki, K. Involvement of cholesterol membrane transporter Niemann-Pick C1-like 1 in the intestinal absorption of lutein. *J. Pharm. Pharm. Sci.* **2012**, *15*, 256–264. [CrossRef] [PubMed]
60. Landschulz, K.; Pathak, R.; Rigotti, A.; Krieger, M.; Hobbs, H. Regulation of scavenger receptor, class B, type I, a high density lipoprotein receptor, in liver and steroidogenic tissues of the rat. *J. Clin. Invest.* **1996**, *98*, 984–995. [CrossRef] [PubMed]
61. Pussinen, P.J.; Karten, B.; Wintersperger, A.; Reicher, H.; McLean, M.; Malle, E.; Sattler, W. The human breast carcinoma cell line HBL-100 acquires exogenous cholesterol from high-density lipoprotein via CLA-1 (CD-36 and LIMPII analogous 1)-mediated selective cholesteryl ester uptake. *Biochem. J.* **2000**, *349*, 559–566. [CrossRef] [PubMed]
62. Bionaz, M.; Loor, J.J. Gene networks driving bovine milk fat synthesis during the lactation cycle. *BMC Genomics* **2008**, *9*, 366. [CrossRef] [PubMed]
63. Macías, H.; Hinck, L. Mammary gland development. *Wiley Interdiscip. Rev. Dev. Biol.* **2012**, *1*, 533–557. [CrossRef] [PubMed]
64. Zimmer, J.P.; Hammond, B.R.Jr. Possible influences of lutein and zeaxanthin on the developing retina. *Clin. Ophthalmol.* **2007**, *1*, 25–35. [PubMed]

7

Dietary Carotenoids Intake and the Risk of Gastric Cancer: A Case—Control Study in Korea

Ji Hyun Kim [1], Jeonghee Lee [1], Il Ju Choi [2], Young-Il Kim [2], Oran Kwon [3], Hyesook Kim [3] and Jeongseon Kim [1,*]

1 Graduate School of Cancer Science and Policy, National Cancer Center, 323 Ilsan-ro, Ilsandong-gu, Goyang-si, Gyeonggi-do 10408, Korea; 1601009@ncc.re.kr (J.H.K.); jeonghee@ncc.re.kr (J.L.)

2 Center for Gastric Cancer, National Cancer Center Hospital, National Cancer Center, 323 Ilsan-ro, Ilsandong-gu, Goyang-si, Gyeonggi-do 10408, Korea; cij1224@ncc.re.kr (I.J.C.); 11996@ncc.re.kr (Y.-I.K.)

3 Department of Nutritional Science and Food Management, Ewha Womans University, 52, Ewhayeodae-gil, Seodaemun-gu, Seoul 03760, Korea; orank@ewha.ac.kr (O.K.); khs7882@hanmail.net (H.K.)

* Correspondence: jskim@ncc.re.kr;

Abstract: Although the incidence of gastric cancer (GC) has declined, it remains the second most common cancer in Korea. As a class of phytochemicals, carotenoids are fat-soluble pigments that are abundant in fruits and vegetables and have health-promoting properties, including cancer prevention effects. This case-control study investigated the effects of total dietary carotenoids, dietary carotenoid subclasses (α-carotene, β-carotene, β-cryptoxanthin, lutein/zeaxanthin, and lycopene), and foods contributing to the dietary intake of each carotenoid on the risk of GC. Four hundred and fifteen cases and 830 controls were recruited from the National Cancer Center Hospital in Korea between March 2011 and December 2014. A significant inverse association between total dietary carotenoids and GC risk was observed among women (odds ratio (OR) 0.56, 95% confidence interval (CI) 0.32–0.99). A higher intake of dietary lycopene was inversely associated with GC risk overall in the subjects (OR 0.60, 95% CI 0.42–0.85, p for trend = 0.012), men (OR 0.60, 95% CI 0.39–0.93), and women (OR 0.54, 95% CI 0.30–0.96, p for trend = 0.039). This significant association between dietary lycopene intake and GC risk was also observed in the subgroups of *Helicobacter pylori* (*H. pylori*)-positive subjects and those who had ever smoked. Among the major contributing foods of dietary lycopene, consumption of tomatoes and tomato ketchup was inversely associated with GC risk in the overall subjects, men, and women. Based on our findings, a higher intake of dietary lycopene and contributing foods of lycopene (tomatoes and tomato ketchup) may be inversely associated with the risk of GC.

Keywords: carotenoids; lycopene; gastric cancer; *H. pylori*; smoking; case-control study; Korea

---

1. Introduction

According to the GLOBOCAN estimates reported in 2012, although gastric cancer (GC) incidence is declining, it remains the fifth most common cancer worldwide [1]. GC is the second most common cause of cancer in Korea, as the estimated age-standardized incidence rate of GC was 35.8 per 100,000 persons in 2015 [2]. Therefore, the primary prevention of GC is a major priority in public health.

Several risk factors for GC have been identified, such as *Helicobacter pylori* (*H. pylori*) infection and tobacco smoking, which are classified as International Agency for Research on Cancer (IARC) group 1 carcinogens (carcinogenic to humans) [3,4]. Dietary factors are considered modifiable risk factors that account for approximately 35% of all causes of cancer, and therefore dietary factors related to cancer must be identified [5,6].

Differences in the incidence rates of GC subtypes by gender have also been observed [7]. The rate of cardia GC was approximately three times higher in males than in females, whereas the rate of non-cardia GC was two times higher in males than in females [7]. The explanations for the higher rates of GC in males are not known, but might be due to the male predominance of *H. pylori* infection, one of the major risk factors for GC [8]. This phenomenon is found in adults worldwide [8]. The higher incidence rate of GC in males might also be due to the higher consumption of tobacco [9]. However, the predominance of males in the male to female ratio were similar in both smokers and non-smokers; therefore, the higher rates of GC in males might not be completely explained by the smoking history [9].

According to the third expert report from the Continuous Update Project (CUP) published by the World Cancer Research Fund (WCRF) International in 2018, the intake of certain types of foods (e.g., fruits) might be closely related to the risk of GC [10]. Carotenoids are fat-soluble pigments that are highly abundant in fruits and vegetables, and belong to a class of phytochemicals that have health-promoting properties [11–13]. Among the more than 40 carotenoids that are derived from a variety of food sources, six types of primary dietary carotenoids are usually detected in human blood plasma (α-carotene, β-carotene, β-cryptoxanthin, lutein, zeaxanthin, and lycopene), suggesting the selective intestinal absorption of these carotenoids [11,12,14].

Several epidemiological studies have been conducted to determine the associations between dietary carotenoids and the risk of GC. However, until now, few studies have been conducted and the results of previous studies are conflicting. Thus, a clear association between dietary carotenoids intake and the risk of GC has not been identified to date. Dietary α-carotene intake was inversely associated with GC risk in some studies [15–18], whereas no significant associations were observed in other studies [19–21]. Dietary β-carotene intake was associated with a reduced risk of GC in some studies [15,16,18,22–24], while other studies did not report a significant association [17,19–21,25,26]. Studies that analyzed dietary β-cryptoxanthin intake did not identify a significant association with the risk of GC [16–18,21]. Dietary lutein/zeaxanthin intake was not significantly associated with the risk of GC [15–17,19,20]. Dietary lycopene intake was inversely associated with the risk of GC in one study [17], whereas other studies have found no association [15,16,18–21,26].

Accordingly, this case-control study aims to investigate the effects of total dietary carotenoids, dietary carotenoid subclasses (α-carotene, β-carotene, β-cryptoxanthin, lutein/zeaxanthin, and lycopene), and the contributing foods of each dietary carotenoid on the risk of GC.

2. Materials and Methods

2.1. Study Population

The subjects were recruited from the National Cancer Center Hospital in Korea between March 2011 and December 2014. Cases were subjects who had been histologically diagnosed with early GC within the preceding three months at the Center for GC. Early GC was defined as GC restricted to the mucosa or submucosa with or without lymph node metastasis, regardless of the tumor size [27]. Patients in the case group did not have advanced GC, diabetes mellitus, severe systemic/mental disease, or a history of cancer within the past five years, and women who were pregnant or currently breastfeeding were also excluded. Controls were subjects who underwent health-screening examinations at the Center for Cancer Prevention and Detection at the same hospital.

Among the 1727 subjects (500 cases and 1227 controls) who agreed to participate in the study, 26 cases and 30 controls were excluded due to an incomplete self-administered questionnaire or semi-quantitative food frequency questionnaire (SQFFQ). Of the 1671 subjects remaining, 5 cases and 10 controls were excluded due to the implausibility of a total energy intake of <500 kcal or ≥ 4000 kcal. Of the 1656 subjects remaining, cases and controls were matched at a ratio of 1:2 by the distribution of age within 5 years and gender. Ultimately, a total of 1245 subjects (415 cases and 830 matched controls; 810 men and 435 women) were selected for this study (Figure 1). Written informed consent was obtained from all participants, and the study protocol was approved by the Institutional Review Board of the National Cancer Center [IRB Number: NCCNCS-11-438].

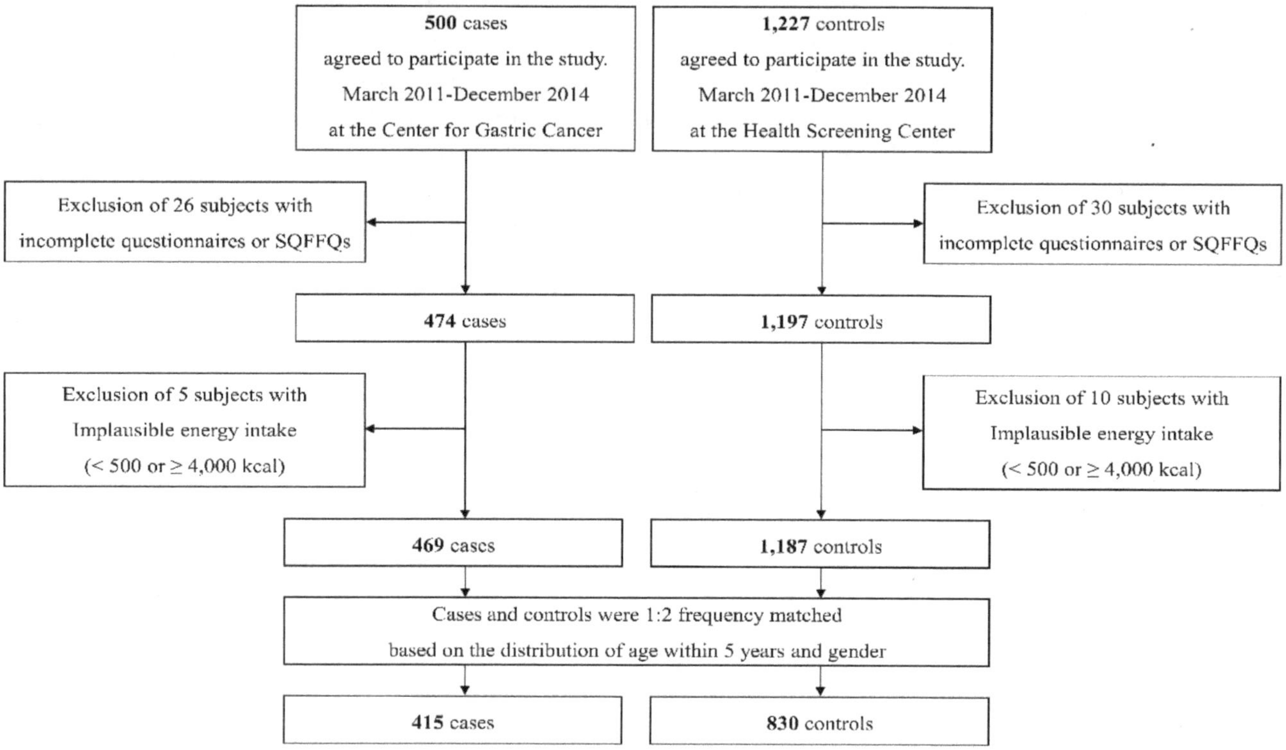

Figure 1. Flow chart of the study subjects. SQFFQ: semi-quantitative food frequency questionnaire.

2.2. Data Collection and Management

Participants were asked to complete a self-administered questionnaire that included demographic, lifestyle, and medical history information. Dietary intake was collected from the 106-item SQFFQ, which has been previously reported to be reliable and valid [28]. The study participants in the case group were surveyed with the self-administered questionnaire and SQFFQ by interviewers who were trained beforehand. Participants in the control group were initially asked to complete the survey by themselves, and interviewers asked any questions with missing answers from the self-completed survey during the second round of the survey.

After collecting the dietary information, the amount of each food item consumed was calculated using CAN-PRO 4.0 (Computer Aided Nutritional Analysis Program, The Korean Nutrition Society, Seoul, Korea). The 106 items of the SQFFQ were classified into 663 detailed food items. The overlapping food items were excluded, and 410 food items remained for the analysis. Then, the above food consumption information was merged with the database of carotenoid contents. The carotenoid database used in our study was composed of the United States Department of Agriculture (USDA) carotenoid database [29] and the Food Functional Composition Table provided by the Korea National Academy of Agricultural Science (NAAS) [30]. Additionally, by referring to the recipes from the NAAS Agricultural and Food Integrated Information System, information on seasoned vegetables and kimchi was also included. In total, this database contained 2903 food items. In terms of the carotenoid subclasses, it contained the five main carotenoids, namely, α-carotene, β-carotene, β-cryptoxanthin, lutein/zeaxanthin, and lycopene, and total carotenoids was defined as the sum of the five main carotenoid subclasses.

In terms of matching, except for meat, poultry, seafood, and dairy products, which rarely contain carotenoids (137 food items), the carotenoid database included 98.5% of all food items reported in the SQFFQ. Four food items were excluded due to a lack of information on the carotenoid content. The validity of the SQFFQ for dietary carotenoid intake has been tested using three-day dietary records from 207 people as a gold standard. The crude, energy-adjusted, and energy-adjusted and de-attenuated correlation coefficients for total carotenoids were 0.189, 0.244, and 0.307, respectively.

A rapid urease test (Pronto Dry; Medical Instruments Corporation, Solothurn, Switzerland) was conducted to examine the *H. pylori* infection status.

2.3. Statistical Analysis

To compare the general characteristics between cases and controls, Student's *t*-test was used for continuous variables and the chi-square test was used for categorical variables. A contribution analysis was conducted to select the foods contributing to total dietary carotenoids and the carotenoid subclasses. The food items contributing to total dietary carotenoids or carotenoid subclasses that represented up to 90% of the cumulative contribution were selected. All types of dietary carotenoids and their contributing foods were adjusted for total energy intake using the regression residual method [31]. Dietary carotenoids and their contributing foods were categorized by tertiles for the analysis based on the distribution of controls. The lowest tertile of each carotenoid and the foods contributing to dietary intake of each carotenoid were used as references. Odds ratios (ORs) and 95% confidence intervals (CIs) were calculated across the tertiles of dietary carotenoids and their contributing foods using the logistic regression model, after controlling for potential confounding factors. To test for trends, the median values of each tertile category of dietary carotenoids and their contributing foods were used as continuous variables. Model 1 was adjusted for age (as a continuous variable). Model 2 was adjusted for age, total caloric intake (as a continuous variable), a first-degree family history of GC (yes or no), smoking status (current, ex-, or non-smoker), regular exercise status (yes or no), education level (middle school or less, high school, or college or more), occupation (professional and administrative, office and sales/service, labor and agricultural, others, and unemployed), and monthly household income in units of 10,000 won/month (<200, 200–400, or ≥400). Model 3 was adjusted for the *H. pylori* infection status (yes or no) and the variables included in model 2. In the overall subjects, models 1, 2, and 3 were additionally adjusted for gender.

In the stratified analysis according to *H. pylori* infection status, model 1 was adjusted for age and gender. Model 2 was adjusted for age, gender, total caloric intake (as a continuous variable), a first-degree family history of GC (yes or no), smoking status (current, ex-, or non-smoker), regular exercise status (yes or no), education level (middle school or less, high school, or college or more), occupation (professional and administrative, office and sales/service, labor and agricultural, others, and unemployed), and monthly household income in units of 10,000 won/month (<200, 200–400, or ≥400). In the stratified analysis according to smoking status (ever-smoker and non-smoker), model 1 was adjusted for age and gender. Model 2 was adjusted for age, gender, total caloric intake (as a continuous variable), a first-degree family history of GC (yes or no), *H. pylori* infection status (yes or no), regular exercise status (yes or no), education level (middle school or less, high school, or college or more), occupation (professional and administrative, office and sales/service, labor and agricultural, others, and unemployed), and monthly household income in units of 10,000 won/month (<200, 200–400, or ≥400).

All statistical analyses were performed using SAS software (version 9.4, SAS Institute, Cary, NC, USA), and a two-sided *p*-value less than 0.05 was considered statistically significant.

3. Results

Table 1 describes the general characteristics of the 415 patients with early GC and 830 controls. Participants in the case group tended to have a higher proportion of *H. pylori* infection ($p < 0.001$) and first-degree family history of GC ($p = 0.001$), a lower percentage of those who had never smoked ($p < 0.001$) and those who exercise regularly ($p < 0.001$), a lower level of education ($p < 0.001$), a different occupational distribution ($p = 0.001$), and a lower level of monthly household income ($p < 0.001$) than those in the control group. Both men and women in the case group had a higher proportion of *H. pylori* infection, a lower proportion of those who never smoked and those who exercise regularly, a lower education level, a different occupational distribution, and a lower level of monthly household income than those in the control group. Additionally, men in the case group had a higher percentage of first-degree family history of GC than the men in the control group.

Table 2 describes the comparison of the consumption of total energy, total dietary carotenoids, and carotenoid subclasses. Subjects in the case group consumed more energy ($p < 0.001$), less total carotenoids ($p = 0.003$), less β-carotene ($p = 0.018$), less β-cryptoxanthin ($p = 0.007$), and less lycopene ($p < 0.001$) than subjects in the control group. Both men and women in the case group consumed less lycopene than the controls. Additionally, men in the case group consumed more energy, and women in the case group consumed less total carotenoids and β-cryptoxanthin compared to controls.

Table 3 shows the ORs and corresponding 95% CIs according to tertiles of total dietary carotenoids and carotenoid subclasses. Among women, higher total carotenoid intake was inversely associated with GC risk (model 2: OR 0.56, 95% CI 0.32–0.99), but the significant association disappeared in model 3, which was additionally adjusted for *H. pylori* infection. A higher lycopene intake was inversely associated with the risk of GC in the overall subjects (model 3: OR 0.60, 95% CI 0.42–0.85, p for trend = 0.012), men (model 3: OR 0.60, 95% CI 0.39–0.93), and women (model 2: OR 0.54, 95% CI 0.30–0.96, p for trend = 0.039).

Because dietary lycopene intake was significantly associated with GC risk in the overall subjects, a further analysis was performed on lycopene intake. Table 4 shows the ORs and 95% CIs of GC according to tertiles of dietary lycopene intake stratified by *H. pylori* infection status. Among the *H. pylori*-positive subjects, higher lycopene intake was inversely associated with the risk of GC (model 2: OR 0.61, 95% CI 0.42–0.90, p for trend = 0.037). When stratified by gender, higher intake of dietary lycopene was associated with a decreased risk of GC among *H. pylori*-positive males (model 2: OR 0.57, 95% CI 0.36–0.91, p for trend = 0.043) (Table S1). Table 5 shows the ORs and 95% CIs of GC according to tertiles of dietary lycopene intake stratified by smoking status (ever-smoker and non-smoker). Subjects who currently smoke or previously smoked were combined as ever-smokers. Among ever-smokers, a significantly reduced risk of GC was observed for the subjects who consumed greater amounts of dietary lycopene (model 2: OR 0.39, 95% CI 0.23–0.65, p for trend = 0.001). When stratified by gender, higher lycopene intake was inversely associated with the risk of GC among males who has ever smoked (model 2: OR 0.45, 95% CI 0.27–0.73, p for trend = 0.005) (Table S2).

Table 6 shows the comparison of the consumption of foods contributing to the dietary intake of lycopene. Compared to controls, cases consumed less tomato in the overall subjects ($p < 0.001$), men ($p = 0.001$), and women ($p < 0.001$); consumed less tomato ketchup in the overall subjects ($p < 0.001$), men ($p = 0.001$), and women ($p < 0.001$); and consumed less watermelon in the overall subjects ($p = 0.004$) and women ($p = 0.028$). Table 7 shows the associations between foods contributing to dietary lycopene intake and the risk of GC. A higher tomato intake was associated with a decreased risk of GC in the overall subjects (model 3: OR 0.59, 95% CI 0.41–0.85, p for trend = 0.016), men (model 3: OR 0.58, 95% CI 0.37–0.92, p for trend = 0.043), and women (model 2: OR 0.47, 95% CI 0.25–0.87, p for trend = 0.010). Higher tomato ketchup intake was associated with a decreased risk of GC in the overall subjects (model 3: OR 0.55, 95% CI 0.38–0.80, p for trend = 0.005), men (model 3: OR 0.62, 95% CI 0.39–0.97), and women (model 2: OR 0.47, 95% CI 0.25–0.88, p for trend = 0.011).

Table 1. General characteristics of the study subjects [a].

	Total (n = 1245)			Men (n = 810)			Women (n = 435)		
	Controls (n = 830)	Cases (n = 415)	p [b]	Controls (n = 540)	Cases (n = 270)	p [b]	Controls (n = 290)	Cases (n = 145)	p [b]
Age (years)	53.7 ± 9.0	53.8 ± 9.3	0.892	54.8 ± 8.4	54.9 ± 8.7	0.905	51.6 ± 9.8	51.7 ± 10.0	0.942
<50	285 (34.3)	139 (33.5)	0.816	153 (28.3)	77 (28.5)	>0.999	132 (45.5)	62 (42.8)	0.658
≥50	545 (65.7)	276 (66.5)		387 (71.7)	193 (71.5)		158 (54.5)	83 (57.2)	
Male, n (%)	540 (65.1)	270 (65.1)	>0.999						
BMI (kg/m^2)	23.9 ± 2.9	23.9 ±3.0	0.627	24.4 ± 2.7	24.2 ± 3.0	0.390	23.1 ± 3.1	23.2 ± 3.0	0.533
<23	314 (37.8)	159 (38.3)	0.975	161 (29.8)	91 (33.7)	0.509	153 (52.8)	68 (46.9)	
23–25	249 (30.0)	122 (29.4)		170 (31.5)	78 (28.9)		79 (27.2)	44 (30.3)	
≥25	266 (32.1)	133 (32.1)		209 (38.7)	101 (37.4)		57 (19.7)	32 (22.1)	
***H. pylori* infection**									
Positive	486 (58.6)	382 (92.1)	<0.001	333 (61.7)	252 (93.3)	<0.001	153 (52.8)	130 (89.7)	<0.001
Negative	320 (38.6)	33 (8.0)		187 (34.6)	18 (6.7)		133 (45.9)	15 (10.3)	
First-degree family history of GC									
Yes	103 (12.4)	82 (19.8)	0.001	74 (13.7)	60 (22.2)	0.003	29 (10.0)	22 (15.2)	0.155
No	725 (87.4)	332 (80.0)		464 (85.9)	209 (77.4)		261 (90.0)	123 (84.8)	
Smoking status, n (%)									
Current-smoker	162 (19.5)	128 (30.8)	<0.001	157 (29.1)	121 (44.8)	<0.001	5 (1.7)	7 (4.8)	0.021
Ex-smoker	284 (34.2)	119 (28.7)		277 (51.3)	110 (40.7)		7 (2.4)	9 (6.2)	
Non-smoker	384 (46.3)	167 (40.2)		106 (19.6)	39 (14.4)		278 (95.9)	128 (88.3)	
Alcohol intake									
Current-drinker	534 (64.3)	254 (61.2)	0.243	404 (74.8)	193 (71.5)	0.282	130 (44.8)	61 (42.1)	0.819
Ex-drinker	60 (7.2)	41 (9.9)		47 (8.7)	33 (12.2)		13 (4.5)	8 (5.5)	
Non-drinker	236 (28.4)	119 (28.7)		89 (16.5)	44 (16.3)		147 (50.7)	75 (51.7)	
Regular exercise									
Yes	466 (56.1)	147 (35.4)	<0.001	303 (56.1)	109 (40.4)	<0.001	163 (56.2)	38 (26.2)	<0.001
No	361 (43.5)	268 (64.6)		234 (43.3)	161 (59.6)		127 (43.8)	107 (73.8)	
Education, n (%)									
Middle school or less	119 (14.3)	142 (34.2)	<0.001	71 (13.2)	91 (33.7)	<0.001	48 (16.6)	51 (35.2)	<0.001
High school	253 (30.5)	174 (41.9)		140 (25.9)	112 (41.5)		113 (39.0)	62 (42.8)	
College or more	426 (51.3)	97 (23.4)		301 (55.7)	66 (24.4)		125 (43.1)	31 (21.4)	
Marital status, n (%)									
Married	716 (86.3)	361 (87.0)	0.674	478 (88.5)	243 (90.0)	0.553	238 (82.1)	118 (81.4)	>0.999
Others	113 (13.6)	52 (12.5)		61 (11.3)	26 (9.6)		52 (17.9)	26 (17.9)	

Table 1. *Cont.*

	Total (n = 1245)			Men (n = 810)			Women (n = 435)		
	Controls (n = 830)	Cases (n = 415)	p [b]	Controls (n = 540)	Cases (n = 270)	p [b]	Controls (n = 290)	Cases (n = 145)	p [b]
Occupation, n (%)									
Professional, administrative	156 (18.8)	70 (16.9)	0.001	117 (21.7)	59 (21.9)	0.010	39 (13.5)	11 (7.6)	0.002
Office, sales and service	266 (32.1)	122 (29.4)		203 (37.6)	81 (30.0)		63 (21.7)	41 (28.3)	
Laborer, agricultural	128 (15.4)	104 (25.1)		111 (20.6)	83 (30.7)		17 (5.9)	21 (14.5)	
Others, unemployed	277 (33.4)	117 (28.2)		106 (19.6)	46 (17.0)		171 (59.0)	71 (49.0)	
Monthly household income, 10,000 won/month, n (%)									
<200	149 (18.0)	133 (32.1)	<0.001	85 (15.7)	85 (31.5)	<0.001	64 (22.1)	48 (33.1)	0.016
200–400	341 (41.1)	148 (35.7)		232 (43.0)	106 (39.3)		109 (37.6)	42 (29.0)	
>400	273 (32.9)	96 (23.1)		168 (31.1)	55 (20.4)		105 (36.2)	41 (28.3)	
Histological subtype of GC (Lauren's classification)									
Intestinal	-	158 (38.1)	-	-	132 (48.9)	-	-	26 (17.9)	-
Diffuse	-	164 (39.5)		-	77 (28.5)		-	87 (60.0)	
Mixed	-	59 (14.2)		-	40 (14.8)		-	19 (13.1)	
Indeterminate	-	4 (1.0)		-	3 (1.1)		-	1 (0.7)	

Missing data are included in the total %. [a] Values are presented as the means ± standard deviations (SD) or n (%); [b] p-values for continuous variables and categorical variables were calculated using Student's t-test and the chi-square test, respectively. BMI: body mass index; GC: gastric cancer.

Table 2. Comparison of the consumption of total energy, total dietary carotenoids, and carotenoid subclasses [a].

	Total (n = 1245)			Men (n = 810)			Women (n = 435)		
	Controls (n = 830)	Cases (n = 415)	p [b]	Controls (n = 540)	Cases (n = 270)	p [b]	Controls (n = 290)	Cases (n = 145)	p [b]
Total energy intake (kcal)	1713.6 ± 545.5	1924.1 ± 612.9	<0.001	1760.6 ± 541.5	2038.5 ± 634.8	<0.001	1626.0 ± 543.1	1711.1 ± 507.0	0.116
Total carotenoid intake (μg/day)									
Total carotenoids	12,121.5 ± 7762.4	10,799.2 ± 6987.1	0.003	10,785.7 ± 6632.5	9990.7 ± 6294.5	0.102	14,608.7 ± 9014.1	12,304.7 ± 7927.0	0.009
α-Carotene	947.5 ± 913.8	925.3 ± 966.0	0.692	839.8 ± 805.4	833.1 ± 861.7	0.913	1148.0 ± 1059.9	1096.9 ± 1118.1	0.642
β-Carotene	5075.9 ± 3276.2	4632.6 ± 3009.4	0.018	4529.7 ± 2682.8	4226.4 ± 2568.0	0.124	6093.1 ± 3971.2	5388.9 ± 3582.4	0.073
β-Cryptoxanthin	393.7 ± 438.8	330.5 ± 364.6	0.007	310.0 ± 269.7	314.3 ± 390.1	0.872	549.6 ± 615.7	360.6 ± 310.5	<0.001
Lutein/Zeaxanthin	3531.7 ± 2584.6	3455.2 ± 2764.4	0.631	3256.6 ± 2200.2	3268.1 ± 2726.8	0.952	4044.0 ± 3119.2	3803.7 ± 2809.2	0.435
Lycopene	2218.0 ± 3847.2	1439.0 ± 2135.7	<0.001	1869.8 ± 3433.0	1312.1 ± 2110.4	0.005	2866.4 ± 4452.9	1675.3 ± 2169.5	<0.001

[a] Adjusted for total energy intake using the residuals method; [b] p-values were calculated using Student's t-test.

Table 3. Odds ratios (ORs) and 95% confidence intervals (CIs) of gastric cancer (GC) according to the tertiles of total dietary carotenoids and carotenoid subclasses [a].

	Median Intake (μg/day)	No. of Controls/Cases	Model 1		Model 2		Model 3	
			OR	(95% CI)	OR	(95% CI)	OR	(95% CI)
Total Carotenoids								
Total (n = 1245)								
T1	6064.75	276/162	1.00		1.00		1.00	
T2	10,171.44	277/146	0.88	(0.67–1.17)	0.98	(0.71–1.34)	1.01	(0.72–1.42)
T3	17,946.94	277/107	0.64	(0.47–0.86)	0.75	(0.53–1.06)	0.79	(0.55–1.15)
p for trend [b]			0.003		0.082		0.185	
Men (n = 810)								
T1	5603.87	180/106	1.00		1.00		1.00	
T2	8921.20	180/88	0.83	(0.58–1.17)	0.95	(0.63–1.43)	1.09	(0.70–1.68)
T3	15,850.62	180/76	0.71	(0.49–1.02)	0.78	(0.51–1.20)	0.84	(0.54–1.33)
p for trend [b]			0.073		0.236		0.386	
Women (n = 435)								
T1	7151.14	96/74	1.00		1.00		1.00	
T2	12,377.35	97/38	0.50	(0.31–0.81)	0.51	(0.30–0.88)	0.51	(0.29–0.91)
T3	21,678.14	97/33	0.43	(0.26–0.71)	0.56	(0.32–0.99)	0.65	(0.35–1.18)
p for trend [b]			0.001		0.051		0.169	
α-Carotene								
Total (n = 1245)								
T1	321.92	276/151	1.00		1.00		1.00	
T2	665.17	277/136	0.90	(0.67–1.19)	0.99	(0.71–1.36)	0.94	(0.67–1.33)
T3	1527.25	277/128	0.84	(0.62–1.12)	0.99	(0.71–1.38)	1.00	(0.70–1.41)
p for trend [b]			0.269		0.969		0.957	
Men (n = 810)								
T1	291.35	180/100	1.00		1.00		1.00	
T2	587.52	180/78	0.78	(0.54–1.12)	0.95	(0.63–1.44)	0.95	(0.61–1.48)
T3	1404.67	180/92	0.92	(0.65–1.31)	0.98	(0.65–1.48)	0.95	(0.61–1.47)
p for trend [b]			0.879		0.972		0.839	
Women (n = 435)								
T1	427.91	96/52	1.00		1.00		1.00	
T2	853.57	97/42	0.80	(0.49–1.31)	0.84	(0.48–1.48)	0.83	(0.46–1.50)
T3	1704.44	97/51	0.97	(0.60–1.57)	1.48	(0.85–2.58)	1.49	(0.83–2.70)
p for trend [b]			0.961		0.113		0.125	
β-Carotene								
Total (n = 1245)								
T1	2574.39	276/162	1.00		1.00		1.00	
T2	4339.20	277/134	0.82	(0.61–1.08)	0.81	(0.58–1.11)	0.84	(0.60–1.18)
T3	7353.32	277/119	0.71	(0.53–0.96)	0.77	(0.55–1.08)	0.85	(0.59–1.22)
p for trend [b]			0.030		0.158		0.426	

Table 3. *Cont.*

	Median Intake (μg/day)	No. of Controls/Cases	Model 1		Model 2		Model 3	
			OR	(95% CI)	OR	(95% CI)	OR	(95% CI)
Men (n = 810)								
T1	2447.55	180/100	1.00		1.00		1.00	
T2	3791.98	180/93	0.93	(0.65–1.32)	1.00	(0.67–1.50)	1.10	(0.72–1.70)
T3	6504.49	180/77	0.76	(0.53–1.10)	0.76	(0.49–1.17)	0.89	(0.56–1.41)
p for trend [b]			0.136		0.179		0.535	
Women (n = 435)								
T1	3178.03	96/68	1.00		1.00		1.00	
T2	5104.57	97/35	0.50	(0.31–0.83)	0.52	(0.30–0.92)	0.53	(0.29–0.97)
T3	8683.53	97/42	0.60	(0.37–0.97)	0.73	(0.42–1.25)	0.79	(0.44–1.41)
p for trend [b]			0.062		0.351		0.551	
β-Cryptoxanthin								
Total (n = 1245)								
T1	128.90	276/170	1.00		1.00		1.00	
T2	270.81	277/136	0.79	(0.60–1.05)	0.90	(0.66–1.24)	0.94	(0.67–1.32)
T3	594.01	277/109	0.62	(0.46–0.84)	0.79	(0.56–1.10)	0.77	(0.54–1.10)
p for trend [b]			0.003		0.172		0.142	
Men (n = 810)								
T1	116.88	180/104	1.00		1.00		1.00	
T2	229.41	180/86	0.83	(0.58–1.18)	0.86	(0.57–1.30)	0.96	(0.62–1.49)
T3	483.12	180/80	0.77	(0.54–1.10)	0.85	(0.56–1.29)	0.92	(0.59–1.43)
p for trend [b]			0.180		0.502		0.717	
Women (n = 435)								
T1	180.27	96/68	1.00		1.00		1.00	
T2	369.16	97/46	0.67	(0.42–1.07)	0.92	(0.54–1.57)	0.84	(0.47–1.48)
T3	851.83	97/31	0.45	(0.27–0.75)	0.60	(0.34–1.07)	0.55	(0.30–1.02)
p for trend [b]			0.003		0.076		0.054	
Lutein/Zeaxanthin								
Total (n = 1245)								
T1	1716.04	276/152	1.00		1.00		1.00	
T2	2832.71	277/135	0.88	(0.66–1.17)	0.93	(0.67–1.28)	1.00	(0.71–1.41)
T3	5188.69	277/128	0.83	(0.62–1.12)	0.87	(0.63–1.22)	0.91	(0.64–1.30)
p for trend [b]			0.245		0.440		0.575	
Men (n = 810)								
T1	1676.82	180/91	1.00		1.00		1.00	
T2	2691.75	180/89	0.98	(0.68–1.40)	1.18	(0.78–1.79)	1.41	(0.91–2.20)
T3	4679.81	180/90	0.99	(0.69–1.41)	1.03	(0.68–1.58)	1.13	(0.72–1.76)
p for trend [b]			0.954		0.996		0.788	

Table 3. *Cont.*

	Median Intake (μg/day)	No. of Controls/Cases	Model 1		Model 2		Model 3	
			OR	(95% CI)	OR	(95% CI)	OR	(95% CI)
Women (n = 435)								
T1	1894.17	96/61	1.00		1.00		1.00	
T2	3268.31	97/39	0.63	(0.38–1.03)	0.60	(0.35–1.05)	0.64	(0.36–1.15)
T3	5678.59	97/45	0.71	(0.44–1.17)	0.83	(0.48–1.45)	0.82	(0.45–1.47)
p for trend [b]			0.240		0.636		0.602	
Lycopene								
Total (n = 1245)								
T1	327.68	276/209	1.00		1.00		1.00	
T2	1105.49	277/112	0.53	(0.40–0.70)	0.67	(0.49–0.92)	0.67	(0.48–0.94)
T3	3666.52	277/94	0.44	(0.33–0.59)	0.57	(0.41–0.80)	0.60	(0.42–0.85)
p for trend [b]			<0.001		0.003		0.012	
Men (n = 810)								
T1	268.48	180/138	1.00		1.00		1.00	
T2	934.05	180/65	0.47	(0.33–0.68)	0.51	(0.34–0.78)	0.55	(0.35–0.86)
T3	2963.59	180/67	0.49	(0.34–0.69)	0.60	(0.40–0.91)	0.60	(0.39–0.93)
p for trend [b]			0.001		0.056		0.062	
Women (n = 435)								
T1	442.87	96/69	1.00		1.00		1.00	
T2	1528.34	97/46	0.66	(0.41–1.05)	0.77	(0.45–1.31)	0.81	(0.46–1.42)
T3	4843.59	97/30	0.43	(0.26–0.72)	0.54	(0.30–0.96)	0.60	(0.32–1.11)
p for trend [b]			0.002		0.039		0.113	

[a] Total dietary carotenoids and carotenoid subclasses were categorized into tertiles according to the distribution of the control groups: Total carotenoids for overall subjects (T1: 7932.26, T2: 7932.26–13,062.36, and T3: ≥13,062.36), men (T1: <7393.71, T2: 7393.71–11,605.58, and T3: ≥11,605.58), and women (T1: <10,177.56, T2: 10,177.56–16,039.47, and T3: ≥16,039.47); α-carotene for overall subjects (T1: <480.37, T2: 480.37–956.11, and T3: ≥956.11), men (T1: <435.49, T2: 435.49–799.48, and T3: ≥799.48), and women (T1: <587.17, T2: 587.17–1160.14, and T3: ≥1160.14); β-carotene for overall subjects (T1: <3370.16, T2: 3370.16–5327.21, and T3: ≥5327.21), men (T1: <3165.51, T2: 3165.51–4843.61, and T3: ≥4843.61), and women (T1: <4238.05, T2: 4238.05–6436.30, and T3: ≥6436.30); β-cryptoxanthin for overall subjects (T1: <190.36, T2: 190.36–381.30, and T3: ≥381.30), men (T1: <166.94, T2: 166.94–322.32, and T3: ≥322.32), and women (T1: <254.69, T2: 254.69–510.98, and T3: ≥510.98); lutein/zeaxanthin for overall subjects (T1: <2242.79, T2: 2242.79–3,707.97, and T3: ≥3707.97), men (T1: <2122.45, T2: 2122.45–3379.04, and T3: ≥3379.04), and women (T1: <2507.60, T2: 2507.60–4218.61, and T3: ≥4218.61); and lycopene for overall subjects (T1: <683.61, T2: 683.61–1881.13, and T3: ≥1881.13), men (T1: <574.69, T2: 574.69–1590.15, and T3: ≥1590.15), and women (T1: <898.55, T2: 898.55–2572.63, and T3: ≥2572.63). [b] To test for a trend across tertiles, the median intake for each tertile category was used as a continuous variable. Model 1: Adjusted for age; Model 2: Adjusted for age, total caloric intake, family history of GC, smoking status, regular exercise, education level, occupation, and monthly household income; Model 3: Additionally adjusted for *H. pylori* infection. In the overall subjects, models 1, 2, and 3 were additionally adjusted for gender.

Table 4. ORs and 95% CIs of GC according to tertiles of dietary lycopene intake stratified by *H. pylori* infection status [a].

	Median Intake (µg/day)	*H. pylori*-Positive (n = 868)					*H. pylori*-Negative (n = 353)				
		No. of Controls/Cases	Model 1		Model 2		No. of Controls/Cases	Model 1		Model 2	
			OR	(95% CI)	OR	(95% CI)		OR	(95% CI)	OR	(95% CI)
Lycopene											
Total (n = 1221)											
T1	327.68	169/194	1.00		1.00		100/15	1.00		1.00	
T2	1105.49	166/100	0.52	(0.37–0.72)	0.60	(0.42–0.86)	102/12	0.75	(0.33–1.69)	1.23	(0.48–3.18)
T3	3666.52	151/88	0.49	(0.35–0.69)	0.61	(0.42–0.90)	118/6	0.30	(0.11–0.81)	0.50	(0.16–1.54)
p for trend [b]			<0.001		0.037			0.017		0.168	

[a] Dietary lycopene intake was categorized into tertiles according to the distribution of the control group among overall subjects (T1: <683.61, T2: 683.61–1881.13, and T3: ≥1881.13). [b] To test for trend across tertiles, the median intake for each tertile category was used as a continuous variable. Model 1: Adjusted for age and gender; Model 2: Adjusted for age, gender, total caloric intake, family history of GC, smoking status, regular exercise, education level, occupation, and monthly household income.

Table 5. ORs and 95% CIs of GC according to tertiles of dietary lycopene intake stratified by smoking status [a].

	Median Intake (µg/day)	Ever-Smoker (n = 693) [b]					Non-Smoker (n = 551)				
		No. of Controls/Cases	Model 1		Model 2		No. of Controls/Cases	Model 1		Model 2	
			OR	(95% CI)	OR	(95% CI)		OR	(95% CI)	OR	(95% CI)
Lycopene											
Total (n = 1244)											
T1	327.68	166/138	1.00		1.00		110/70	1.00		1.00	
T2	1105.49	152/63	0.49	(0.34–0.71)	0.49	(0.31–0.77)	125/49	0.61	(0.39–0.96)	0.88	(0.52–1.48)
T3	3666.52	128/46	0.40	(0.26–0.60)	0.39	(0.23–0.65)	149/48	0.49	(0.32–0.77)	0.75	(0.45–1.27)
p for trend [c]			<0.001		0.001			0.006		0.307	

[a] Dietary lycopene intake was categorized into tertiles according to the distribution of the control group among overall subjects (T1: <683.61, T2: 683.61–1881.13, and T3: ≥1881.13). [b] Subjects who currently smoke or previously smoked were combined as ever-smokers. [c] To test for trend across tertiles, the median intake for each tertile category was used as a continuous variable. Model 1: Adjusted for age and gender; Model 2: Adjusted for age, gender, total caloric intake, family history of GC, *H. pylori* infection, regular exercise, education level, occupation, and monthly household income.

Table 6. Comparison of the consumption of lycopene contributing foods [a].

Food Consumption (g/day)	Cumulative (%) [b]	Total (n = 1245) Controls (n = 830)	Total Cases (n = 415)	Total p [c]	Men (n = 810) Controls (n = 540)	Men Cases (n = 270)	Men p [c]	Women (n = 435) Controls (n = 290)	Women Cases (n = 145)	Women p [c]
Watermelon	34.56	21.02 ± 69.39	13.45 ± 21.73	0.004	15.25 ± 36.47	11.27 ± 21.19	0.050	31.75 ± 105.62	17.50 ± 22.22	0.028
Tomato	66.68	32.61 ± 90.50	14.71 ± 31.94	<0.001	27.01 ± 91.31	12.68 ± 32.60	0.001	43.05 ± 88.19	18.50 ± 30.43	<0.001
Tomato ketchup	90.26	5.64 ± 15.31	2.62 ± 5.67	<0.001	4.71 ± 15.51	2.28 ± 5.79	0.001	7.38 ± 14.81	3.25 ± 5.40	<0.001

[a] Adjusted for total energy intake using the residuals method. [b] Food items contributing to dietary lycopene intake that represented up to 90% of the cumulative contribution were selected. [c] p-values were calculated using Student's t-test.

Table 7. ORs and 95% CIs of GC according to tertiles of the consumption of lycopene contributing foods.

	Range (g/day)	Median Intake (g/day)	No. of Controls/Cases	Model 1 OR	Model 1 (95% CI)	Model 2 OR	Model 2 (95% CI)	Model 3 OR	Model 3 (95% CI)
Watermelon									
Total (n = 1245)									
T1	<3.91	1.47	276/188	1.00		1.00		1.00	
T2	3.91–13.59	7.23	277/116	0.61	(0.46–0.81)	0.75	(0.54–1.04)	0.73	(0.52–1.03)
T3	≥13.59	29.32	277/111	0.58	(0.43–0.77)	0.77	(0.55–1.07)	0.71	(0.50–1.02)
p for trend [a]				0.002		0.233		0.130	
Men (n = 810)									
T1	<3.16	1.30	180/121	1.00		1.00		1.00	
T2	3.16–10.63	5.34	180/75	0.62	(0.44–0.88)	0.75	(0.50–1.13)	0.78	(0.51–1.20)
T3	≥10.63	24.63	180/74	0.61	(0.43–0.87)	0.84	(0.56–1.27)	0.78	(0.50–1.21)
p for trend [a]				0.034		0.657		0.391	
Women (n = 435)									
T1	<6.14	2.50	96/63	1.00		1.00		1.00	
T2	6.14–22.08	11.35	97/42	0.66	(0.41–1.07)	0.80	(0.46–1.40)	0.83	(0.46–1.51)
T3	≥22.08	43.54	97/40	0.63	(0.39–1.02)	0.76	(0.44–1.34)	0.77	(0.42–1.39)
p for trend [a]				0.117		0.421		0.440	
Tomato									
Total (n = 1245)									
T1	<4.70	1.70	276/217	1.00		1.00		1.00	
T2	4.70–20.12	10.15	277/120	0.55	(0.41–0.72)	0.66	(0.48–0.90)	0.66	(0.47–0.91)
T3	≥20.12	47.87	277/78	0.34	(0.25–0.47)	0.54	(0.38–0.77)	0.59	(0.41–0.85)
p for trend [a]				<0.001		0.002		0.016	

Table 7. *Cont.*

	Range (g/day)	Median Intake (g/day)	No. of Controls/Cases	Model 1		Model 2		Model 3	
				OR	(95% CI)	OR	(95% CI)	OR	(95% CI)
Men (n = 810)									
T1	<4.03	1.33	180/144	1.00		1.00		1.00	
T2	4.03–16.68	8.75	180/72	0.50	(0.35–0.71)	0.67	(0.45–1.00)	0.64	(0.42–0.99)
T3	≥16.68	35.92	180/54	0.37	(0.26–0.54)	0.57	(0.37–0.88)	0.58	(0.37–0.92)
p for trend [a]				<0.001		0.022		0.043	
Women (n = 435)									
T1	<6.13	2.74	96/67	1.00		1.00		1.00	
T2	6.13–30.90	14.03	97/54	0.79	(0.50–1.25)	0.98	(0.58–1.65)	0.97	(0.56–1.68)
T3	≥30.90	63.63	97/24	0.34	(0.20–0.60)	0.47	(0.25–0.87)	0.57	(0.30–1.12)
p for trend [a]				<0.001		0.010		0.084	
Tomato ketchup									
Total (n = 1245)									
T1	<0.84	0.30	276/217	1.00		1.00		1.00	
T2	0.84–3.58	1.81	277/123	0.56	(0.42–0.74)	0.66	(0.49–0.90)	0.66	(0.48–0.92)
T3	≥3.58	8.34	277/75	0.33	(0.24–0.45)	0.51	(0.36–0.72)	0.55	(0.38–0.80)
p for trend [a]				<0.001		0.001		0.005	
Men (n = 810)									
T1	<0.71	0.24	180/140	1.00		1.00		1.00	
T2	0.71–2.98	1.52	180/75	0.54	(0.38–0.76)	0.72	(0.49–1.08)	0.69	(0.45–1.06)
T3	≥2.98	6.45	180/55	0.39	(0.27–0.57)	0.61	(0.40–0.94)	0.62	(0.39–0.97)
p for trend [a]				<0.001		0.039		0.067	
Women (n = 435)									
T1	<1.08	0.50	96/67	1.00		1.00		1.00	
T2	1.08–5.19	2.43	97/54	0.79	(0.50–1.25)	0.97	(0.58–1.64)	0.96	(0.56–1.67)
T3	≥5.19	10.94	97/24	0.34	(0.20–0.60)	0.47	(0.25–0.88)	0.58	(0.30–1.12)
p for trend [a]				<0.001		0.011		0.089	

[a] Adjusted for total energy intake using the residuals method. Model 1: Adjusted for age; Model 2: Adjusted for age, total caloric intake, family history of GC, smoking status, regular exercise, education level, occupation, and monthly household income; Model 3: Additionally adjusted for *H. pylori* infection. In the overall subjects, models 1, 2, and 3 were additionally adjusted for gender.

4. Discussion

In our study, an inverse association was observed between higher dietary lycopene intake and the risk of GC in the overall subjects. This significant association remained in the subgroups of gender, *H. pylori*-positive subjects, and those who had ever smoked. The protective effect of dietary lycopene intake on the risk of GC among *H. pylori*–positive subjects and those who had ever smoked was particularly evident in males. Among the contributing foods of dietary lycopene, tomatoes and tomato ketchup exerted protective effects on the risk of GC.

However, previous epidemiological studies of the association between dietary lycopene intake and the risk of GC revealed that lycopene intake is less likely to be associated with GC risk. Among the five case-control studies regarding dietary lycopene intake, a significantly reduced GC risk was observed in only one study conducted in Uruguay (OR 0.37, 95% CI 0.19–0.73) [17]. In other studies, conducted in the US [20], Spain [19], Poland [15], and Italy [16], no significant association was observed. No significant associations between dietary lycopene intake and the risk of GC were observed in three cohort studies conducted in the Netherlands [21], Sweden [18], and in male participants who smoked in Finland [26]. Furthermore, in a meta-analysis that included only studies with validated food frequency questionnaires (FFQs), no statistically significant association was observed between higher dietary lycopene intake with the risk of GC [32]. Another meta-analysis of five case-control studies did not identify any association between higher dietary lycopene intake and the risk of GC [33].

The possible explanation for this trend is that dietary sources and trends of consumption differ among countries and, thus, do not perfectly overlap between studies. Another potential contributing factor is that the studies utilized diverse carotenoid content databases to estimate the consumption of dietary carotenoids, which were linked to various FFQ models. The carotenoid content of each food item was estimated using a different food composition database, such as the USDA database [20,24], the Nutrition Coding Center Nutrient Data System from the University of Minnesota [23], both American and Polish databases [15], Swedish [18,25], Italian [16], North American [17], Spanish [19], Finnish [26], and Dutch databases [21].

In our study, nine lycopene-containing food items were included, in order from the largest contribution to dietary lycopene intake: Watermelons, tomatoes, tomato ketchup, hamburgers, pizza, persimmons, red cabbage, carrots, and pepper powder (data not shown). Three of the nine food items were selected as the primary foods contributing to dietary lycopene intake. Unlike other dietary carotenoid subclasses and total carotenoids, which consist of contributing foods that were different from other studies, foods contributing to dietary lycopene intake were consistent with those from other studies because they included tomatoes and tomato-based products. Tomatoes and tomato-based products accounted for 81.2% of all dietary sources of lycopene in the US, and tomato-based soups and stews accounted for 3.8% [34]. Similarly, in European countries, tomatoes and tomato-based products constituted the major foods contributing to dietary lycopene intake: Tomatoes (25%), canned tomatoes (16%), and pizza (16%) in France; canned tomatoes (23%), tomato soup (17%), and pizza (16%) in Ireland; tomatoes (21%), canned tomatoes (20%), and pizza (15%) in the UK; tomato soup (29%), tomatoes (16%), and pizza (16%) in the Netherlands; and tomatoes (55%) and tomato puree (42%) in Spain [35]. On the other hand, in a previous study conducted in Korea, watermelons, tomatoes, and tomato ketchup contributed to 53.6%, 36.9%, and 5.7% of lycopene intake, respectively [36]. In our study, the major contributors of dietary lycopene intake were the same, but the only difference was the contribution percentage of each food item: 34.56% for watermelons, 32.12% for tomatoes, and 23.58% for tomato ketchup. Although the proportion of each food item that contributed to dietary intake of lycopene differed, the foods contributing to lycopene overlapped, indicating that some country-specific trends in the food items that contribute to lycopene intake might exist.

Among the foods that contribute to dietary lycopene intake, tomatoes and tomato ketchup were significantly associated with the risk of GC. The lycopene content (mg lycopene/100 g) of tomato ketchup is greater than fresh tomatoes [37–39]. Lycopene from fresh tomatoes is not readily bioavailable, and thus, by processing tomatoes, the bioavailability of lycopene is increased due to a breakdown of the tissue matrix [40]. This characteristic is due to the structure of the lycopene molecule: Lycopene in raw tomatoes is mainly in the *trans*-isomer form, but, during heat processing, the structure undergoes isomerization to a *cis* form and is thereby more efficiently absorbed [40]. This result is consistent with our finding that the intake of both tomatoes and tomato ketchup were inversely associated with the risk of GC.

Previously, several epidemiological studies on tomato consumption and the risk of GC have been conducted. In a case-control study conducted in the US, an inverse association was observed among only African Americans (OR 0.56, 95% CI 0.34–0.90), but not in Caucasians [41]. In a case-control study conducted in Sweden, a significant inverse association was observed between higher tomato intake (consumed more than 2.9 times per month) during adolescence (OR 0.36, 95% CI 0.23–0.58, p for trend < 0.0001) [42]. However, other case-control studies conducted in Spain [43], Sweden [22], Japan [44], and the US [45] did not identify any significant associations. In a cohort study conducted in the Netherlands, a borderline positive association was found between tomato consumption and non-cardia GC risk (relative risk (RR) per 25 g/day increase in the amount of tomatoes consumed: 1.13, 95% CI 1.00–1.28) [46]. However, when a meta-analysis was conducted with those seven studies listed above that have validated FFQs, tomato consumption was significantly associated with a decreased risk of GC (OR 0.73, 95% CI 0.60–0.90), with moderate heterogeneity (I^2 = 47.92%) [32]. This finding is consistent with our results because we also observed the protective effects of tomatoes and tomato ketchup on the risk of GC.

In our study, lycopene was inversely associated with the risk of GC, and the association remained significant in *H. pylori*-positive subjects and those who had ever smoked. There is a possible explanation of those risk factors and the effect of lycopene on GC prevention. Smoking, inflammation, and *H. pylori* infection may increase oxidative stress in the gastrointestinal tract, which leads to DNA damage, extracellular signal-regulated kinase (ERK) activation and p53 induction, decreased activities of antioxidant enzymes (glutathione, GSH; glutathione-S-transferase, GST; and glutathione peroxidase, GPx), and impaired immune function [46]. Lycopene might scavenge reactive oxygen species (ROS) and stimulate antioxidant enzyme activities, which protect gastric mucosa from oxidative stress-induced ERK activation, p53 induction, cell cycle disturbances, and impaired immune function, thereby, preventing gastric carcinogenesis [47]. Lycopene might scavenge ROS and stimulate antioxidant enzyme activities, which protect the gastric mucosa from oxidative stress-induced ERK activation, p53 induction, cell cycle disturbances, and impaired immune function, thereby, preventing gastric carcinogenesis [47].

However, regarding contributing foods, it would be presumptuous to assume that certain foods are representative of a specific nutrient, and to conclude that a food item protects against GC because of the specific nutrient. Foods contributing to dietary carotenoid intake are mostly fruits and vegetables, but they are also good sources of bioactive phytochemicals [48]. In a Spanish case-control study, a higher intake of dietary flavonoids, particularly kaempferol, exerted a protective effect on the risk of GC, while no significant association was observed for carotenoids [19]. Tomatoes are rich in carotenoids, but they also contain lower concentrations of polyphenols, such as hydroxycinnamic acids, flavanones, flavonols, anthocyanins, and flavonol glycosides [49]. In addition, tomatoes are a relatively rich source of vitamin C [32]. In vivo and in vitro studies have suggested that bioactive compounds in tomatoes may work additively or synergistically to reduce the growth of cancer cells [12]. However, since both higher dietary lycopene consumption and higher tomato intake were inversely associated with the risk of GC in our study, we may still suggest a possible effect of dietary lycopene intake by consuming tomatoes and tomato ketchup, which contributed to 55.7% of the total lycopene intake.

Our study has certain strengths: (1) A comprehensive and validated 106-item SQFFQ was used; (2) the study participants in the case group were surveyed by trained interviewers. Subjects in the control group were initially asked to complete the survey by themselves, and trained interviewers asked any questions with missing answers in a second session. Therefore, the quality of data was improved; (3) the carotenoid database included the contents of kimchi and seasoned vegetables, and covered 98.5% of all items reported in the SQFFQ; (4) information on the prevalence of *H. pylori* infection and smoking status, which are known risk factors for GC according to the IARC, were available [3,4]; and (5) to our knowledge, this is the first study conducted in Korea to investigate the association between dietary carotenoids and GC risk.

Several limitations should also be mentioned: (1) In this hospital-based, case-control study, selection bias might have occurred because the controls were those who had participated in the health screening. Subjects who chose to undergo screening may have had healthier lifestyles and dietary habits (e.g., greater consumption of fruits and vegetables) than individuals who did not choose to undergo screening; thus, the controls might be less representative of the general population; (2) our findings might be prone to recall bias because subjects were required to report their dietary intake for the past 12 months, which is a relatively long period. Additionally, when the SQFFQ was assessed, cases had already received a confirmed diagnosis; thus, the recall ability may have differed between cases and controls. However, in our study, cases were only patients who were diagnosed with early GC. Thus, compared to advanced GC cases, the influence of dietary changes on GC symptoms will be negligible. Moreover, cases with other health factors that might have affected their diet (subjects with diabetes mellitus, a severe systematic/mental disease, a history of cancer within five years, and women who were pregnant or currently breastfeeding) were excluded. Therefore, the recall bias in this study might be minimal; and (3) the sample size was relatively small in our study; in particular, few *H. pylori*-negative subjects and subjects with cardia GC were included. However, the higher percentage of cases with non-cardia GC among the overall GC incidence is a unique trend in Asian countries, including Korea [7]; nevertheless, a larger sample size is needed to increase the statistical power.

5. Conclusions

Based on our findings, higher dietary lycopene intake might be inversely associated with the risk of GC in the overall subjects. The association remained significant in the subgroups of gender, *H. pylori*-positive subjects, and those who had ever smoked. Foods contributing to dietary lycopene that exerted protective effects on the risk of GC were tomatoes and tomato ketchup. Further studies with larger sample sizes, including sufficient numbers of *H. pylori*-negative subjects and patients with cardia GC, are needed.

Author Contributions: Formal analysis, J.L. and J.H.K.; Writing original draft, J.H.K.; Data curation, I.J.C., O.K., J.K., H.K. and J.L.; Investigation, I.J.C. and Y.-I.K.; Methodology, I.J.C., Y.-I.K. and J.K.; Funding acquisition, J.K. and O.K.; Project administration, J.K.; Supervision, J.K.

References

1. Ferlay, J.; Soerjomataram, I.; Dikshit, R.; Eser, S.; Mathers, C.; Rebelo, M.; Parkin, D.M.; Forman, D.; Bray, F. Cancer incidence and mortality worldwide: Sources, methods and major patterns in GLOBOCAN 2012. *Int. J. Cancer* **2015**, *136*, E359–E386. [CrossRef] [PubMed]
2. Jung, K.W.; Won, Y.J.; Kong, H.J.; Lee, E.S.; Kim, C.H.; Yoo, C.I.; Park, J.H.; Nam, H.S.; Huh, J.S.; Youm, J.H.; et al. Cancer statistics in Korea: Incidence, mortality, survival, and prevalence in 2015. *Cancer Res. Treat.* **2018**, *50*, 303–316. [CrossRef] [PubMed]
3. International Agency for Research on Cancer, Schistosomes, Liver Flukes and *Helicobacter pylori*: IARC Monographs on the Evaluation of Carcinogenic Risks to Humans. Volume 61. Available online: https://monographs.iarc.fr/ENG/Monographs/vol61/mono61.pdf (accessed on 31 March 2018).
4. International Agency for Research on Cancer, Tobacco Smoke and Involuntary Smoking: IARC Monographs on the Evaluation of Carcinogenic Risks to Humans. Volume 83. Available online: https://monographs.iarc.fr/ENG/Monographs/vol83/mono83.pdf (accessed on 31 March 2018).

5. Doll, R.; Peto, R. The causes of cancer: Quantitative estimates of avoidable risks of cancer in the United States today. *J. Natl. Cancer Inst.* **1981**, *66*, 1192–1308. [CrossRef]
6. Willett, W.C. Diet, nutrition, and avoidable cancer. *Environ. Health Perspect.* **1995**, *103*, 165–170. [CrossRef] [PubMed]
7. Colquhoun, A.; Arnold, M.; Ferlay, J.; Goodman, K.; Forman, D.; Soerjomataram, I. Global patterns of cardia and non-cardia gastric cancer incidence in 2012. *Gut* **2015**, *64*, 1881–1888. [CrossRef] [PubMed]
8. De Martel, C.; Parsonnet, J. *Helicobacter pylori* infection and gender: A meta-analysis of population-based prevalence surveys. *Dig. Dis. Sci.* **2006**, *51*, 2292–2301. [CrossRef] [PubMed]
9. Freedman, N.; Derakhshan, M.; Abnet, C.; Schatzkin, A.; Hollenbeck, A.; McColl, K. Male predominance of upper gastrointestinal adenocarcinoma cannot be explained by differences in tobacco smoking in men versus women. *Eur. J. Cancer* **2010**, *46*, 2473–2478. [CrossRef] [PubMed]
10. World Cancer Research Fund International. *Diet, Nutrition, Physical Activity and Stomach Cancer*; World Cancer Research Fund International: London, UK, 2018.
11. Stange, C. *Carotenoids in Nature: Biosynthesis, Regulation and Function*; Springer Nature: Basel, Switzerland, 2016.
12. Tanumihardjo, S.A. *Carotenoids and Human Health*; Humana Press: New York, NY, USA, 2013.
13. Wardlaw, G.M.; Smith, A.M.; Lindeman, A.K. *Contemporary Nutrition: A Functional Approach*; McGraw-Hill: New York, NY, USA, 2010; Volume 2.
14. Tanaka, T.; Shnimizu, M.; Moriwaki, H. Cancer chemoprevention by carotenoids. *Molecules* **2012**, *17*, 3202–3242. [CrossRef] [PubMed]
15. Lissowska, J.; Gail, M.H.; Pee, D.; Groves, F.D.; Sobin, L.H.; Nasierowska Guttmejer, A.; Sygnowska, E.; Zatonski, W.; Blot, W.J.; Chow, W.H. Diet and stomach cancer risk in Warsaw, Poland. *Nutr. Cancer* **2004**, *48*, 149–159. [CrossRef] [PubMed]
16. Pelucchi, C.; Tramacere, I.; Bertuccio, P.; Tavani, A.; Negri, E.; La Vecchia, C. Dietary intake of selected micronutrients and gastric cancer risk: An Italian case-control study. *Ann. Oncol.* **2008**, *20*, 160–165. [CrossRef] [PubMed]
17. De S., E.; Boffetta, P.; Brennan, P.; Deneo Pellegrini, H.; Carzoglio, J.; Ronco, A.; Mendilaharsu, M. Dietary carotenoids and risk of gastric cancer: A case-control study in Uruguay. *Eur. J. Cancer Prev.* **2000**, *9*, 329–334.
18. Larsson, S.C.; Bergkvist, L.; Näslund, I.; Rutegård, J.; Wolk, A. Vitamin A, retinol, and carotenoids and the risk of gastric cancer: A prospective cohort study. *Am. J. Clin. Nutr.* **2007**, *85*, 497–503. [CrossRef] [PubMed]
19. Garcia Closas, R.; Gonzalez, C.A.; Agudo, A.; Riboli, E. Intake of specific carotenoids and flavonoids and the risk of gastric cancer in Spain. *Cancer Cause Control* **1999**, *10*, 71–75. [CrossRef]
20. Harrison, L.E.; Zhang, Z.F.; Karpeh, M.S.; Sun, M.; Kurtz, R.C. The role of dietary factors in the intestinal and diffuse histologic subtypes of gastric adenocarcinoma: A case-control study in the US. *Cancer* **1997**, *80*, 1021–1028. [CrossRef]
21. Botterweck, A.A.; Van den Brandt, P.A.; Goldbohm, R.A. Vitamins, carotenoids, dietary fiber, and the risk of gastric carcinoma: Results from a prospective study after 6.3 years of follow-up. *Cancer* **2000**, *88*, 737–748. [CrossRef]
22. Ekström, A.M.; Serafini, M.; Nyrén, O.; Hansson, L.E.; Ye, W.; Wolk, A. Dietary antioxidant intake and the risk of cardia cancer and noncardia cancer of the intestinal and diffuse types: A population-based case-control study in Sweden. *Int. J. Cancer* **2000**, *87*, 133–140. [CrossRef]
23. Mayne, S.T.; Risch, H.A.; Dubrow, R.; Chow, W.H.; Gammon, M.D.; Vaughan, T.L.; Farrow, D.C.; Schoenberg, J.B.; Stanford, J.L.; Ahsan, H. Nutrient intake and risk of subtypes of esophageal and gastric cancer. *Cancer Epidemiol. Biomark.* **2001**, *10*, 1055–1062.
24. Nomura, A.M.; Hankin, J.H.; Kolonel, L.N.; Wilkens, L.R.; Goodman, M.T.; Stemmermann, G.N. Case-control study of diet and other risk factors for gastric cancer in Hawaii (United States). *Cancer Cause Control* **2003**, *14*, 547–558. [CrossRef]
25. Terry, P.; Lagergren, J.; Ye, W.; Nyrén, O.; Wolk, A. Antioxidants and cancers of the esophagus and gastric cardia. *Int. J. Cancer* **2000**, *87*, 750–754. [CrossRef]
26. Nouraie, M.; Pietinen, P.; Kamangar, F.; Dawsey, S.M.; Abnet, C.C.; Albanes, D.; Virtamo, J.; Taylor, P.R. Fruits, vegetables, and antioxidants and risk of gastric cancer among male smokers. *Cancer Epidemiol. Biomark.* **2005**, *14*, 2087–2092. [CrossRef] [PubMed]

27. Hamilton, S.R.; Aaltonen, L.A. *World Health Organization Classification of Tumors: Pathology and Genetics of Tumours of the Digestive System*; IARC Press: Lyon, France, 2000.
28. Ahn, Y.; Kwon, E.; Shim, J.; Park, M.; Joo, Y.; Kim, K.; Park, C.; Kim, D. Validation and reproducibility of food frequency questionnaire for Korean genome epidemiologic study. *Eur. J. Clin. Nutr.* **2007**, *61*, 1435–1441. [CrossRef] [PubMed]
29. United States Department of Agriculture, USDA Food Composition Databases. Available online: https://ndb.nal.usda.gov/ndb/nutrients/index (accessed on 31 March 2018).
30. *Tables of Food Functional Composition*, 1st ed.; Korea National Academy of Agricultural Science: Suwon, Korea, 2009.
31. Willett, W.C. *Nutritional Epidemiology*; Oxford University Press: New York, NY, USA, 2013; Volume 3.
32. Yang, T.; Yang, X.; Wang, X.; Wang, Y.; Song, Z. The role of tomato products and lycopene in the prevention of gastric cancer: A meta-analysis of epidemiologic studies. *Med. Hypotheses* **2013**, *80*, 383–388. [CrossRef] [PubMed]
33. Zhou, Y.; Wang, T.; Meng, Q.; Zhai, S. Association of carotenoids with risk of gastric cancer: A meta-analysis. *Clin. Nutr.* **2016**, *35*, 109–116. [CrossRef] [PubMed]
34. Murphy, M.M.; Barraj, L.M.; Herman, D.; Bi, X.; Cheatham, R.; Randolph, R.K. Phytonutrient intake by adults in the United States in relation to fruit and vegetable consumption. *J. Am. Diet Assoc.* **2012**, *112*, 222–229. [CrossRef]
35. O'neill, M.; Carroll, Y.; Corridan, B.; Olmedilla, B.; Granado, F.; Blanco, I.; Van den Berg, H.; Hininger, I.; Rousell, A.; Chopra, M. A European carotenoid database to assess carotenoid intakes and its use in a five-country comparative study. *Br. J. Nutr.* **2001**, *85*, 499–507. [CrossRef] [PubMed]
36. Lee, H.S.; Cho, Y.H.; Park, J.; Shin, H.R.; Sung, M.K. Dietary intake of phytonutrients in relation to fruit and vegetable consumption in Korea. *J. Acad. Nutr. Diet* **2013**, *113*, 1194–1199. [CrossRef] [PubMed]
37. Alda, L.M.; Gogoasa, I.; Bordean, D.M.; Gergen, I.; Alda, S.; Moldovan, C.; Nita, L. Lycopene content of tomatoes and tomato products. *J. Agroaliment. Process. Technol.* **2009**, *15*, 540–542.
38. Tonucci, L.H.; Holden, J.M.; Beecher, G.R.; Khachik, F.; Davis, C.S.; Mulokozi, G. Carotenoid content of thermally processed tomato-based food products. *J. Agric. Food Chem.* **1995**, *43*, 579–586. [CrossRef]
39. Story, E.N.; Kopec, R.E.; Schwartz, S.J.; Harris, G.K. An update on the health effects of tomato lycopene. *Annu. Rev. Food Sci. Technol.* **2010**, *1*, 189–210. [CrossRef] [PubMed]
40. Rao, A.; Waseem, Z.; Agarwal, S. Lycopene content of tomatoes and tomato products and their contribution to dietary lycopene. *Food Res. Int.* **1998**, *31*, 737–741. [CrossRef]
41. Correa, P.; Fontham, E.; Pickle, L.W.; Chen, V.; Lin, Y.; Haenszel, W. Dietary determinants of gastric cancer in south Louisiana inhabitants. *J. Natl. Cancer Inst.* **1985**, *75*, 645–654. [PubMed]
42. Hansson, L.E.; Nyrén, O.; Bergström, R.; Wolk, A.; Lindgren, A.; Baron, J.; Adami, H.O. Diet and risk of gastric cancer. A population-based case-control study in Sweden. *Int. J. Cancer* **1993**, *55*, 181–189. [CrossRef] [PubMed]
43. González, C.A.; Sanz, J.M.; Marcos, G.; Pita, S.; Brullet, E.; Saigi, E.; Badia, A.; Riboli, E. Dietary factors and stomach cancer in Spain: A multi-centre case-control study. *Int. J. Cancer* **1991**, *49*, 513–519. [CrossRef] [PubMed]
44. Takezaki, T.; Gao, C.M.; Wu, J.Z.; Ding, J.H.; Liu, Y.T.; Zhang, Y.; Li, S.P.; Su, P.; Liu, T.K.; Tajima, K. Dietary protective and risk factors for esophageal and stomach cancers in a low-epidemic area for stomach cancer in Jiangsu Province, China: Comparison with those in a high-epidemic area. *Jpn. J. Cancer Res.* **2001**, *92*, 1157–1165. [CrossRef] [PubMed]
45. Navarro Silvera, S.A.; Mayne, S.T.; Risch, H.; Gammon, M.D.; Vaughan, T.L.; Chow, W.H.; Dubrow, R.; Schoenberg, J.B.; Stanford, J.L.; West, A.B. Food group intake and risk of subtypes of esophageal and gastric cancer. *Int. J. Cancer* **2008**, *123*, 852–860. [CrossRef] [PubMed]
46. Steevens, J.; Schouten, L.J.; Goldbohm, R.A.; Van den Brandt, P.A. Vegetables and fruits consumption and risk of esophageal and gastric cancer subtypes in the Netherlands cohort study. *Int. J. Cancer* **2011**, *129*, 2681–2693. [CrossRef] [PubMed]
47. Kim, M.J.; Kim, H. Anticancer effect of lycopene in gastric carcinogenesis. *J. Cancer Prev.* **2015**, *20*, 92–96. [CrossRef] [PubMed]
48. Rao, A.V.; Rao, L.G. Carotenoids and human health. *Pharmacol. Res.* **2007**, *55*, 207–216. [CrossRef] [PubMed]

8

Serum Lutein is Related to Relational Memory Performance

Corinne N. Cannavale [1], Kelsey M. Hassevoort [2,3], Caitlyn G. Edwards [4], Sharon V. Thompson [4], Nicholas A. Burd [4,5], Hannah D. Holscher [4,5,6], John W. Erdman Jr. [4,6], Neal J. Cohen [1,2,3,7] and Naiman A. Khan [1,4,5,*]

1 Neuroscience Program, University of Illinois at Urbana-Champaign, Champaign, IL 61801, USA; cannava2@illinois.edu (C.N.C.); njc@illinois.edu (N.J.C.)

2 Beckman Institute for Advanced Science and Technology, University of Illinois at Urbana-Champaign, Champaign, IL 61801, USA; kelseyhassevoort@gmail.com

3 Center for Brain Plasticity, University of Illinois at Urbana-Champaign, Champaign, IL 61801, USA

4 Division of Nutritional Sciences, University of Illinois at Urbana-Champaign, Champaign, IL 61801, USA; cgedwar2@illinois.edu (C.G.E.); svthomp2@illinois.edu (S.V.T.); naburd@illinois.edu (N.A.B.); hholsche@illinois.edu (H.D.H.); jwerdman@illinois.edu (J.W.E.J.)

5 Department of Kinesiology and Community Health, University of Illinois at Urbana-Champaign, Champaign, IL 61801, USA

6 Department of Food Science and Human Nutrition, University of Illinois at Urbana-Champaign, Champaign, IL 61801, USA

7 Department of Psychology, University of Illinois at Urbana-Champaign, Champaign, IL 61801, USA

* Correspondence: nakhan2@illinois.edu;

Abstract: Dietary carotenoids, plant pigments with anti-oxidant properties, accumulate in neural tissue and are often found in lower concentrations among individuals with obesity. Given previous evidence of negative associations between excess adiposity and memory, it is possible that greater carotenoid status may confer neuroprotective effects among persons with overweight or obesity. This study aimed to elucidate relationships between carotenoids assessed in diet, serum, and the macula (macular pigment optical density (MPOD)) and relational memory among adults who are overweight or obese. Adults aged 25–45 years ($N = 94$) completed a spatial reconstruction task. Task performance was evaluated for accuracy of item placement during reconstruction relative to the location of the item during the study phase. Dietary carotenoids were assessed using 7-day diet records. Serum carotenoids were measured using high-performance liquid chromatography. Hierarchical linear regression analyses were used to determine the relationship between carotenoids and task performance. Although initial correlations indicated that dietary lutein, beta-carotene, and serum beta-carotene were positively associated with memory performance, these relationships were not sustained following adjustment for age, sex, and BMI. Serum lutein remained positively associated with accuracy in object binding and inversely related to misplacement error after controlling for covariates. Macular carotenoids were not related to memory performance. Findings from this study indicate that among the carotenoids evaluated, lutein may play an important role in hippocampal function among adults who are overweight or obese.

Keywords: obesity; hippocampus; nutrition; overweight; carotenoids

---

1. Introduction

Overweight and obesity are conditions that increase metabolic risk and are characterized by a body mass index (BMI) greater than 25 kg/m^2 [1]. Obesity can lead to a variety of metabolic and cardiovascular concerns such as type 2 diabetes, non-alcoholic fatty liver disease, and cardiovascular disease [1]. According to the National Health and Nutrition Examination Survey (NHANES) data from 2015–2016, approximately 40% of adults in the United States have obesity, with women having a slightly higher prevalence than men (41.1% vs. 37.9%) [1]. In addition to the cardiometabolic concerns that accompany obesity, excess fat mass or adiposity, as well as the associated metabolic complications, have been associated with poorer cognitive function and brain structure [2]. One specific brain region thought to be affected by obesity and other associated disorders is the hippocampus [2–4]. The hippocampus is a highly plastic region of the brain, which may explain why hippocampal-dependent memory function can be susceptible to behavior modulation through environmental factors [5,6]. Obesity, as well as a "western" diet characterized by high saturated fat and added sugar intake, has been related to poorer hippocampal function [3,4]. However, research examining the influence of specific dietary components on relational memory among individuals with overweight or obesity has been limited.

Relational memory is a hippocampal-dependent process that involves the flexible binding of arbitrary elements within an episode, and the subsequent reactivation of these relations [7]. In a practical sense, relational memory allows us to put a name to a face or re-tell the story of a trip in any order one chooses. One approach for assessing relational memory is to use a spatial reconstruction task. Spatial reconstruction tasks require participants to return objects to locations they have previously studied. This task design requires the participant to encode the arbitrary relationships between objects and locations (or other objects) within each trial and subsequently use these bindings to reconstruct the studied display successfully. Previous studies have shown that obesity and diet are associated with relational memory performance; however, this has not yet been thoroughly investigated [4,8].

Carotenoids have been recently found to have relevance for hippocampal-dependent memory performance [7]. Carotenoids are plant pigments that represent red, yellow, and orange color, and can be found in egg yolks and a variety of fruits and vegetables such as avocados, carrots, sweet potatoes, spinach, and other leafy green vegetables [9]. Previous studies have shown that, among the numerous carotenoids in nature, only a handful accumulate in human neural tissue. These include lutein, beta-carotene, beta-cryptoxanthin, and zeaxanthin, all of which accumulate in all cortices and the hippocampus in humans and non-human primates [10–12]. However, lutein accumulation in neural tissue is up to 5-fold greater than other carotenoids, inferring a potentially unique role for this carotenoid in cognitive function and brain health [10]. Further, lutein, its stereoisomer, zeaxanthin, and the lutein intermediate *meso*-zeaxanthin, collectively belonging to a group known as xanthophylls, selectively accumulate in the macula of the human eye. The structural properties of xanthophylls allow them to serve as blue light filters and antioxidants in the eye and protect retinal tissue from photo-oxidative damage [9,13,14]. Opportunely, the macular concentration of lutein, zeaxanthin, and *meso*-zeaxanthin can be non-invasively assessed as macular pigment optical density (MPOD) [15]. Macular xanthophylls have previously been related to brain carotenoid concentrations in non-human primates [16]. These macular carotenoids, assessed through MPOD, are also positively associated with relational memory performance in children and with intellectual ability and executive function in adults [7,17,18]. Additionally, higher MPOD scores have been associated with better memory performance assessed using a delayed recall task [11,19]. However, given that MPOD represents a composite metric of all three xanthophylls in the retina, it is incorrect to isolate carotenoid-related cognitive benefits to lutein alone. Individual carotenoid quantification in serum provides an opportunity to study the influence of lutein in a manner that would be separable from other carotenoids in vivo. While serum does not provide a direct assessment of neuronal lutein, it provides us with a more precise measure of individual carotenoids than what is determined using MPOD or dietary assessment. In previous studies quantifying serum lutein rather than the composite MPOD measure, it was shown that serum lutein mediated the relationship between the parahippocampal cortex and crystallized intelligence [20]. Serum lutein is also associated with multiple domains of cognition, including memory [11]. However, a potential limitation of relying on serum alone is that the content in serum is transient and may not reflect xanthophyll status in neural tissue. Therefore, additional studies that assess both MPOD and serum carotenoids are necessary to clarify the impact of lutein and other carotenoids on relational memory. To our knowledge, there have been no previous studies investigating associations between both MPOD and serum xanthophylls on relational memory abilities among adults with overweight or obesity. Accordingly, this study aimed to understand whether dietary, serum, or macular levels of carotenoids were associated with relational memory function in adults that are overweight and obese. We hypothesized that macular carotenoids, assessed as MPOD, would be positively associated with relational memory performance. Additionally, we anticipated that a greater serum concentration of lutein would be associated with greater relational memory performance.

2. Materials and Methods

2.1. Participants

Eligible participants were adults aged 25–45 years who were overweight or obese (BMI $\geq$ 25 kg/m^2) and no prior history of physician-diagnosed metabolic or gastrointestinal disease (e.g., Crohn's Disease, Diabetes, CVD, etc.), or neurological or cognitive disorders. Participants were also excluded if they were using any tobacco products.

2.2. Ethical Approval

At the first appointment, participants were informed of the overall procedure and written informed consent was obtained before collection of any data. The University of Illinois Institutional Review Board approved consent before recruitment, and the study was conducted following the Declaration of Helsinki.

2.3. Procedure

Data were collected over the course of two appointments. At the first appointment, participants were screened using medical history and demographic questionnaires. The second appointment followed a 10-h overnight fast. The participants subsequently underwent adiposity assessment using dual-energy X-ray absorptiometry (DXA) (Hologic, Bedford, MA, USA) and IQ was assessed using the Kaufman brief intelligence test-2 (KBIT-2). A spatial reconstruction task was administered to assess hippocampal-dependent relational memory ability. Fasted blood was collected at the conclusion of the appointment and serum lutein levels were determined using high-performance liquid chromatography. All participants were provided with a 7-day diet record to document their regular carotenoid intake, which was completed within one week of relational memory assessment.

2.4. Relational Memory Assessment

Hippocampal-dependent relational memory ability was evaluated through a computerized spatial reconstruction task (Figure 1). This task was completed using Presentation Software (Neurobehavioral Systems, Berkeley, CA, USA). Participants were first shown 6 abstract shapes in the center of the screen to introduce the shapes used for the reconstruction phase. After 6 s, the stimuli disappeared and reappeared in a randomized array on the screen. The identities of the objects were then masked by small squares and participants had 18 s to click the boxes and one-by-one learn the locations of each shape. The boxes then disappeared and, after a 2 s fixation, they reappeared at the top of the screen. Participants were instructed to reconstruct the array they previously studied. Reconstruction was self-paced and, once the participant was satisfied with their reconstruction, they moved on to the subsequent trial, for a total of 20 trials (4 blocks of 5). Each participant's performance was assessed using two error metrics: misplacement and object-location binding (Figure 2). Misplacement was calculated as the average measure of distance (in pixels) between the objects' studied and reconstructed locations, with a higher score indicating poorer performance. Object-location binding was defined as the number of times the participant correctly placed an item within a pre-defined radius around its studied location. For each trial, a participant received a score of 0–6 for this metric, with a higher score indicating better performance, and performance was averaged across trials. More detailed explanations of these error metrics can be found in Horecka et al. (2018) [21].

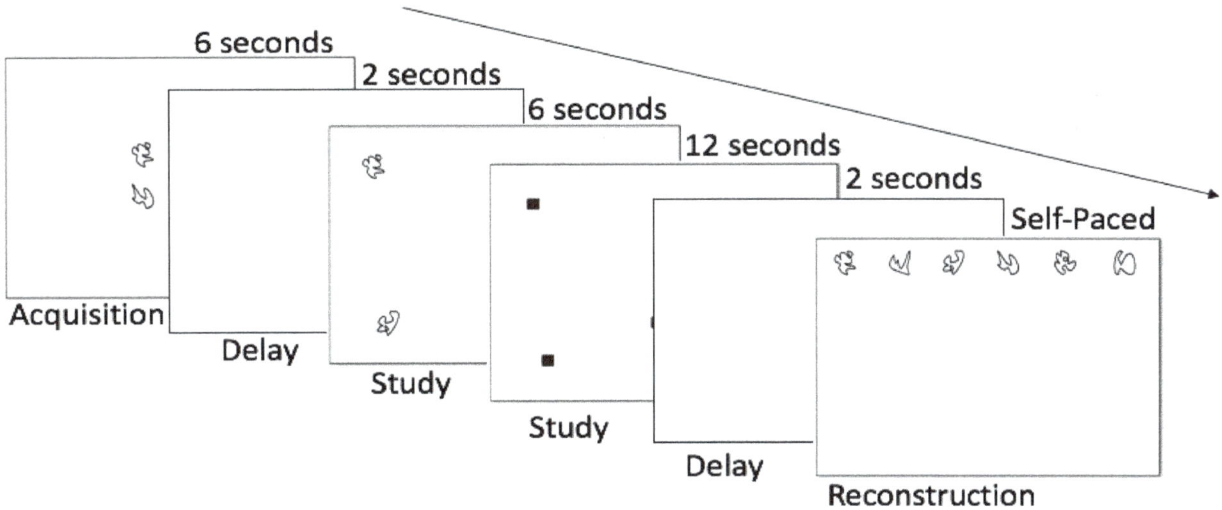

Figure 1. Spatial reconstruction task description.

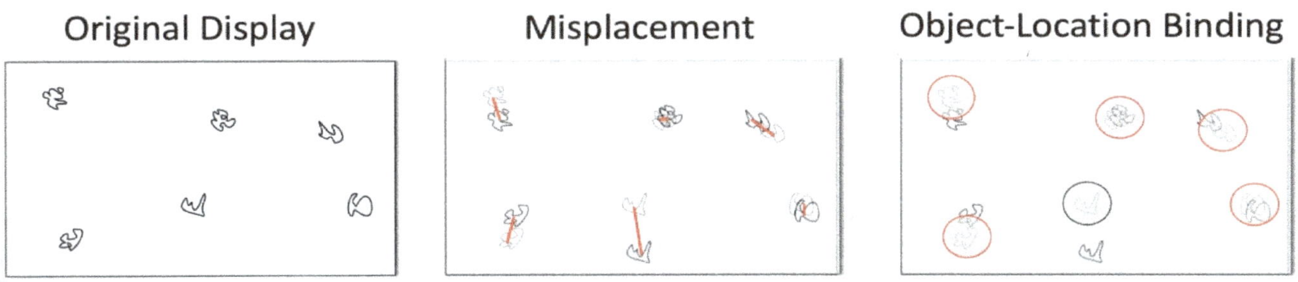

Figure 2. Spatial reconstruction task error metrics.

2.5. Intelligence Assessment

The KBIT-2 was administered by a trained staff member to estimate IQ. The assessment is comprised of 3 subtests: verbal knowledge, matrices, and riddles. Correct answers are given a score of 1 and each subtest score is then transformed to a standardized score normed for ages 4–90 years [22,23]. The verbal knowledge subtest includes 60 questions where the participant chooses which of six images is most associated with a word or question spoken by the researcher. The matrices subtest has 46 logic problems where the participant must choose an image that is most associated with a single stimulus picture or which picture best completes the pattern of a 2×2, 2×3 or 3×3 matrix. The riddle subtest consists of 48 riddles spoken by the researcher where the participant gives a single word response.

2.6. Dietary Assessment

All participants recorded regular dietary intake for 7 days in a provided food diary after instruction by a trained staff member. Diet record data were recorded and analyzed using the Nutrition Data System for Research (NDSR) 2015 (Minneapolis, MN, USA) by trained research staff. There was not enough dietary information in the available nutrient databases to extract levels of individual xanthophylls; therefore, dietary lutein and zeaxanthin were ascertained as an aggregate measure (i.e., lutein + zeaxanthin). Consumption amounts of lutein + zeaxanthin, beta-carotene, and beta-cryptoxanthin were extracted from NDSR.

2.7. Serum Carotenoid Assessment

Serum carotenoid levels were assessed using high-performance liquid chromatography (HPLC). Serum carotenoids were extracted using 3 consecutive hexane extraction processes using a previously published protocol [24]. Briefly, the hexane layers were combined, dried under nitrogen, taken up into 90% MTBE, 8% methanol, and 2% ammonium acetate in water solution (1.5% solution) and then analyzed for carotenoid concentrations using the Alliance HPLC system (e2695 Separation Module) equipped with 2998 photodiode array detector (Waters, Milford, MA, USA) and a reverse-phase C30 column (4.6 × 150 nm, 3 micron, YMC, Wilmington, NC, USA). Serum levels of carotenoids previously found in human neural tissue were assessed including lutein, zeaxanthin, beta-carotene, and cryptoxanthin.

Carotenoid standards were obtained from Carotenature, Ostermundigen, Switzerland. For quantification, standard curves were run for each carotenoid, and serum carotenoids were quantified by use of the following extinction coefficients (all 1% solution): lutein 2550 in ethanol; zeaxanthin 2540 in ethanol; beta carotene 2592 in hexane; cryptoxanthin 2565 in hexane. The Erdman laboratory routinely participates in the National Institutes for Standards and Testing micronutrient proficiency testing program, and our serum carotenoid values for blinded serum samples consistently were within 1–2 SD of the medians.

2.8. Retinal Carotenoid Assessment

MPOD was assessed using a macular densitometer (Macular Metrics Corporation, Rehoboth, MA, USA) via a customized hetero-flicker photometry (cHFP) technique). This two-step process first required participants to focus on a flickering stimulus in their central line of vision, where the macular pigment is at its highest concentration, and 7 degrees parafoveally, where the macular pigment is at its lowest concentration. The stimulus flickered between 460 nm and 570 nm wavelengths at a rate that has been optimized for the width of the null zone for the participant. Participants then adjusted the radiance to identify the point at which they could not detect a flicker (the null flicker zone). MPOD was calculated by subtracting the foveal from the parafoveal log sensitivity measurements after normalizing at 570 nm. More detailed information on the principles behind this technique were described in Wooten, et al. (1999) [25].

2.9. Weight Status and Adiposity

Height and weight were measured three times using a stadiometer (model 240; SECA, Hamburg, Germany) and a digital scale (WB-300 Plus; Tanita, Tokyo, Japan) while participants were wearing light clothing and no shoes. Mean height and weight values were used to calculate BMI. Whole body adiposity (%Fat) was measured using a Hologic Horizon W bone densitometer (software version 13.4.2, Bedford, MA, USA) DXA scanner.

2.10. Statistical Analysis

All statistical analyses were conducted using SPSS 2016 v24 (IBM Corp., Armonk, NY, USA). Normality was assessed using the Shapiro-Wilk test and variables that did not display normal distribution were log transformed. Pearson's correlations were run to determine initial relationships between hippocampal task performance, carotenoids, MPOD, Age, Sex, and %Fat. Hierarchical linear regression modeling was used to further investigate the relationships between carotenoids with statistically significant correlations to relational memory metrics. Step 1 of each regression model included covariates that were found to be significantly related to the dependent, relational memory, variable via bivariate correlations. Separate step 2′s were conducted for each carotenoid found to be related to the respective dependent variable from bivariate correlations. A one-tailed approach was used due to the positive directionality of our hypothesis and outcomes seen in the previous literature [17,18,20,26].

3. Results

Descriptive statistics for participant demographics can be found in Table 1.

Table 1. Participant characteristics and memory performance.

Variable	Mean ± SD
Sex, F/M	45, 54
Age, years	34.9 ± 6.1
BMI, kg/m^2	33.3 ± 6.6
Fat, %	40.2 ± 8.42
Intelligence Quotient	107 ± 12.1
Macular Pigment Optical Density	0.438 ± 0.20
Dietary Lutein + Zeaxanthin, mcg/day	2283 ± 3382
Serum Lutein, μmol/L	0.129 ± 0.06
Misplacement, pixels	219.3 ± 77.0
Object-location binding	2.67 ± 0.83

Bivariate correlations revealed that misplacement was positively related to age ($r = 0.33$, $p = 0.001$) and %Fat ($r = 0.19$, $p = 0.03$), and inversely related to IQ ($r = -0.37$, $p < 0.001$). Further, misplacement was negatively associated with dietary lutein + zeaxanthin ($r = -0.22$, $p = 0.02$) and serum lutein ($r = -0.25$, $p = 0.005$) concentrations. Similarly, dietary and serum beta-carotene were negatively associated with misplacement ($r = -0.24$, $p = 0.01$; $r = -0.20$, $p = 0.03$). Object-location binding was negatively related to age ($r = -0.25$, $p = 0.007$) and positively related to IQ ($r = 0.32$, $p = 0.001$). Object-location binding was not associated with %Fat ($r = -0.11$, $p = 0.1$), likely due to the decreased range of performance. Additionally, object-location binding was positively associated with dietary lutein + zeaxanthin ($r = 0.21$, $p = 0.02$), serum lutein ($r = 0.22$, $p = 0.02$), and dietary beta-carotene ($r = 0.20$, $p = 0.03$). No other carotenoids were statistically significantly related to relational memory measures in either diet or serum (all p's > 0.09).

MPOD was not related to relational memory measures (all p's > 0.4), nor was it related to dietary lutein + zeaxanthin ($p > 0.1$). MPOD was, however, related to serum lutein ($r = 0.30$, $p = 0.002$), dietary ($r = 0.20$, $p = 0.03$) and serum ($r = 0.25$, $p = 0.007$) beta-carotene, serum cryptoxanthin ($r = 0.29$, $p = 0.007$), and serum zeaxanthin ($r = 0.22$, $p = 0.017$). Bivariate correlations are summarized in Table 2.

Table 2. Bivariate correlations (Pearson's r) between relational memory, participant characteristics, and carotenoids.

	Misplacement	Object-Location Binding
Age	0.33 **	−0.25 **
Sex	−0.17	0.10
%Fat	0.19 *	−0.11
IQ	−0.37 **	0.32 **
Dietary L + Z	−0.21 *	0.21 *
Dietary Beta-Carotene	−0.24 **	0.20 *
Dietary Beta-Cryptoxanthin	−0.06	0.05
MPOD	−0.110	0.083
Serum Lutein	−0.266 **	0.223 *
Serum Zeaxanthin	−0.027	0.002
Serum Beta-Carotene	−0.202 *	0.137
Serum Cryptoxanthin	−0.103	0.076

* $p < 0.05$, ** $p < 0.01$.

Misplacement was modeled using hierarchical linear regression modeling with dietary lutein + zeaxanthin, serum lutein, and dietary and serum beta-carotene. Each carotenoid was modeled in a separate step 2. Step 1 of each misplacement model controlled for covariates that were statistically significantly related to misplacement in bivariate correlations (Age, %Fat, IQ).

Statistically significant regressions for misplacement can be found in Table 3. Serum lutein was the only carotenoid significantly related to misplacement after covariate adjustment ($\beta = -0.15$, $p = 0.05$). Dietary lutein + zeaxanthin ($\beta = -0.07$, $p = 0.2$), dietary beta-carotene ($\beta = -0.07$, $p = 0.2$), and serum beta-carotene ($\beta = -0.05$, $p = 0.3$) were no longer related after controlling for covariates in step 1.

Table 3. Hierarchical linear regression modeling of misplacement and carotenoids.

Step & Variable		β	ΔR^2
Step 1	Age	0.179 **	0.142 **
	%Fat	0.019	
	IQ	−0.363 **	
Step 2	Serum Lutein	−0.152 *	0.207 *

* $p < 0.05$, ** $p < 0.01$.

Object-location binding was modeled with serum lutein, dietary lutein + zeaxanthin, and dietary beta-carotene. Similarly, serum lutein was the only carotenoid that was still statistically significantly related to object-location binding after controlling for covariates in step 1 ($\beta = 0.16$, $p = 0.05$). Dietary lutein + zeaxanthin ($\beta = 0.10$, $p = 0.1$), and dietary beta-carotene ($\beta = 0.08$, $p = 0.2$) were no longer related to object-location binding after covariates were accounted for. This model is described in Table 4.

Table 4. Hierarchical linear regression modeling of object-location binding and carotenoids.

Step & Variable		β	ΔR^2
Step 1	Age	0.290 **	0.142 **
	IQ	−0.197 *	
Step 2	Serum Lutein	0.159 *	0.166 *

* $p < 0.05$, ** $p < 0.01$.

4. Discussion

The present work examined the relationship between carotenoids in the macula, diet, and serum, and their relationship with hippocampal-dependent relational memory performance. Given previous literature indicating that lutein disproportionately accumulates in neural tissue, including the hippocampus, we anticipated that serum and macular lutein concentrations, in particular, would be related to relational memory. Herein, the results indicated that higher serum, but not macular, lutein concentrations were positively associated with greater relational memory performance on a spatial reconstruction task. Although dietary lutein + zeaxanthin and both dietary and serum beta-carotene were correlated with performance, these relationships did not persist after covariate adjustment. Taken together, these findings provide additional evidence that serum carotenoid status may impact memory performance among adults who are overweight or obese.

There are many potential roles lutein may play in the brain. One proposed mechanism, which is relevant in our sample, is that lutein can modulate inflammatory and oxidative stress pathways [13,14]. Participants with overweight or obesity are more susceptible to oxidative and inflammatory stress due to the higher levels of chronic inflammation associated with excess adipose tissue [27,28]. Inflammation and oxidative stress can be mitigated by fruit and vegetable intake, foods that are often rich in carotenoids [27]. Inflammation is detrimental to hippocampal function, specifically by inhibiting long term potentiation, the molecular mechanism for memory formation [29]. In the retina, lutein is protective against age-related macular degeneration by reducing oxidative stress [13,14]. Thus, we hypothesize that lutein may play a similar role in the hippocampus.

Previous studies have shown that elevated serum lutein concentrations are positively associated with multiple realms of cognition, particularly in brain regions where lutein is known to deposit. A recent MRI study found that the parahippocampal cortex mediates the relationships between serum lutein concentrations and fluid intelligence [20]. Additionally, serum lutein concentrations were positively related to delayed recall memory task performance, controlled oral word association tests, and the Weshler adults intelligence scale-III similarities subtest [11]. Vishwanathan et al. did not observe similar relationships with delayed recall and serum lutein + zeaxanthin in their sample [19]. Our results in comparison to these studies indicate that lutein, in particular, may impact cognition in participants with overweight or obesity. When lutein is assessed as a combined metric (dietary, MPOD, serum L + Z), significant associations have not been found. Our results, however, display a strong association with lutein assessed independently of zeaxanthin.

Contrary to our *a priori* hypothesis, macular xanthophylls, assessed by MPOD, were not related to relational memory performance. This was surprising given previous work linking MPOD to relational memory in children, and in older adults which has shown positive associations between other memory forms (e.g., delayed recall) and MPOD [19]. However, our finding may differ from the previous literature due to the weight status of our participants. It is thought that increased adipose tissue, owing to its capacity to store carotenoids, may limit carotenoid availability for other tissues (e.g., retina), which may contribute to this disparity. Though the current body of literature has displayed positive relationships between MPOD and relational memory or executive function, these samples were mainly healthy weight [7,18,26,30,31]. Nevertheless, our team has previously shown that MPOD is associated with intellectual abilities among persons who are overweight or obese [17]. Therefore, it is possible that the relationship between MPOD and cognitive function among persons with overweight or obesity may be domain-dependent. While previous adult studies have displayed relationships with memory function and MPOD, the memory assessments used primarily assessed item-memory and therefore may not have depended on the hippocampus to the extent the spatial reconstruction task does [18,26,30,31]. Additionally, we may have failed to observe the relationship between MPOD and memory due to limitations in the technique we used to assess MPOD. Previous work has shown that, while macular pigmentation is densest at the foveal pit at two sites, we were unable to assess the complete spatial distribution of xanthophylls in the macula, thus, limiting our ability to link macular lutein to memory performance. Additional research studies examining the impact of the spatial profiles of the xanthophylls in the macula on memory function are necessary to characterize the impact of macular lutein to hippocampal function comprehensively. Nevertheless, this work suggests that serum lutein is unique among carotenoids in its relationship with memory. Future studies should assess both blood and macular carotenoids to further elucidate this relationship in a larger and more diverse population.

While we found significant correlations between memory performance and serum lutein concentrations, there are some limitations worth considering. While spatial reconstruction tasks have been shown to elicit the hippocampus, hippocampal-dependent cognition can also be assessed via other tasks/paradigms that could inform the specific memory processes that benefit from lutein. Second, relative to a previously studied Midwest sample, our serum lutein concentrations were lower when compared to the population average (0.28 μmol/L ± 0.13 versus 0.129 μmol/L ± 0.06) [32]. This, however, may be explained by the higher BMI of our sample. Finally, this study design was cross-sectional, providing no insights into the causal mechanisms that may underlie the carotenoid and relational memory relationship. Intervention studies are necessary to understand whether improvement in lutein status does, in fact, positively influence hippocampal-dependent relational memory performance.

5. Conclusions

This study aimed to understand the relationship between dietary, serum, and macular carotenoids, and relational memory. Our results revealed that serum lutein was significantly related to two metrics of relational memory performance even after adjusting for significant covariates. While this study was correlational, it lays the groundwork for subsequent research in this area. Further intervention studies where carotenoids are assessed in the macula and serum must be conducted to better understand this relationship, particularly in participants withoverweight or obesity.

Author Contributions: N.A.K., C.N.C, and K.M.H analyzed the data. C.N.C., C.G.E., and S.V.T. were involved in data collection. N.A.B., H.D.H., and N.A.K. conceived, designed, and acquired funding for the study. N.A.B was responsible for blood sample collection. J.W.E.J. supervised serum carotenoid analyses. N.J.C. and K.M.H. designed the spatial reconstruction task. All authors contributed to the writing of the manuscript draft.

References

1. Hales, C.M.; Carroll, M.D.; Fryar, C.D.; Ogden, C.L. Prevalence of Obesity Among Adults and Youth: United States, 2015–2016. *NCHS Data Brief* **2017**, *288*, 1–8.
2. Burkhalter, T.M.; Hillman, C.H. A Narrative Review of Physical Activity, Nutrition, and Obesity to Cognition and Scholastic Performance across the Human Lifespan. *Adv. Nutr.* **2011**, *2*, 201S–206S. [CrossRef] [PubMed]
3. Kanoski, S.E.; Davidson, T.L. Western diet consumption and cognitive impairment: Links to hippocampal dysfunction and obesity. *Physiol. Behav.* **2011**, *103*, 59–68. [CrossRef] [PubMed]
4. Khan, N.A.; Baym, C.L.; Monti, J.M.; Raine, L.B.; Drollette, E.S.; Scudder, M.R.; Moore, R.D.; Kramer, A.F.; Hillman, C.H.; Cohen, N.J. Central adiposity is negatively associated with hippocampal-dependent relational memory among overweight and obese children. *J. Pediatr.* **2015**, *166*, 302–308. [CrossRef]
5. Dupret, D.; Revest, J.-M.; Koehl, M.; Ichas, F.; De Giorgi, F.; Costet, P.; Abrous, D.N.; Piazza, P.V. Spatial Relational Memory Requires Hippocampal Adult Neurogenesis. *PLoS ONE* **2008**, *3*, e1959. [CrossRef]
6. Monti, J.M.; Cooke, G.E.; Watson, P.D.; Voss, M.W.; Kramer, A.F.; Cohen, N.J. Relating Hippocampus to Relational Memory Processing across Domains and Delays. *J. Cogn. Neurosci.* **2014**, *27*, 234–245. [CrossRef]
7. Hassevoort, K.M.; Khazoum, S.E.; Walker, J.A.; Barnett, S.M.; Raine, L.B.; Hammond, B.R.; Renzi-Hammond, L.M.; Kramer, A.F.; Khan, N.A.; Hillman, C.H.; et al. Macular Carotenoids, Aerobic Fitness, and Central Adiposity Are Associated Differentially with Hippocampal-Dependent Relational Memory in Preadolescent Children. *J. Pediatr.* **2017**, *183*, 108–114. [CrossRef]
8. Baym, C.L.; Khan, N.A.; Monti, J.M.; Raine, L.B.; Drollette, E.S.; Moore, R.D.; Scudder, M.R.; Kramer, A.F.; Hillman, C.H.; Cohen, N.J. Dietary lipids are differentially associated with hippocampal-dependent relational memory in prepubescent children. *Am. J. Clin. Nutr.* **2014**, *99*, 1026–1032. [CrossRef]
9. Abdel-Aal, E.-S.; Akhtar, H.; Zaheer, K.; Ali, R. Dietary Sources of Lutein and Zeaxanthin Carotenoids and Their Role in Eye Health. *Nutrients* **2013**, *5*, 1169–1185. [CrossRef] [PubMed]
10. Vishwanathan, R.; Kuchan, M.J.; Sen, S.; Johnson, E.J. Lutein and Preterm Infants With Decreased Concentrations of Brain Carotenoids. *J. Pediatr. Gastroenterol. Nutr.* **2014**, *59*, 659–665. [CrossRef]
11. Johnson, E.J.; Vishwanathan, R.; Johnson, M.A.; Hausman, D.B.; Davey, A.; Scott, T.M.; Green, R.C.; Miller, L.S.; Gearing, M.; Woodard, J.; et al. Relationship between Serum and Brain Carotenoids, α-Tocopherol, and Retinol Concentrations and Cognitive Performance in the Oldest Old from the Georgia Centenarian Study. *J. Aging Res.* **2013**, *2013*, 951786. [CrossRef]
12. Erdman, J.; Smith, J.; Kuchan, M.; Mohn, E.; Johnson, E.; Rubakhin, S.; Wang, L.; Sweedler, J.; Neuringer, M. Lutein and Brain Function. *Foods* **2015**, *4*, 547–564. [CrossRef]
13. Seddon, J.M.; Ajani, U.A.; Sperduto, R.D.; Hiller, R.; Blair, N.; Burton, T.C.; Farber, M.D.; Gragoudas, E.S.; Haller, J.; Miller, D.T.; et al. Dietary Carotenoids, Vitamins A, C, and E, and Advanced Age-Related Macular Degeneration. *JAMA* **1994**, *272*, 1413–1420. [CrossRef]
14. Kamoshita, M.; Toda, E.; Osada, H.; Narimatsu, T.; Kobayashi, S.; Tsubota, K.; Ozawa, Y. Lutein acts via multiple antioxidant pathways in the photo-stressed retina. *Sci. Rep.* **2016**, *6*, 30226. [CrossRef]
15. Beatty, S.; Nolan, J.; Kavanagh, H.; O'Donovan, O. Macular pigment optical density and its relationship with serum and dietary levels of lutein and zeaxanthin. *Arch. Biochem. Biophys.* **2004**, *430*, 70–76. [CrossRef] [PubMed]

16. Vishwanathan, R.; Neuringer, M.; Snodderly, D.M.; Schalch, W.; Johnson, E.J. Macular lutein and zeaxanthin are related to brain lutein and zeaxanthin in primates. *Nutr. Neurosci.* **2013**, *16*, 21–29. [CrossRef] [PubMed]
17. Khan, N.A.; Walk, A.M.; Edwards, C.G.; Jones, A.R.; Cannavale, C.N.; Thompson, S.V.; Reeser, G.E.; Holscher, H.D. Macular xanthophylls are related to intellectual ability among adults with overweight and obesity. *Nutrients* **2018**, *10*, 396. [CrossRef] [PubMed]
18. Renzi, L.M.; Dengler, M.J.; Puente, A.; Miller, L.S.; Hammond, B.R. Relationships between macular pigment optical density and cognitive function in unimpaired and mildly cognitively impaired older adults. *Neurobiol. Aging* **2014**, *35*, 1695–1699. [CrossRef] [PubMed]
19. Vishwanathan, R.; Iannaccone, A.; Scott, T.M.; Kritchevsky, S.B.; Jennings, B.J.; Carboni, G.; Forma, G.; Satterfield, S.; Harris, T.; Johnson, K.C.; et al. Macular pigment optical density is related to cognitive function in older people. *Age Ageing* **2014**, *43*, 271–275. [CrossRef]
20. Zamroziewicz, M.K.; Paul, E.J.; Zwilling, C.E.; Johnson, E.J.; Kuchan, M.J.; Cohen, N.J.; Barbey, A.K. Parahippocampal Cortex Mediates the Relationship between Lutein and Crystallized Intelligence in Healthy, Older Adults. *Front. Aging Neurosci.* **2016**, *8*, 297. [CrossRef]
21. Horecka, K.M.; Dulas, M.R.; Schwarb, H.; Lucas, H.D.; Duff, M.; Cohen, N.J. Reconstructing relational information. *Hippocampus* **2018**, *28*, 164–177. [CrossRef]
22. Naugle, R.I.; Chelune, G.J.; Tucker, G.D. Validity of the Kaufman Brief Intelligence Test. *Psychol. Assess.* **1993**, *5*, 182–186. [CrossRef]
23. Wang, J.-J.; Kaufman, A.S. Changes in Fluid and Crystallized Intelligence Across the 20- to 90-Year Age Range on the K-Bit. *J. Psychoeduc. Assess.* **1993**, *11*, 29–37. [CrossRef]
24. Jeon, S.; Neuringer, M.; Kuchan, M.J.; Erdman, J.W. Relationships of carotenoid-related gene expression and serum cholesterol and lipoprotein levels to retina and brain lutein deposition in infant rhesus macaques following 6 months of breastfeeding or formula feeding. *Arch. Biochem. Biophys.* **2018**, *654*, 97–104. [CrossRef]
25. Wooten, B.R.; Hammond, B.R., Jr.; Land, R.I.; Snodderly, D.M. A Practical Method for Measuring Macular Pigment Optical Density. *Invest. Ophthalmol. Vis. Sci.* **1999**, *40*, 2481–2489.
26. Renzi-Hammond, L.; Bovier, E.; Fletcher, L.; Miller, L.; Mewborn, C.; Lindbergh, C.; Baxter, J.; Hammond, B. Effects of a Lutein and Zeaxanthin Intervention on Cognitive Function: A Randomized, Double-Masked, Placebo-Controlled Trial of Younger Healthy Adults. *Nutrients* **2017**, *9*, 1246. [CrossRef] [PubMed]
27. Kaulmann, A.; Bohn, T. Carotenoids, inflammation, and oxidative stress—Implications of cellular signaling pathways and relation to chronic disease prevention. *Nutr. Res.* **2014**, *34*, 907–929. [CrossRef] [PubMed]
28. Dandona, P. Inflammation: The link between insulin resistance, obesity and diabetes. *Trends Immunol.* **2004**, *25*, 4–7. [CrossRef]
29. Dantzer, R.; O'Connor, J.C.; Freund, G.G.; Johnson, R.W.; Kelley, K.W. From inflammation to sickness and depression: When the immune system subjugates the brain. *Nat. Rev. Neurosci.* **2008**, *9*, 46–56. [CrossRef] [PubMed]
30. Lindbergh, C.A.; Renzi-Hammond, L.M.; Hammond, B.R.; Terry, D.P.; Mewborn, C.M.; Puente, A.N.; Miller, L.S. Lutein and Zeaxanthin Influence Brain Function in Older Adults: A Randomized Controlled Trial. *J. Int. Neuropsychol. Soc.* **2018**, *24*, 77–90. [CrossRef]
31. Johnson, E.J. Role of lutein and zeaxanthin in visual and cognitive function throughout the lifespan. *Nutr. Rev.* **2014**, *72*, 605–612. [CrossRef] [PubMed]
32. Curran-Celentano, J.; Hammond, B.R.; Ciulla, T.A.; Cooper, D.A.; Pratt, L.M.; Danis, R.B. Relation between dietary intake, serum concentrations, and retinal concentrations of lutein and zeaxanthin in adults in a Midwest population. *Am. J. Clin. Nutr.* **2001**, *74*, 796–802. [CrossRef] [PubMed]

9

Skin Carotenoids in Public Health and Nutricosmetics: The Emerging Roles and Applications of the UV Radiation-Absorbing Colourless Carotenoids Phytoene and Phytofluene

Antonio J. Meléndez-Martínez *, Carla M. Stinco and Paula Mapelli-Brahm

Food Colour & Quality Laboratory, Area of Nutrition & Food Science, Universidad de Sevilla, 41012 Seville, Spain; cstinco@us.es (C.M.S.); pmapelli@us.es (P.M.-B.)
* Correspondence: ajmelendez@us.es;

Abstract: In this work, the importance of dietary carotenoids in skin health and appearance is comprehensively reviewed and discussed. References are made to their applications in health-promoting and nutricosmetic products and the important public health implications that can be derived. Attention is focused on the colourless UV radiation (UVR)-absorbing dietary carotenoids phytoene and phytofluene, which are attracting increased interest in food science and technology, nutrition, health and cosmetics. These compounds are major dietary carotenoids, readily bioavailable, and have been shown to be involved in several health-promoting actions, as pinpointed in recent reviews. The growing evidence that these unique UVR-absorbing carotenoids with distinctive structures, properties (light absorption, susceptibility to oxidation, rigidity, tendency to aggregation, or even fluorescence, in the case of phytofluene) and activities can be beneficial in these contexts is highlighted. Additionally, the recommendation that the levels of these carotenoids are considered in properly assessing skin carotenoid status is made.

Keywords: colourless carotenoids; cosmeceuticals; functional foods; nutraceuticals; nutricosmetics; photoprotection; phytoene; phytofluene; public health

---

1. Introduction

Epithelial tissues like those that form the skin are essential to protect the human body from diverse aggressions. The skin is the largest organ of the human body and consists of several layers and structures. It is an essential physical barrier that protects us from the external environment (radiation, xenobiotics, microorganisms, etc.) but also intervenes in essential processes. Examples are thermoregulation, metabolism, the homeostasis of fluids, sensing, or the production of vitamin D and other important compounds [1–5].

Given its importance at different levels, damage to the skin lead to disorders of different natures that can eventually lead to diseases, for instance those derived from infections or even skin cancers, with consequent negative effects in terms of well-being and associated healthcare costs. Skin appearance is also important for individuals at various levels, since some attributes (pigmentation, colour uniformity, wrinkling, elasticity, etc.) have a significant influence on attractiveness judgements, and skin signalling has been associated to aspects ranging from mating choices to socioeconomic status [6–10].

Within this context, protection of the skin against sunlight and other sources of radiation (for example tanning lamps) is of great relevance, as excessive exposure in particular to UV radiation (UVR) can lead to photosensitivity, sunburn, photoaging, immunosuppresive effects, or even development of skin cancer, disorders with associated negative health and aesthetic outcomes [11].

The role of nutrition in skin health and appearance is undeniable and long-known. In this context, several terms are commonly used and sometimes overlap, such as cosmetics, cosmeceuticals, nutricosmetics, functional foods, or nutraceuticals. Although there is no broad standard consensus definition, the term "nutricosmetics" is associated with the oral consumption of products containing food components (e.g., vitamins, peptides, polysaccharides, polyphenols, coenzyme Q10, polyunsaturated fatty acids, and carotenoids) for cosmetic purposes. Thus, the term is clearly linked to concepts like 'beauty pills', 'beauty from within', 'beauty foods', 'nutraceuticals for skin care', or 'oral cosmetics' [5,12–14].

Carotenoids are natural dietary products ingested from foods, as additives, or from supplements, among other products [15,16]. Some carotenoids can be consistently found in human plasma, milk, and various tissues, including the skin, with major carotenoids usually being lutein, zeaxanthin, β-cryptoxanthin, α-carotene, β-carotene, lycopene, phytoene, and phytofluene [17]. Apart from their role as natural colourants, carotenoids have been important in nutrition because some of them function as provitamin A, and evidence has accumulated over the last 30 years that carotenoids may contribute to decreasing the risk of developing various non-communicable diseases including several types of cancers, cardiovascular disease, and skin or eye disorders, among others [18–21]. This is the main source of their indisputable value in the context of functional foods, nutraceuticals and related products.

The UVR-absorbing colourless carotenoids phytoene and phytofluene are rarities in the carotenoid family and have been largely ignored in studies dealing with food science and technology, nutrition, public health, and cosmetics. This is surprising since recent comprehensive reviews have indicated that they are major dietary carotenoids (found in widely consumed products, including tomatoes, carrots, citrus, and derivatives), readily bioavailable (they are present as major carotenoids in plasma, human milk, skin and other tissues) and involved in several health-promoting actions, as revealed by various studies. Notably, evidence is accumulating that they could be involved in the health benefits traditionally associated to lycopene [22–24]. Being the unique major dietary carotenoids absorbing maximally in the UV region and possessing other distinctive characteristics within the carotenoid family, research, and applications in the use of these carotenoids for the promotion of health and cosmetics is a live and expanding area recently featuring in the carotenoid field.

2. Structure and Functions of the Skin

Epithelial tissues, including the skin, are essential for survival since they protect from physical, chemical, and microbial damage and intervening in homeostasis [3].

2.1. Skin Structure

The skin is the largest organ of the human body with a surface area of 1.5–2 m^2 and accounting for about 15% of the total body weight of an adult. It is composed of epidermis, dermis, subcutaneous fat and structures like hair follicles, as well as sweat and sebaceous glands. The different layers that are distinguished in the epidermis are characterized by the state of differentiation of keratinocytes, the most numerous cells in this skin layer. The outermost epidermis layer is the stratum corneum, with a thickness of 10 μm to 30 μm. The cells in this external layer are called corneocytes and lack nuclei and cytoplasmic organelles. Below the stratum corneum there are keratinocytes (~95% of epidermal cells), melanocytes, Langerhans cells and Merkel cells [1,4,5].

The dermis is made up of ~60% water and has a thickness ranging from 0.5–5 mm depending on the location. In it, two main layers are distinguished: the papillary dermis (rich in blood vessels and nerve endings); and the reticular dermis, the main part of the dermis that is in contact with the subcutis. The main dermal cells are fibroblasts, mast cells, plasma cells, lymphocytes, dermal dendritic cells and histiocytes. The dermis also contains interstitial materials, including collagen fibres (~70–90% of the dermis dry weight), elastic tissue or ground substance (that together form part of the so-called extracellular matrix proteins complex) as well as sweat pores and hair follicles. It is estimated that in the dermis there are 1.5–6 million sweat glands, which are of two types, namely eccrine (from which most thermoregulatory sweating and sweat fluid comes from) and apocrine. Within the dermis, different types of mechanoreceptors can also be found [1,4,5].

The hypodermis or subcutis is the most internal layer of the skin and contains cells known as lipocytes. It is estimated that almost 80% of all body fat is deposited in the subcutis (in non-obese individuals) [1,4,5].

2.2. Skin Functions

The skin is an essential physical barrier that protects the body from the external environment (radiation, xenobiotics, microorganisms, etc.), the epidermis being fundamental for this function. The dermis confers mechanical strength and elasticity to the skin and the subcutis acts as insulation and mechanical protection and contributes to thermoregulation [1,4,5]

In relation to the protection against radiation, it is to be noted that the degree of light penetration in the skin is wavelength-dependent. Thus, the longer the wavelength (and the lower the energy of the radiation), the deeper is the penetration. Long wave UVA (320–400 nm) can penetrate the whole dermis but the more energetic medium wave UVB (280–320 nm) mainly reaches only as deep as the epidermis. The shortwave UVC (200–280 nm) is absorbed by the ozone layer and does not reach the Earth's surface. Visible radiation (approximately 400–770 nm) penetrates into subcutaneous tissue. [5,11,25,26] (Figure 1).

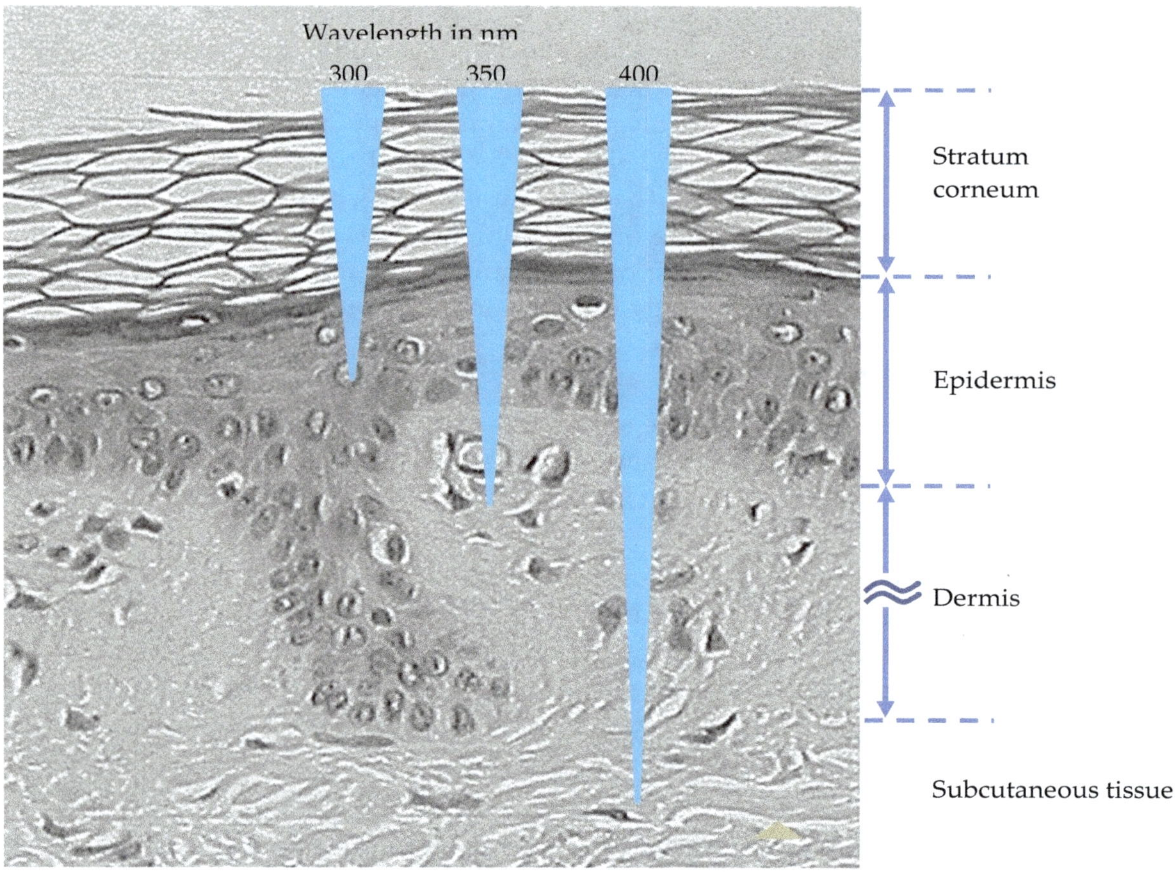

Figure 1. Skin penetration depth of different wavelenghts.

Protection against UV light is of great importance to prevent lesions of different gravity, some of which may lead to an undesirable appearance. For instance, excessive exposure to sunlight or artificial sources of UV light, a situation commonly associated with tanning, lead to adverse effects. These can be categorized into different disorders, including sunburn, immunosuppression, photocarcinogenesis, and photoaging. The latter is characterized by collagen proteolysis that results in signs such as wrinkles. Other signs of photoaging are teleangiectasia (dilated and deformed microvasculature) or hyper-pigmentation [11], all of them undesirable signs from an aesthetic point of view.

Concerning the barrier function of the skin, the stratum corneum has a prominent role as a water-proof, relatively impermeable barrier that is key in preventing the entry of diverse xenobiotics [2] However, many compounds can absorb through the stratum corneum, from which derives the existence of a wide variety of pharmaceutical and cosmetic products intended for topical application [27–30].

The skin also play key roles in vital processes such as thermoregulation, metabolism and the homeostasis of fluids. In relation to the latter, the skin, particularly the water-impermeable stratum corneum, helps reduce water loss and, therefore, dehydration. The skin also contributes to innate and adaptive immunity. For instance, substances produced in keratinocytes or derived from the sweat can exhibit antimicrobial activity against a wide variety of bacteria, viruses, and fungi. Additionally, the skin's Langerhans cells act in the immune response against threats. Regarding the role of skin in the regulation of body temperature, the regulation of body temperature and heat loss is effected by sweating and the vasodilatation and vasoconstriction of vascular plexi. Dissipation of excess heat occurs mostly through the skin, by means of the production of sweat from plasma and the subsequent heat transfer to the environment (perspiration) [1,2].

The skin is also important for sensory perception due to the presence of abundant free nerve endings and end-corpuscles. Thus, different kinds of mechanoreceptors (including Merkel's disks, Meissner's corpuscles, Ruffini's endings, Pacinian corpuscles and, in some locations, Krause's end bulbs) are present [31–33].

Skin is important for the synthesis of vitamin D and, therefore, has a role in bone synthesis, calcium metabolism and other processes associated with the vitamin. More specifically, the epidermis is considered the major source of vitamin D for humans, as ultraviolet radiation (specifically UVB) can lead to the conversion of 7-dehydrocholesterol to vitamin D. Furthermore, the keratinocytes contain the enzymes required to further convert the vitamin into 1,25 dihydroxyvitamin D, its active form. The layer of subcutaneous fat is important to provide insulation and for mechanical protection, acting as a cushion. Finally, this layer has a role as an energy reserve and in the secretion of hormones [1,4,5,34].

The properties of the skin, related to its functions and individual quality of life, are dependent on manifold factors of varying nature, such as the ones summarized in Figure 2 [4]. Most of the factors related to the individual are congenital. In this regard, it is considered that some factors, notably ethnicity and gender, influence the skin's properties to a lesser degree. The Fitzpatrick–Pathak skin type, a classification of six different types of skin based on their response to sun exposure (Table 1), has a marked impact on protection against radiation and photoaging, which features reduced hydration and elasticity. Factors dependent on the skin characteristics can vary markedly depending on the body site considered. Additionally, the presence or penetration of different substances may have a marked effect on the skin properties. Indeed, the cosmetic and pharmaceutical industries have made use of the skin's capacity to absorb such substances [4].

Table 1. Characteristics of the different types of skin according to the Fitzpatrick–Pathak classification.

		Characteristics [a]	
Skin type [a]	**Colour [b]**	**Sunburn**	**Tan**
I	White	Yes	No
II	White	Yes	Minimal
III	White	Yes	Yes
IV	White	No	Yes
V	Brown	No	Yes
VI	Black	No	Yes

[a] Based on the responses to a verbal questionnaire related to the response of the skin to initial sun exposure, i.e., three minimum erythema doses (MEDs) or about 45–60 min of noon exposure in northern latitudes in the early summer. [b] Colour of the unexposed skin. From Fitzpatrick [35].

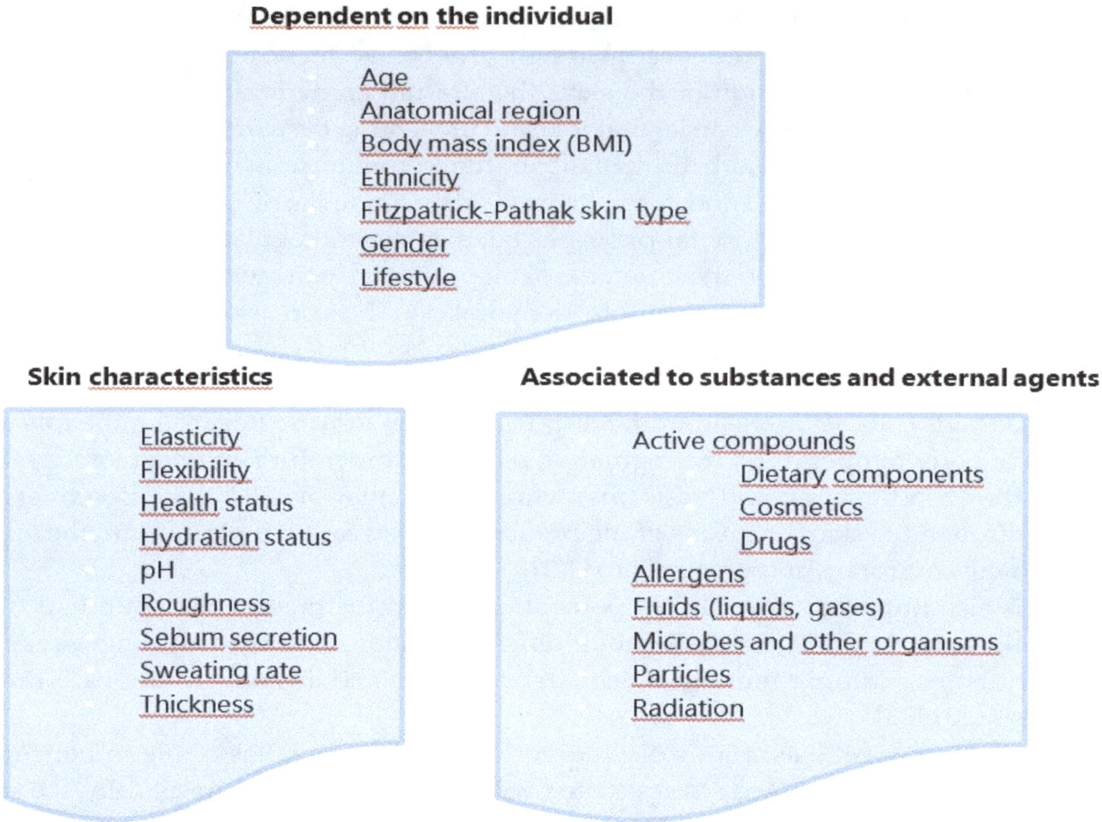

Figure 2. Factors affecting skin properties. Adapted from Dąbrowska et al. [4].

3. Skin Disorders

It is estimated that over one thousand disorders involving the skin have been described (infections, drug reactions, psoriasis, eczema, urticaria, acne vulgaris, pityriasis rubra pilaris, Darier's disease, ichthyosis, lichen ruber, and different skin cancers, including basal cell carcinoma, squamous cell carcinoma, or melanoma, etc.) and that 1/5 of all patient referrals to general practitioners involve skin pathologies. From this it can be inferred that skin disorders involve an important economic cost to both the citizens and the healthcare services [1,28].

3.1. UV Radiation Types and Consequences of Exposure

UV radiation (UVR) can be categorized into three types as a function of wavelengths, namely UVA (320–400 nm, accounting for ~95% of the UV radiation reaching the earth), UVB (280–320 nm, accounting for ~5%), and UVC (200–280 nm), the latter not reaching the surface of our planet [26].

Exposure to UV radiation may lead to the production of reactive oxygen species (ROS), a generic term used to refer to both oxygen radicals and also some non-radical derivatives of oxygen, including the deleterious singlet oxygen, $^1O_2$. This is generated from O_2 by an input of energy rearranging the electrons. Due to continuous exposure to light, this non-radical ROS may be easily formed in the skin or even the eye, where they can directly damage lipids, proteins and even DNA [36]. This compound and/or UVA are thought to be able to regulate the expression of a wide variety of genes, including genes intervening in the cell cycle, apoptosis or photoaging (such as matrix metalloproteases or heme oxygenase). UVB can also cause sunburn and lead to the appearance of mutations and skin cancer through direct interaction with DNA [11]. Interestingly, UVA light is not filtered by window glass (unlike UVB light) and it is estimated that half of UVA exposure takes place in the shade [26].

Some of the skin's mechanisms for protection against UVR are increasing the thickness of epidermis; DNA repair mechanisms; programmed cell death; antioxidant enzymes; and skin pigmentation [26]. There is also ample evidence that dietary components, among which carotenoids, may have a protective role in some cases [11,37,38]. UVR can also increase sensitivity to some drugs, e.g., corticoids, and have beneficial effects beyond the induction of vitamin D synthesis. Thus, UVR may be positive for the treatment of skin pathologies, including psoriasis, morphea, scleroderma, vitiligo, or atopic dermatitis [5].

3.2. Skin Disorders Associated to UVR

Depending on the intensity and the continuity, exposure to UVR may lead to disorders of different nature and severity, such as photosensitivity disorders, photocarcinogenesis, sunburn, photoaging, and even photoimmune modulation.

3.2.1. Photosensitivity Disorders

One example of photosensitivity disorder is erythropoietic protoporphyria. This is an uncommon inborn haematological disease that leads to increased levels of protoporphyrin in plasma, red globules, skin and faeces. Protoporphyrin is an endogenous photosensitizer. Upon exposure to light can eventually favour the formation of ROS that cause cellular damage and leads to photosensitivity clinical symptoms. Specifically, the patients experience itching, burning, and pain in the skin exposed to sunlight after even only minutes of exposure, followed by edema, erythema, and purpura [11,39–41]. Apart from porphyrins, other endogenous compounds (for instance, flavins or amino acids) act as sensitizing molecules [38].

The first classification of skin based on the skin response to the sun was based exclusively on the phenotype (hair and eye colour) [42]. However, it was soon realized that it was not fully valid since people with the same hair or eye phenotype had very different responses to the sun. Therefore, Fitzpatrick developed a new classification based on the responses of people to a brief and simple questionnaire, about the response of the skin to sun exposure. Based on this questionnaire six types of skin were eventually defined. The first four types correspond to white skins and were defined by Fitzpatrick [42]. The last two types are made up of skins that do not suffer sunburn and get suntanned after the initial sun exposure and whose colours before the sun exposure are brown (Type V) or black (Type VI) (Table 1). Types V and VI were defined by Fitzpatrick [43] and Pathak [44]. It is considered that the higher the phototype, the higher the melanin levels and the lower the risk of skin cancer [5].

3.2.2. Sunburn

Sunburn, or erythema solare, is the acute inflammatory reaction of the skin, originated by an excessive exposure to natural of artificial UV radiation. The effectiveness of UV in causing sunburn is wavelength-dependent, decreasing with longer wavelengths. In this sense it has been estimated that it takes 1000 times more UVA relative to UVB to produce the same erythemal response. Therefore, it is commonly assumed that sunburn is caused by UVB, which induces cytokine-mediated processes and neuroactive and vasoactive mediators in the skin, resulting in inflammatory responses [5].

The classical symptom of this disorder is the reddening of the skin and vasodilation of cutaneous blood vessels, although blisters and ablation of the epidermis can appear in more severe episodes. The sunburn episode occurs approximately 4 h after exposure and reaches the peak in the interval 8–24 h. Normally, it disappears in approximately one day, although the persistence of the erythema depends on age and skin type. Thus, it is considered that sunburn lasts longer (up to several days) in older individuals and those with fairer skin. Sunburn cells are keratinocytes undergoing apoptosis [11,25,26].

Minimal erythema dose (MED) refers to the minimal dose of UVB required to cause sunburn and is markedly dependent on the skin type. This parameter is used to evaluate the protection factor of sun screens [11].

3.2.3. Photoaging

The structural and functional decline of skin is categorized into two main categories, namely aging due to the passage of time (intrinsic or chronological aging) or to external factors (extrinsic aging). The latter includes skin aging due to chronic exposure to high UVR (or photoaging) and other agents, namely smoking, pollution, sleep deprivation and poor nutrition [45]. Intrinsic and extrinsic aging can be superimposed. However, chronological aging and photoaging display some differences histologically and are sometimes clinically distinguishable. Chronological aging is clinically associated with increased fragility and loss of elasticity, and photoaging with elasticity loss, irregular pigmentation, dryness and wrinkling, signs mostly derived from the degradation of proteins of the extracellular matrix and aberrations in the production of melanin (leading to the appearance of spots or irregular skin tone). Skin aging in general has an impact on manifold characteristics, processes and functions (regenerative capability, pigmentation, thermoregulation, the strength and resiliency conferred by the collagenous extracellular matrix, etc.) converging into increased skin fragility and susceptibility to diseases [2,5].

UVA has a prominent role in photoaging. This radiation favours the production of ROS that may eventually cause mutations in the mitochondrial DNA, leading to defects in the cell energy metabolism that result in further inductions of ROS. Additionally, singlet oxygen can also upregulate matrix metalloproteases directly, leading to further damage to the extracellular matrix and the formation of wrinkles and skin sagging [11,46]. Other features of photoaging include pigmented lesions (actinic lentigines or "age spots", ephelides or "freckles", and pigmented solar and seborrhoeic keratosis), teleangiectasia (a widening and deformation of the fine capillaries in skin), dryness and inelasticity. Photoaging signs are more common in locations that are more frequently exposed to UVR like the face, neck, forearms, or the back of the hands [2,11].

Besides UVR, both near-infrared (NIR, IRA: 760–1440 nm and IRB: 1440–3000 nm) and visible light (400–760 nm) may also be involved in the development of photoaging. More specifically, it is estimated that the solar radiation energy received at the surface of the Earth is divided in this way: 6.8% UV (0.5% UVB, 6.3% UVA), 38.9% VIS, and 54.3% NIR [47]. NIR can generate ROS in the skin and contribute to photoaging [48]. Analogously, visible light may also cause the generation of ROS in the skin [49].

3.2.4. Photoimmune Modulation

There is consistent evidence that excessive UVR induces a number of immunological changes to the immune system [11]. Both UVA and UVB have been shown to be able to cause local and systemic immunosuppressive effects. For example, after UVR exposure, the Langerhans cells (epidermal antigen-presenting dendritic cells produced in the bone marrow) undergo functional and morphological changes leading to their depletion. Exposure to UVR may also result in T cell tolerance [1,5,26].

3.2.5. Photocarcinogenesis

Photocarcinogenesis refers to events initiated by the exposure to solar or artificial light that eventually lead to the development of skin cancer [50]. UVB is thought to be absorbed directly by DNA, causing DNA base structural damage, for instance formation of cyclobutane pyrimidine dimers and pyramidine-pyrimidone photodimers, which may eventually cause mutations and cancer. UVA is considered to provoke indirect DNA damage through the generation of ROS resulting in single-strand breaks and in DNA–protein crosslinks. Indeed, DNA absorbs maximally in the range of UV wavelengths from 245–290 nm, implicating UVB as a primary mutagen. Overall, UVR can cause alterations in DNA integrity and homeostasis, and affect genes, including oncogenes and tumour suppressor genes [5,26].

4. Skin Beauty

From evidence referred to in different sections of this and other works, it is arguable that the skin reflects health-status as well as intrinsic and extrinsic aging. Also, that apart from serving diverse essential functions, the skin is very important in terms of beauty and appeal. Some key attributes of skin appearance (for instance colour, texture, or elasticity) have been long known to be affected by nutritional status, and even by micronutrients or other minor food components of nutritional interest. Thus, vitamin C deficiency can cause various alterations in epithelial tissues, including impaired wound healing or skin fragility, since this vitamin is involved in collagen synthesis and antioxidant protection. Furthermore, it is well-known that retinoic acid (a form of vitamin A) and derivatives modulate the expression of genes involved in cellular differentiation and proliferation at the skin level, hence their many therapeutic and cosmetic applications. Furthermore, increases of dietary intakes of fruits and vegetables may cause perceptible changes in the yellowness of the skin, whilst excessive provitamin A (usually β-carotene) or lycopene may lead to increased skin pigmentation [5,30,51–55].

4.1. Colour and Other Parameters Associated to Skin Beauty

4.1.1. Colour

The main skin pigment is melanin. However, there also exist other chromophore-containing molecules that contribute to skin colouration, including oxyhemoglobin, deoxyhemoglobin, and carotenoids [26]. The distribution of carotenoids across the different skin layers and anatomical regions is not uniform. The highest levels are usually found in the stratum corneum especially close to the skin surface [56,57]. Oxyhemoglobin and deoxyhemoglobin are especially important in the papillary dermis, which is rich in blood vessels [1]. Melanin is a term used to refer to a group of natural pigments that also confer colour to the hair. There are two types of melanin, namely, eumelanin (dark brown-black insoluble polymer) and pheomelanin (light red-yellow sulphur-containing polymer). Melanin is synthesized in melanosomes, special organelles within the melanocytes in the basal layer of the epidermis, and then distributed to surrounding keratinocytes. The biosynthesis of melanin (melanogenesis) can be induced by diverse factors (α-melanocyte-stimulating hormone, stem cell factor, endothelin-1, nitric oxide, adrenocorticotropic hormone, prostaglandins, thymidine dinucleotide, or histamine) that eventually lead to the expression of genes codifying for microphthalmia-associated transcription factor (MITF). This is a master regulator of melanogenesis that, among other actions related to melanogenesis, upregulates the melanogenesis enzymes tyrosinase (TYR), tyrosine-related protein-1 (TRP-1), and tyrosine-related protein-2 (TRP-2). Of these three enzymes, TYR is thought to be the only one exclusively necessary for melanogenesis. The amino acid L-tyrosine acts as a substrate for the enzyme and is generally transported into the melanosome by facilitated diffusion. Skin pigmentation is regarded to be one important photoprotective factor as melanin, besides functioning as a broadband UV absorbent, seems to protect against oxidation. Evidence is accumulating that UVR-induced damage and its repair are also signals for the induction of the synthesis of melanin. Many epidemiological studies point to the fact that there is a lower incidence of skin cancer in individuals with darker skin relative to those with fair skin [1,2,10,26,58].

The number of melanocytes across different ethnicities is very similar. Indeed, the differences in skin melanin-related colour are mainly attributed to the size and distribution pattern of melanosomes, their contents in eumelanin and phaeomelanin, and to metabolic and tyrosinase activity within the melanocytes. For example, there is evidence that East Asians have a yellowish skin colour due to a higher proportion of phaeomelanin to eumelanin, and a spherical rather than ellipsoidal arrangement of the clustered pigments. Likewise, other studies indicated that the most fair-skinned ethnical groups (including European, Chinese, and Mexican) have about half the amount of melanin in their epidermis in comparison to the most darkly pigmented groups (including sub-Saharan African and Indian ethnicities) and that the size of melanosomes seems to vary across these groups, so that the largest melanosomes are found in sub-Saharan African individuals, followed in turn by Indian, Mexican, Chinese, and Europeans [9].

Interestingly, independently of the ethnicity group, there is evidence that the melanin volume fraction in the epidermis is positively correlated with the mean dose of surface solar UV-radiation received at the geographical location of the group in question [9].

Skin pigmentation and colour homogeneity are well-known to have a significant influence on attractiveness judgements, above all in women, since they can convey information about age, health status and social status, with some cultural differences [6–9].

4.1.2. Other Skin Aesthetic Parameters

Physical appeal in general and facial attractiveness in particular, are well-known to be largely associated with health, mate choices, and social status, such that youthful appearance confers advantages, including socioeconomic ones. Thus, there is constant interest in skin rejuvenation, mostly of the face, which is permanently exposed and perceived by others. In this context, there is evidence in the scientific and technical literature that skin structure conducive to a youthful appearance is a very important attribute of attractiveness, along with such others as facial symmetry and proportions [8,10]. Thus, the cosmetic industry aims to fight signs impairing youthful appearance like loss of elasticity, wrinkles and folds, dryness, or pigmentation disorders (spots, uneven colour, sallowness), which are associated with aging in general [2,5,10,59].

4.2. Geographic and Ethnic Differences

Regarding aesthetic preferences, the cosmetic industry must take into account aspects as diverse as differences in preferences across ethnicities or even environmental factors. Thus, it is well-known that many Asians (above all of the east) have preference for fair skin, whereas Caucasians prefer tanned skin, which in both cases is often associated to better health or economic status. Skin tone is an attribute of beauty of current great relevance for some population groups like African American individuals, since there is evidence that skin colouration in individuals of colour has a deep impact in the way they are perceived. Thus, some studies indicate that individuals of colour with lighter skin are perceived more favourably compared to others with darker skins. Additionally, that among African Americans, African American women with lighter skin tones are perceived as more attractive than their darker skinned counterparts [60–63]. Additionally, the environmental differences across geographical regions (for instance tropical vs. temperate) have an important impact on skin characteristics (colour, photosensitivity, hydration, etc.), so that cosmetics must be conceived, designed, and customized accordingly [64].

5. Functional Foods, Nutraceuticals, Cosmetics, Cosmeceuticals, and Nutricosmetics: Definitions and Concepts

The interest of scientists, physicians, pharmacists and other professionals in the impact of nutrition on skin is not new. However, the growing interest of citizens in health-promoting products and the consequent expansion of functional foods and nutraceuticals in different industries experienced in the last 30–40 years have also had an impact on the cosmetic sector. In this context, there is a series of terms, interrelated to a greater or lesser extent, which are commonly used in those industries.

Although there is no consensus definition for the term "functional foods", at least in Europe, there is a widely accepted working definition stemming from the concerted action "Functional Food Science in Europe" (FUFOSE), as follows:

(1) "A food that beneficially affects one or more target functions in the body beyond adequate nutritional effects in a way that is relevant to either an improved state of health and well-being and/or reduction of risk of disease"; (2) "not a pill, a capsule or any form of dietary supplement"; (3) "consumed as part of a normal food pattern" [65].

Stephen DeFelice (founder of the Foundation for Innovation in Medicine, FIM) is usually credited with the coining of the term "nutraceutical" some 30 years ago. According to him "a nutraceutical is any substance that is a food or part of a food and provides medical or health benefits, including the prevention and treatment of disease. Such products may range from isolated nutrients, dietary supplements and specific diets to genetically engineered designer foods, herbal products, and processed foods such as cereals, soups and beverages" [66]. Although it refers to products at the intersection between foods and drugs (sometimes they are referred to as "pharma-foods") there is no consensus definition or legal frame for "nutraceuticals" either [67].

According to Regulation (EC) No 1223/2009 of the European Parliament and of the Council of 30 November 2009 on cosmetic products, "'cosmetic product' means any substance or mixture intended to be placed in contact with the external parts of the human body (epidermis, hair system, nails, lips and external genital organs) or with the teeth and the mucous membranes of the oral cavity with a view exclusively or mainly to cleaning them, perfuming them, changing their appearance, protecting them, keeping them in good condition or correcting body odours." [68]. The US Federal Food, Drug, and Cosmetic Act (FD&C Act) defines "cosmetics" as "(1) articles intended to be rubbed, poured, sprinkled, or sprayed on, introduced into, or otherwise applied to the human body or any part thereof for cleansing, beautifying, promoting attractiveness, or altering the appearance, and (2) articles intended for use as a component of any such articles; except that such term shall not include soap" [69].

According to Saint-Leger [70], the composite term "cosmeceuticals", which also lacks consensus definition and legal identity to date, was coined by Mr. R. E. Reed (as President of the Society of Cosmetic Chemists) in 1962. According to this allegedly first definition, a cosmeceutical was a scientifically designed product meeting rigid chemical, physical and medical standards, intended for external application to the human body, which produces useful, desired results and has desirable aesthetic properties [70].

There is no consensus definition of "nutricosmetics" either, although this term is commonly used to refer to products containing food components that are intended for cosmetic purposes and are administered orally. Thus, the term is also associated to concepts like "inside-out approach" "beauty pills", "beauty from within", "beauty foods", "nutraceuticals for skin care", or "oral cosmetics" [12–14]. Common food components used in these products are vitamins, peptides, polysaccharides, polyphenols, coenzyme Q10, polyunsaturated fatty acids, and carotenoids [5].

6. Dietary Carotenoids

Carotenoids are widespread isoprenoid compounds that appeared very early in the history of life on earth. Their structures, physicochemical properties and activities have evolved so that they play key roles in photosynthesis, communication between species through colour signalling, nutrition, and health and other processes [21,71].

6.1. Basics on Dietary Carotenoids

6.1.1. Sources and Intakes

The main dietary sources of carotenoids are fruits and vegetables [15]. However, carotenoids are also present in other components of the diet, like herbs, legumes or cereals [72], algae [73,74], foods of animal origin (egg yolk, mammals' milk and tissues, seafood) [75–79] additives (colourants) [80,81] and in the form of supplements [16,82].

The diets of humans usually contain ~50 carotenoids, although not all of them are found at detectable levels in humans [17,21]. The normal dietary intakes of major carotenoids in various countries, as recently reviewed, are within the range 0–10 mg/day [21].

6.1.2. Presence in Plasma, Other Biological Fluids and Tissues

Traditionally, it has been considered that the main dietary carotenoids are lutein, zeaxanthin, β-cryptoxanthin, α-carotene, β-carotene and lycopene. These, along with phytoene and phytofluene are usually the major carotenoids in human fluids and tissues [15,17,83–85], at typical levels in the range of 0–2 μmol/L (plasma) and 0–1 nmol/g (tissues) [84,86].

6.1.3. Health-Promoting Biological Actions

Provitamin A carotenoids are key in the fight against vitamin A deficiency, a global health problem leading to different manifestations (xerophthalmia, negative effects on growth, compromised immunity, etc.) and that is responsible for large numbers of child mortality [87,88]. In addition, evidence has accumulated over the last 30 years that carotenoids contribute to decreasing the risk of developing non-communicable diseases like several kind of cancers, cardiovascular disease, bone, skin, neurological, metabolic or eye disorders [18,19,54,89–96]. The importance of carotenoids in the context of functional foods, nutraceuticals and related products for health promotion is therefore undeniable.

6.2. The "Undercover" Colourless Carotenoids Phytoene and Phytofluene

Phytoene and phytofluene are carotenoid rarities since they are colourless. They are very important from a biosynthetic point of view because they are precursors of the rest of the carotenoids; hence, they have been thoroughly studied in relation to their biosynthesis. The typical committed step of carotenoid biosynthesis within the isoprenoid route is the condensation of two C_{20} molecules to form (15Z)-phytoene, the major geometrical isomer of this carotenoid in most carotenogenic organisms [21,97].

Surprisingly, phytoene and phytofluene have been largely ignored in food science and technology, nutrition, health or cosmetics, relative to the other major carotenoids found in human fluids and tissues (lutein, zeaxanthin, β-cryptoxanthin, α-carotene, β-carotene, lycopene). This is probably largely due to a considerable lack of analytical data compared to these latter carotenoids. This in turn is attributable to their lack of colour. Indeed, before the advent of modern detectors attached to liquid chromatography (like diode-arrays allowing the simultaneous monitoring of different wavelengths, or mass spectrometry detectors) their lack of colour made their analysis more difficult, since they absorb mainly UV radiation rather than visible light like virtually all the rest of carotenoids [23]. Currently, there is a fast-expanding interest in these colourless carotenoids because the critical analysis of the literature in recent reviews [22–24] has revealed that:

- They are present in widely consumed foods;
- Their intakes and levels in plasma and tissues are comparable (or even superior in some cases) to those of other major dietary carotenoids; and
- They are involved in biological actions that result in health and cosmetic benefits.

6.2.1. Distinctive Chemical Features among Carotenoids

The system of conjugated double bonds (c.d.b.), that is, of alternate single and double bonds, is the main structural characteristic of carotenoids. It is the main feature responsible for their physicochemical characteristics (light-absorbing properties, shape or reactivity) and activities [98]. Phytoene and phytofluene are linear hydrocarbons with three and five c.d.b., respectively (Figure 3). Since their polyene chain is markedly shorter than that of other dietary carotenoids (for instance lutein contains 10 c.d.b., zeaxanthin, lycopene and β-carotene 11 c.d.b., and astaxanthin and canthaxanthin 13 c.d.b.) (Figure 3), both colourless carotenoids are expected to exhibit important differences in some physico-chemical properties and biological actions, compared to other carotenoids [23].

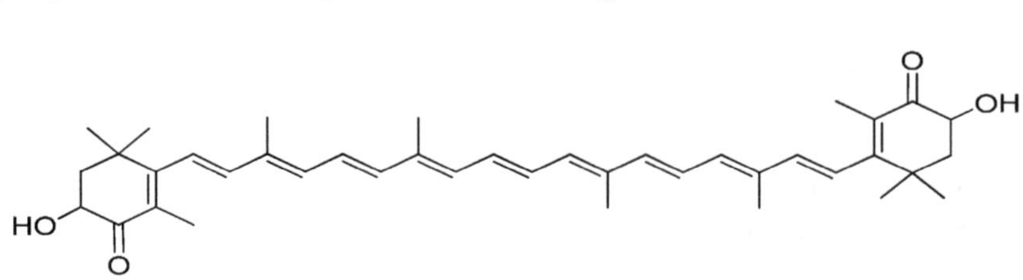

Astaxanthin (13 c.d.b.)

Figure 3. *Cont.*

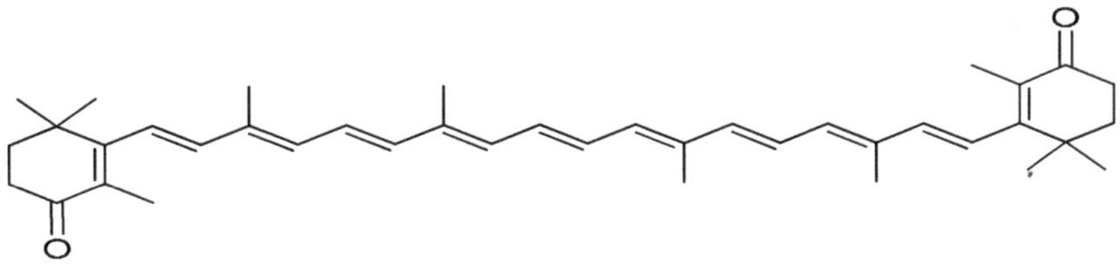

Canthaxanthin (13 C.D.B.)

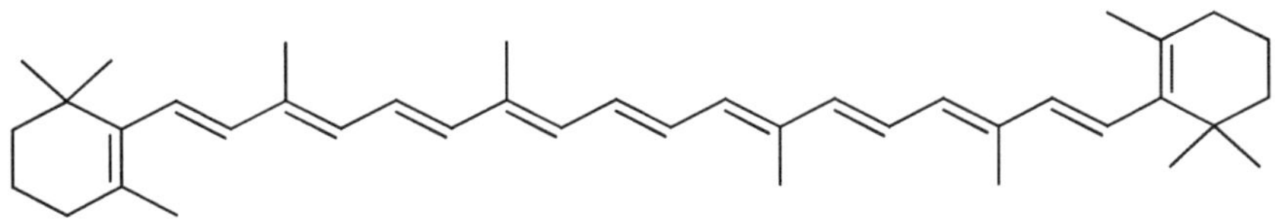

β-Carotene (11 c.d.b.)

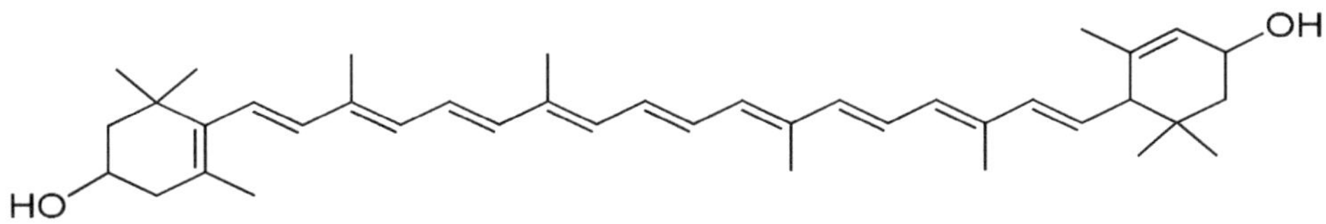

Lutein (10 c.d.b.)

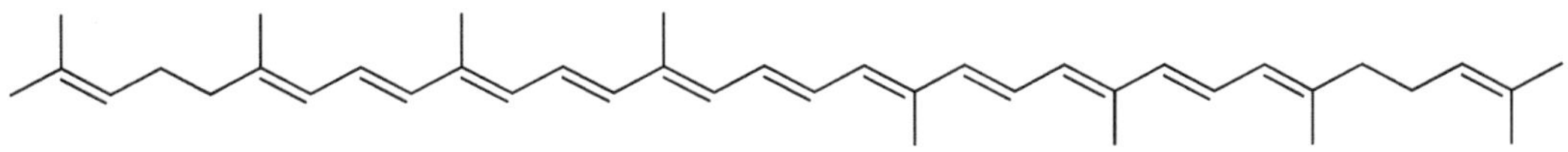

Lycopene (11 c.d.b.)

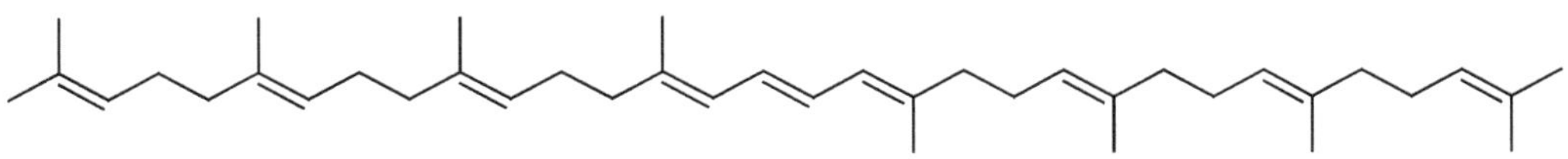

Phytoene (3 c.d.b.)

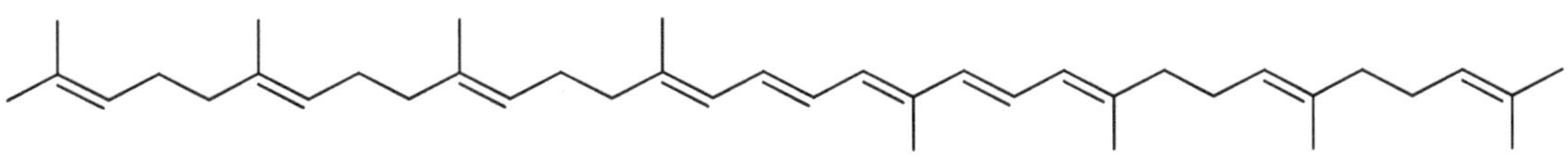

Phytofluene (5 c.d.b.)

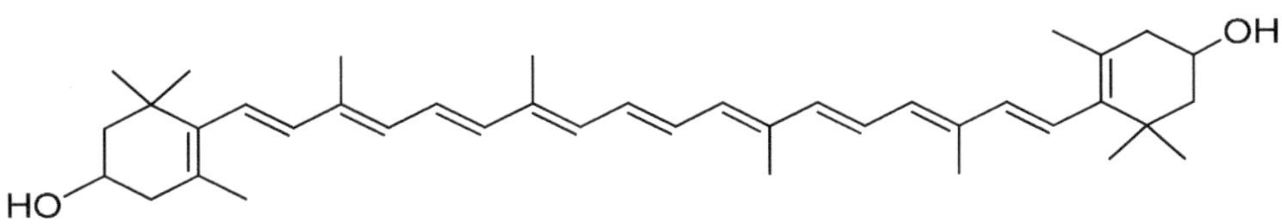

Zeaxanthin (11 c.d.b.)

Figure 3. Chemical structures of some carotenoids of interest for skin health and appearance.

UV Light Absorption

Due to their shorter polyene chain, phytoene and phytofluene absorb maximally in the UV region and are colourless (Table 2). Indeed, it is accepted that 7 c.d.b. are needed for a carotenoid to exhibit appreciable colour [99]. More specifically, phytoene absorbs maximally in the UVB region (280–320) and phytofluene in the UVA region (320–400 nm), unlike virtually the rest of carotenoids in general, including the main carotenoids being studied in relation to skin health and appearance in particular (Table 2) [23]. Their UV–VIS spectra are shown in Figure 4.

Table 2. Absorption maxima in acetone or petroleum ether, number of conjugated double bonds (c.d.b.) and colour of carotenoids important for skin health and appearance [99,100].

Carotenoid	Colour	c.d.b. (in rings)	Absorption maxima (nm)		
Canthaxanthin	Red	13 (4)		472	
Astaxanthin *	Red	13 (4)		468	
Lycopene	Red	11 (0)	446	474	504
β-Carotene	Orange	11 (2)		454	480
Zeaxanthin	Orange	11 (2)		454	480
Lutein	Yellow	10 (1)	424	448	476
Phytofluene *	Colourless	5 (0)	331	348	367
Phytoene *	Colourless	3 (0)		286	

* Absorption maxima in petroleum ether.

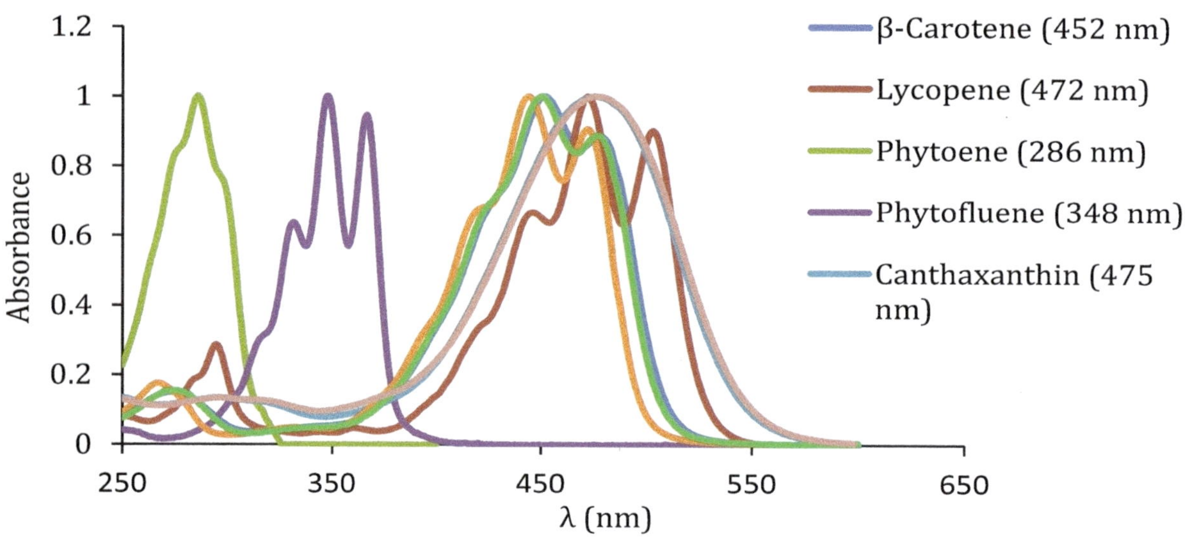

Figure 4. UV–VIS spectra of diverse carotenoids important for photoprotection and cosmetics.

The detection of phytofluene can be enhanced by its intense greenish-white fluorescence. Indeed, it is known to fluorescence at around 510 nm when it is excited with near-UV light [101,102].

Susceptibility to Oxidation

The characteristic long chromophore of c.d.b. of coloured carotenoids is thought to be closely related to their susceptibility to oxidation and antioxidant/prooxidant properties [98]. Being significantly less unsaturated, the colourless carotenoids could be expected to be more stable towards oxidation under certain conditions. In a recent study, the interaction of phytoene, phytofluene and lycopene with the synthetic oxidizing 2,29-azinobis-(3-ethylbenzothiazoline-6-sulfonic acid) (ABTS) radical cation was assessed by Density Functional Theory and ABTS radical cation decolouration assay strategies. The results suggested that the colourless carotenoids (with 3 and 5 c.d.b., respectively, Figure 3) are not as effective antiradicals as lycopene (11 c.d.b., Figure 3) [103]. Although data on the oxidative stability of phytoene and phytofluene in comparison to other carotenoids in tissues are lacking, there is evidence that they could be more stable in food matrices, for example thermally-treated tomato products [104]

Rigidity and Tendency to Aggregation

Their characteristic system of c.d.b. confer carotenoid molecules with rigidity. Since the number of c.d.b. is much lower in phytoene and phytofluene as compared to lycopene for example (another linear carotene), they are expected to adopt shapes notably less rigid relative to most carotenoids in general and lycopene in particular [23,105]. This is expected to have an important impact in terms of their release from the food matrix and incorporation into micelles ("bioaccessibility"). Bioaccessibility is one of the key factors explaining carotenoid bioavailability, since carotenoids must be incorporated into these structures to be taken up by the enterocytes prior to their transfer into the bloodstream [17,106]. In this sense, evidence is accumulating that the bioaccessibility of the colourless carotenoids is markedly higher relative to other carotenoids, probably partly due to their less rigid shape (due to their lower number of c.d.b., but also to their geometrical configuration) and they are less prone to aggregate and form crystals, which are regarded to impair carotenoid release from the food matrix [105,107,108].

Carotenoids undergo geometrical isomerization, so all-*trans* (all-*E*) and *cis* (*Z*) isomers can exist. The shapes and sizes of these isomers vary considerably (Figure 5). Thus, the former are linear and rigid and the latter have a bent shape. The geometrical isomerism in carotenoids is thought to have an impact in their solubility, tendency to aggregation, reactivity, bioavailability, or interaction with enzymes, hence the importance of discerning between geometrical isomers [85,105]. Regarding phytoene and phytofluene, it is thought that the (15Z)-isomer is usually the major isomer [102].

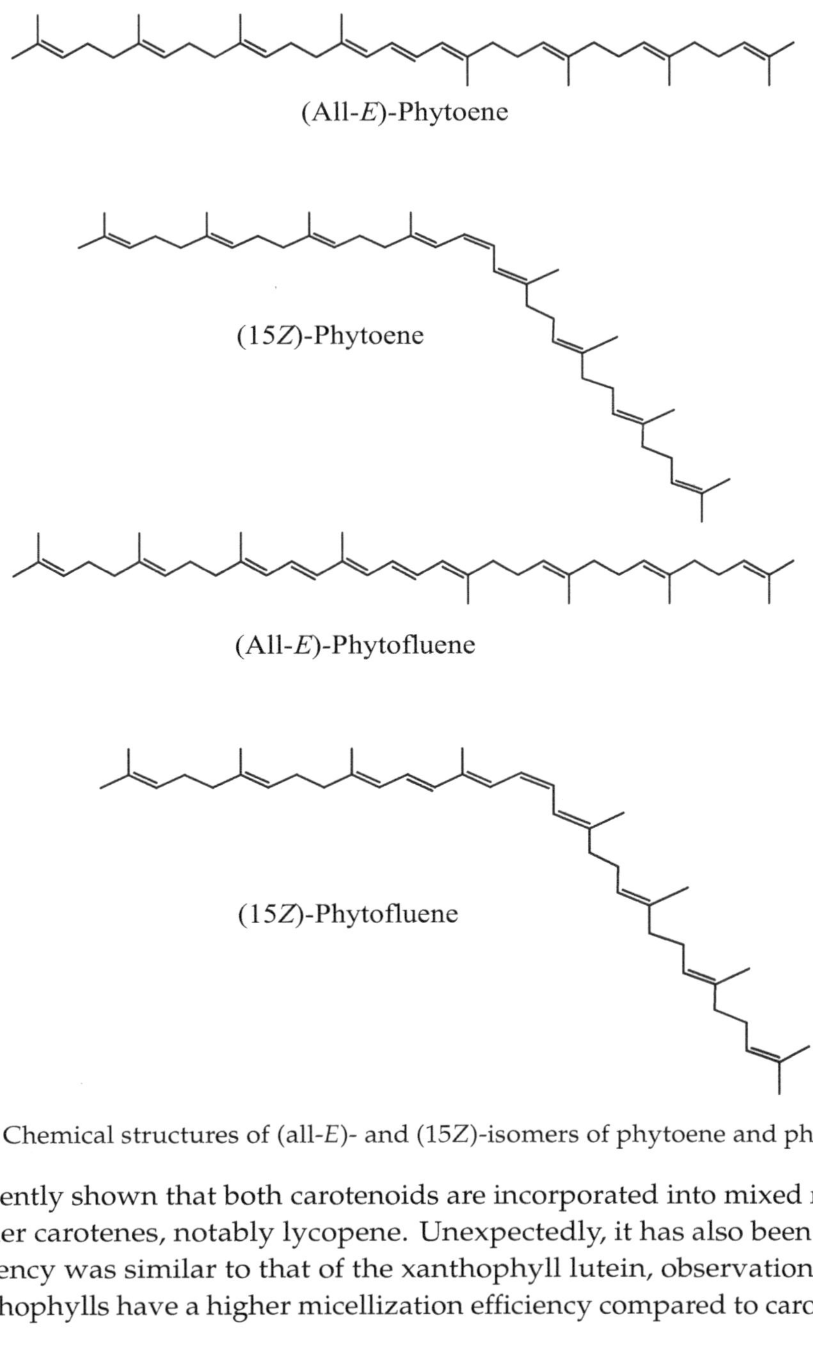

Figure 5. Chemical structures of (all-*E*)- and (15*Z*)-isomers of phytoene and phytofluene.

It has been recently shown that both carotenoids are incorporated into mixed micelles much more efficiently than other carotenes, notably lycopene. Unexpectedly, it has also been observed that their micellization efficiency was similar to that of the xanthophyll lutein, observation that challenges the paradigm that xanthophylls have a higher micellization efficiency compared to carotenes. These results have been attributed to the fact that phytoene and phytofluene were mainly present in the form of *Z*-isomers and/or to these carotenes' higher molecular flexibility, due to their shorter polyene chain [109].

6.2.2. Sources and Intakes

High contents of the colourless carotenoids are found in tomatoes, red grapefruits, watermelon (typically along with lycopene in these three cases), apricot, carrots, and some peppers. Other sources are cantaloupe, banana, melon, oranges, lemon, clementines, avocado, mandarin, nectarine, peach, and exotic fruits (caja, buriti, mamey, marimari, physalis, or gac) [23,24]. The daily dietary intakes of colourless carotenoids was recently assessed in Luxembourg, The percentage intake of phytoene+phytofluene was estimated to be 16% (2.7 mg, especially 2.0 mg for phytoene and 0.7 mg for phytofluene) of total carotenoid intake. Noticeably, the estimated daily intake of lycopene was lower (1.8 mg) than that of phytoene [110].

6.2.3. Presence in Plasma, Other Biological Fluids, and Tissues

Plasma levels of phytoene and phytofluene in the range of 0.04–0.33 μM have been reported [111–113] (Table 3). These compounds are also present in breast milk at comparable levels to the other major carotenoids (in the μg/dL range) [114]. Their presence in several human tissues (lung, breast, liver, prostate, cervix, colon, and skin) has been reported, at ng/g levels [115] (Table 3).

Table 3. Concentration of phytoene and phytofluene in body fluids (μM) and tissues (ng/g).

Body Fluid/ Tissue	Phytoene	Phytofluene	Reference
Blood	0.11 ± 0.01	0.30 ± 0.02	[111]
Blood	0.14 ± 0.08	0.14 ± 0.08	[112]
Blood	0.06 ± 0.04	0.33 ± 0.15	[113]
Blood	0.04	0.17	[114]
Breast	69	416	[115]
Cervix	-	106	[115]
Colon	70	116	[115]
Liver	168	261	[115]
Lung	1275	195	[115]
Milk	0.002	0.016	[114]
Prostate	45	201	[115]

6.2.4. Health-Promoting Biological Actions

Evidence is accumulating that phytoene and phytofluene could be involved in the health benefits traditionally attributed to lycopene, since some reviews suggest that such benefits have usually been observed when tomato products (also containing the colourless carotenoids and other compounds) rather than pure lycopene were used [116,117]. Aside from this, there are studies of different nature (in humans, animals, cell cultures, isolated lipoproteins) indicating that phytoene and phytofluene may be involved, either on their own or together with other compounds, in health-promoting biological actions such as protection against oxidation [118–120], inflammation [121–123], or anticarcinogenic activity [124–128].

6.2.5. Safety of Phytoene and Phytofluene

The safe use of phytoene and phytofluene in topical applications is backed by various evidence, namely in vitro cytotoxicity and genotoxicity studies or human in vivo 48-h patch tests and a longer-term Human Repeat Insult Patch Test [29]. The safety of oral formulations can be presumed. On one hand, these compounds are naturally present in many fruits and vegetables. Indeed, estimated daily intakes of phytoene + phytofluene of ~2.70 mg have been proposed for Luxembourg citizens [110]. Furthermore, several phytoene and phytofluene-rich products, notably tomato-derived, have been regarded as safe for human consumption by different competent bodies, including the US FDA or the European Food Safety Authority (EFSA). More especifically, several tomato products have been categorized as GRAS by the FDA, including tomato pulp powder or concentrated tomato lycopene extract [129,130]. Similarly, EFSA considers colourless carotenoid-containing tomato oleoresins safe for human consumption [131].

7. Carotenoids in the Skin

7.1. Deposition Mechanism

Regarding the delivery and distribution of carotenoids into the skin layers, there appear to be two main pathways, namely 1) diffusion from the adipose tissue, blood and lymph; and 2) secretion through sweat and/or sebaceous glands onto the skin surface and subsequent penetration [56].

Based on the observation that in untreated skin the larger carotenoid fraction is detected in the external part of the stratum corneum, it has been hypothesized that carotenoids are delivered to that location through secretions by eccrine sweat glands and/or sebaceous glands, similarly to what occurs with vitamin E [57]. In relation to this, it has been observed that, upon consumption of carotenoid-rich products, the increase in the dermal level of carotenoids occurs within 1–3 days, whereas the process of stratum corneum renewal takes 2–3 weeks [132]. According to these authors, the deposition of carotenoids in the skin surface requires their diffusion from the blood, hypodermis and the dermis to the epidermis. Then, the carotenoids would be transported from the blood, the hypodermis and the dermis into the sweat glands, and subsequently to the skin surface with sweat. This explanation is consistent with the fact that the highest levels of skin carotenoids are detected in locations with high numbers of sweat glands [132].

It is hypothesized that the subcutaneous tissue is a storage site for carotenoids and that these are loaded into the keratinocytes which are continuously formed at the basal layer and then migrate to the skin surface, transporting along the carotenoids. In this regard, the time the keratinocytes take to travel from the basal layer to the skin surface (ca. six weeks) matches very well with the time supplementation studies with carotenoids take in producing perceived photoprotection [38].

Finally, it is known that the application of carotenoids topically, results in increased levels in the stratum corneum [56].

7.2. Assessment of Skin Carotenoid Levels

To date, the two major strategies to assess dermal carotenoid levels are classical HPLC analysis and non-invasive spectroscopic methods.

7.2.1. HPLC Analysis

The HPLC analysis of skin requires the obtaining of biopsies and a suitable extraction method. Apart from the volunteer's discomfort, this is a time-consuming approach that may also lead to the oxidative loss of carotenoids. Therefore, it is not suitable for high throughput analyses or the analysis of kinetics of carotenoid levels changes in human skin. Some methodologies are found in recent studies for validation of resonance Raman spectroscopy approaches [133,134].

7.2.2. Non-Invasive Spectroscopic Methods

Resonance Raman spectroscopy (RRS) and light reflection spectroscopy (LRS), including the assessment of colour parameters from reflectance measurement are optical methods used for the rapid, almost instantaneous evaluation of carotenoid levels in skin.

They are non-invasive, so that the performance of biopsies is not required, with obvious advantages. Given that skin carotenoids are a biomarker of fruits and vegetables intake, the use of these techniques is very useful to screen large population sets for nutritional and epidemiological purposes in the context of public health. To avoid interferences from other sources of colour in skin, the measurements should be made in areas with minimal melanin content, for example the heel of the palm, the tip of a finger, or the heel of the foot. RRS is a more widely used and thoroughly validated method. LRS is an emerging alternative with some advantages, including higher simplicity, portability and the possibility of quantifying the major tissue chromophores and taking them into account to estimate skin carotenoid levels, made possible through detecting reflection over a wider spectral range, from the near UV to the near IR regions [135].

A major drawback of spectroscopic approaches relative to HPLC analyses is that the former do not take into account the levels of the colourless carotenoids. Thus, in RRS carotenoids are usually excited in the typical maximal absorption band of coloured carotenoids in the blue region of the visible spectrum. LRS results in the calculation of a score for coloured carotenoid compounds absorbing in the 460–520 nm range [135].

Light Reflection Spectroscopy (LRS)

The LRS methodology, which was first applied to the assessment of dermal carotenoids ~20 years ago [136,137] is more simple and requires much smaller devices, some of which are portable. Thus, even a low-power white lamp can be used as a light source and the carotenoid levels are derived from the reflection spectra. Currently, the LRS leads to the calculation of a composite score for all carotenoids absorbing in the 460–520 nm range. Some limitations that this methodology needs to overcome are the interference of the optical properties of the skin (related to autofluorescence, skin hydration, and sweat and sebum production), including those derived from other coloured molecules, namely melanin, haemoglobin, or oxyhemoglobin [138]. Although the technique is not as widely validated as RRS [56,135,139] its use is becoming more popular [140,141].

Another approach based on reflectance measurement consists in measuring colour parameters [135] Indeed, correlations between skin colour parameters and carotenoid levels have been recently reported [142,143]. The assessment of carotenoids from colour parameters derived from reflection spectra has also been widely used in food science and technology to estimate concentrations of a wide diversity of carotenoids [144–147], notably such as those occurring in industrially-processed orange juices, with different chromophores and functional groups [148].

Resonance Raman Spectroscopy (RRS)

Details about the basics of the technique are provided elsewhere [135,139]. RRS methods are based on the use of laser or LED light sources of narrow spectrum' and detects the characteristic vibrational/rotational energy levels of a molecule. The characteristic polyene chain of carotenoids makes them well suited for detection by this method. They are characterized by three intense Stokes lines at 1005 cm^{-1} (due to the rocking motion of the methyl group), 1156 cm^{-1} (owed to a carbon-carbon single-bond stretch vibration of the polyene chain) and 1523 cm^{-1} (carbon–carbon double-bond stretch vibration of the conjugated polyene) [56]. The Raman line intensities have been shown to have good linear correlation with the physiological skin carotenoid levels [134,135,139].

RSS has become a valuable tool for different types of studies, for instance the use of dermal carotenoids as nutritional biomarkers in diverse groups [133,149–151] or the study of associations between carotenoid status and several conditions [152].

7.2.3. Major Skin Carotenoids

It is accepted that, in general, carotenoid levels in the skin reflect those present in plasma [153]. Major human circulating carotenoids (lutein, zeaxanthin, β-cryptoxanthin, β-carotene, lycopene, phytoene, and phytofluene) have been detected in the skin, usually in the range of 0–10 nmol/g wet tissue (Table 4), although higher concentrations are detected in case of dietary supplementation or in carotenodermia [11,113,154]. The presence of other less common carotenoids (α-cryptoxanthin and anhydrolutein) has also been reported [155]. Interestingly, carotenoid esters have been found in the skin, unlike in other tissues. Indeed, it is well-known that esterified xanthophylls are hydrolyzed during digestion and absorbed as free xanthophylls [17,156,157]. Specifically, up to eighteen esters (including both mono- and di-esters) of lutein, zeaxanthin, 2′,3′-anhydrolutein, α-cryptoxanthin, and β-cryptoxanthin have been described in human skin, although at levels considerably lower (pmol/g) than those of free carotenoids [155].

Table 4. Carotenoid concentrations reported in human skin (nmol/g).

Carotenoid	Tissue	Concentration	Reference
α-Carotene	Abdominal skin	0.01	[154]
β-Carotene	Epidermis	0.39	[11]
β-Carotene	Dermis	0.01	[11]
β-Carotene	Epidermis	4.1	[11]
β-Carotene	Dermis	1.3	[11]
β-Carotene	Subcutis	3.5	[11]
β-Carotene	Surface lipid	10.0	[11]
β-Carotene	Comedones	14.5	[11]
β-Carotene	Whole skin	0.09	[11]
β-Carotene	Whole skin	1.41	[11]
β-Carotene	Punch biopsy	8.3	[11]
β-Carotene	Abdominal skin	0.05	[154]
γ-Carotene	Abdominal skin	0.04	[154]
ζ-Carotene	Abdominal skin	0.02	[154]
Lycopene	Abdominal skin	0.13	[154]
Phytoene	Abdominal skin	0.12	[154]
Phytoene	Whole skin	0.12	[115]
Phytofluene	Abdominal skin	0.03	[154]
Phytofluene	Whole skin	0.03	[115]
Total carotenoids	Whole skin	0.17	[113]

7.2.4. Factors Affecting Skin Carotenoid Levels

Obviously, there are important individual differences in the skin carotenoid levels, as a result of the manifold factors affecting carotenoid bioavailability, from dietary patterns to lifestyle and genotypic factors [17,158,159]. The skin levels of antioxidants are known to depend not only on the diet, but also on skin location or type, individual characteristics (gender, age), health status, or stress factors, both environmental and derived from lifestyle [56,132].

Diet

Dermal carotenoid levels can be increased in a relatively short time by dietary means. There is ample evidence that not only supplements, but also fruits and vegetables increase carotenoid skin levels [160–162] and that this may have a noticeable impact in terms of skin colour [55,163]. Occasionally, excessive carotenoid intake leads to carotenodermia, an apparently innocuous phenomenon featuring noticeable orange pigmentation of the skin as a result of elevated carotenoid deposition mainly in the stratum corneum, sweat, and sebum. The condition can be due to high carotenoid intake (normally of β-carotene), metabolic disorders, or familial carotenemia. It is believed that it appears when the serum carotenoid levels are in the range of 2.5 mg/L. Following the cessation of excessive carotenoid ingestion, the possible altered biochemical parameters normalize within several weeks. A similar condition due to very high intakes of lycopene has been sometimes termed lycopenemia [52,53,164].

Skin Location

Concerning carotenoids' distribution in different skin areas, there are marked differences, such that it has been reported that the highest levels can be detected in the forehead and the palm of the hands and lower concentrations are found in the back of the hands, inside the arm or in the dorsal area [57,136]. Additionally, the distribution of carotenoids across skin layers is not homogeneous.

It appears that the maximum levels are found close to the skin surface (depth of ~4–8 μm), and levels decrease at least up to the depth of 30 μm [56,57].

Individual Characteristics

There is evidence that gender and body mass index (BMI) could have an impact on dermal carotenoid status. Thus, a recent study observed higher values in women and volunteers with BMI below 30. Age did not seem to have an effect, except in the case of lycopene [165].

Stress Factors

External stress factors (e.g., radiation) or derived from lifestyle (smoking) or disease (cold, psoriasis or cancer) have been shown to have a negative impact on carotenoid levels in the skin.

Thus, in a classical study, controlled exposure to sunlight was shown to lead to noticeable decreases of circulating and skin carotenoid levels in human volunteers [166]. Exposure to visible blue-violet and infra-red light has also been shown to lead to the decrease of skin carotenoids, likely through the production of ROS [167–169]. In an interesting study the topical administration of β-carotene resulted in a protective effect [169].

As an example of lifestyle factors, it has been observed that, overall, smokers had lower levels of skin carotenoids relative to non-smokers [165].

Psoriasis is an inflammatory disease that affects the skin but can also have impacts at the nutritional level. In a cross-sectional study, it was concluded that patients with psoriasis had lower dermal carotenoid levels as assessed in the palm of the hand. However, the carotenoid levels were not significantly associated with the severity of the disorder [170].

A recent study involving 102 breast cancer patients evaluated possible associations between anxiety and skin carotenoid levels (assessed non-invasively as skin carotenoid score, SCS) as a measure of oxidative stress, since chronic stress has been associated with tumour progression, higher recurrence rates and increased risk of metastasis of this malignancy. The results indicated that higher levels of skin carotenoids were associated with decreased severity of anxiety and other miscellaneous parameters (lower body max index (BMI), higher intakes of fruits and vegetables, Hispanic race, lower educational status, and non-smoking) [171].

7.2.5. Kinetic Aspects

In a very interesting work Darvin et al. [132] evaluated the changes in the levels of β-carotene and lycopene (assessed by resonance Raman spectroscopy) in human skin over one year in relation to diet and exposure to stress factors as assessed via questionnaires. The skin carotenoid levels in all volunteers were noticed to be higher in summer and autumn, which was mainly attributed to the increased intake of fruits and vegetables and decrease occurrence of illnesses. Overall, they concluded that large intakes of fruits and vegetables clearly enhanced the levels of these two carotenoids in the skin, while stress factors (radiation, fatigue, illness, smoking, or alcohol intake) decreased them, probably in relation to the production of reactive oxygen species. The kinetics of the observed rises in carotenoid levels owed to fruit and vegetable intakes, and the corresponding decreases seemed due to stress factors behave differently. The decreases took place relatively quickly (over the course of 2h), while the subsequent recovery usually took up to three days to level. Both increases and decreases in carotenoid levels took place much faster than the subsequent return to basal levels [132].

Another study showed that skin carotenoid levels rose quickly with increased carotenoid intakes, and that such rises were useful to evaluate compliance in intervention studies as soon as two weeks after start of the dietary intervention [161]. Circulating carotenoid levels returned to baseline after three weeks, which is in good agreement with depletion studies showing decreases in blood carotenoids within 2–3 weeks. In the latter, the dermal carotenoid levels did not return to baseline until volunteers returned to their usual diets for ca. one month. The authors argued that this could be due to the fact that skin acts as a storage tissue for carotenoids. This argument agrees with the findings of other authors after a supplementation trial suggesting that the delayed drop in the skin carotenoid levels relative to those in blood may indicate a peripheral buffer function of the skin for carotenoids [172]. The study by Jahns et al. [161] concluded that skin carotenoid levels assessed by RRS was a valid biomarker of change in skin carotenoid status through fruit and vegetable consumption at recommended intake levels in the US, but with a longer half-life relative to blood carotenoids and the additional advantage that the methodology is non-invasive [161].

8. Carotenoids and Photoprotection

8.1. Carotenoids and Protection Against Light in Diverse Organisms and Locations

Carotenoids are used in photosynthesis to aid in collecting light of certain wavelengths and protecting from light-derived damage in photosynthetic organisms, including cyanobacteria, considered to be the most ancient oxygenic photosynthetic organisms and the origin of plant chloroplasts [173]. Other organisms that appeared on earth later, also used them in liaison with light: for instance, they play essential roles (quenching of excited chlorophyll or singlet oxygen, light harvesting, assembly of protein-pigment complexes, among others) in photosynthetic tissues in other organisms. Additionally, they are important for vision, including in functions beyond the role of some carotenoids as precursors of retinal for the visual cycle. For instance, some birds have carotenoid-containing oil droplets, through which light passes before reaching the photoreceptors in the retina. This seems to be a means of filtering shorter (more energetic) visible wavelengths and enhancing the sensitivity and perception of colours [174].

Strikingly, the human macula lutea, the yellow spot in the central part of the retina (with a diameter of 5–6 mm) has the highest local concentration of carotenoids in humans. This area contains the fovea (with a diameter of ~1.5 mm), which is the area with the highest visual acuity. More specifically, only lutein and zeaxanthin (in the form of two stereoisomers (3*R*,3′*R*)-zeaxanthin and (3*R*,3′*S*)-zeaxanthin, the latter of non-dietary origin and also referred to as *meso*-zeaxanthin) of the circulating human carotenoids are found in the macula lutea [175]. *Meso*-zeaxanthin is thought to be formed in vivo from lutein [176]. This selective accumulation is due to the existence of specific transporters for these two carotenoids, such as a Pi isoform of glutathione S-transferase (GSTP1) (which has been shown to be a zeaxanthin-binding protein in the human macula) [177] or a member of the steroidogenic acute regulatory domain (StARD) (which has been demonstrated to bind lutein in the primate retina) [178]. The presence of such high amounts of just two specific carotenoids in this area of the retina, where light reaches with high intensity is unlikely to be fortuitous. Indeed, the macular carotenoids are thought to be important to reduce the risk of developing age-related macular degeneration, maybe, at least in part, by absorbing blue light and, thus, protecting the photoreceptor cell layer from light-induced damage that could be initiated by the formation of reactive oxygen species during a photosensitized reaction [179]. Thus, carotenoids are important in the protection of different organisms against damage caused by light. Consequently, it is reasonable to expect that they can also have such a role in the skin, which is exposed to sunlight on a daily basis.

8.2. Sunscreens vs. Dietary Approaches

When it comes to providing protection from sunlight, sunscreens are usually the method of choice. However, dietary approaches may also be used, which entails additional benefits.

Photoprotection based on dietary components in terms of sun protection factor is regarded to be markedly lower than that achievable by using topical sunscreens. Additionally, whilst the protection conferred by the latter is virtually instantaneous, the intervention studies carried out with coloured carotenoids indicate that it takes 7–10 weeks until the protection against sunburn becomes significant. However, it is argued that the presence of dietary antioxidants and other compounds from the diet is a good and natural strategy to endow the skin with basal defences against photodamage and other aggressions that can also affect appearance [54]. β-carotene has been shown to protect against photodamage caused by visible and infra-red radiations and may be an effective antioxidant in sunscreens [49,169]. However, carotenoids are very unstable compounds, and strategies to overcome this fact are needed for the meaningful formulation of carotenoid-containing products. In this context, as a result of a study in which the topical photoprotection of β-carotene was assessed it was recommended that products intended for topical use should consist of a mixture of antioxidants reflecting those present in the skin rather than single antioxidants [169].

8.3. Mechanisms of Skin Protection by Carotenoids

Apart from possible cosmetic benefits, another great advantage of increasing the intake of carotenoids and other dietary components for photoprotection is that their levels in plasma and other tissues can also be enhanced, with consequent health-promoting benefits. There is ample evidence indicating that carotenoids contribute to decreasing the risk of developing diseases, including cancer, cardiovascular, and metabolic diseases [19,21–24].

Goralczyk and Wertz [11] identified some major mechanisms, among which inhibition of lipid peroxidation, inhibition of UVA-induced expression of heme oxygenase 1, prevention of mitochondrial DNA mutations, inhibition of metalloproteases and photoimmune modulation. Recent experiments in hairless mice subjected to UVB radiation indicated that tangerine tomato carotenoids may exert beneficial effects by attenuating DNA-damage and inflammation, with interesting differences between males and females [180]. Noticeably, new possible mechanisms are hypothesized thanks to the use of omics technologies for the study of changes in gene expressions associated to exposure to carotenoids. In any case, attribution of the effect to a single mechanism does not seem possible, and there may be connections among them in some cases [11].

Further, provitamin A carotenoids are beneficial for the skin through the production of retinoic acid, which plays important roles at this level, as do other retinoids. They are thought to intervene in processes including keratinocyte proliferation, epidermal differentiation and keratinisation, reduction of inflammation or oxidation, or even the enhancement of the penetration of agents administered topically, among many others. Thus, retinoids are applied for different purposes, for example improving wound healing, preventing skin aging or the treatment of acne, psoriasis, or other skin conditions [28,181]. However, this topic will not be discussed in detail in this review.

8.3.1. Inhibition of Lipid Peroxidation

The peroxidation of diverse lipids (importantly free and esterified cholesterol, and polyunsaturated fatty acids) by enzymatic or non-enzymatic means leads to the formation of various products that act as redox signalling molecules. They may have negative effects at the level of structures like membranes or molecules (proteins or DNA bases) that eventually lead to disease states [182].

It is well-known that carotenoids intervene by quenching singlet oxygen or scavenging free radicals, both in solution and in other systems such as membranes or cells, although they can also interact with other antioxidant and non-antioxidant compounds or even act as pro-oxidants under certain conditions [19,46,183,184]. Discussion about the protection by carotenoid-containing products against lipid oxidation is found elsewhere [185].

Interestingly, there is evidence that carotenoids may also be prooxidants depending on factors including their concentration, oxygen tension, exposure to radiation, or interaction with other compounds. The resulting prooxidant effects could be harmful or beneficial [186–188].

8.3.2. Inhibition of UVA-Induced Expression of Heme Oxygenase 1

Heme oxygenase-1 (HO1) is a ubiquitous enzyme that catalyses the first reaction in heme degradation, which eventually leads to the formation of CO, biliverdin, and Fe^{2+}. The enzyme is involved many processes related to the regulation of cell proliferation, differentiation and apoptosis [189]. The expression of the gene codifying the enzyme is inducible. As an example, it is activated via singlet oxygen within the first hours after the exposure of skin fibroblasts to UVA. Some studies in cell cultures involving mainly β-carotene in different formulations suggest that this could be a possible mechanism of carotenoid protection [11].

8.3.3. Prevention of Mitochondrial DNA Mutations

Mutations (typically a ~5000 base pair deletion usually termed "common mutation") at the level of the mitochondrial DNA, are thought to be involved in negative effects including skin chronological and UV-induced aging and carcinogenesis. Indeed, these mutations have been shown to be increased in aged skin. There is evidence from cell culture studies that β-carotene (and/or some oxidative metabolites) could protect fibroblasts by reducing the occurrence of such mutations [11].

8.3.4. Metalloprotease Inhibition

Matrix metalloprotease (MMPs) encoding genes are regarded to be among the most important genes involved in photoaging, whose expression is induced by singlet oxygen. MMPs are members of a family of enzymes (collagenases, gelatinases, stromelysins, some elastases, and aggrecanases) that catalyze the normal degradation of extracellular matrix (ECM) macromolecules including collagens, proteoglycans (aggrecan, decorin, biglycan, fibromodulin, and versican) and accessory ECM proteins like fibronectin [190].

UVR can activate cell-surface growth factors and cytokine receptors by a ligand-independent mechanism. This induces several signalling pathways that result in the stimulation of the transcription factor AP-1, which upregulates genes of several members of the matrix metalloprotease (MMP) family. This increases the proteolysis of proteins of the extracellular matrix, mostly collagen, but also fibronectin, proteoglycans, and elastin, and results in skin elastosis and wrinkling. MMPs are also thought to be important in photocarcinogenesis since they intervene in cell growth, angiogenesis and metastasis. If the high exposure to UVR is chronic, other signs, such as dilated and twisted microvasculature (teleangiectasia) or hyper-pigmentation may appear, these being clinical features of photoaging [5,11].

The use of omics technologies for the overall assessment of changes in the expression of genes in whole genomes is expanding the knowledge of possible biological actions of carotenoids and mechanistic aspects. In this sense, the results of a classical study about overall changes of gene expressions due to treatment of keratinocytes with β-carotene (at physiological dose levels, namely 0.5, 1.5, and 3.0 μmol/L) prior to UVA exposure indicated that carotenoids can act in these cells by modulating the expression of genes related to multiple pathways. More specifically, it was concluded that of the 568 genes whose expression was regulated by UV, the carotene reduced the effect of radiation for 143 and enhanced it for 180 [191]. In this sense, it would not be surprising that carotenoids protect the skin by several of the major mechanisms pinpointed. Thus, a recent study has shown that supplementation with two products containing different carotenoids (lycopene and lutein) results in the modulation of the expression of not only heme-oxygenase 1 and matrix metallopeptidase 1 genes, but also of the intercellular adhesion molecule 1 [192].

8.4. Visible Light-Absorbing Coloured Carotenoids and Photoprotection in Humans

8.4.1. Astaxanthin

Astaxanthin is a xanthophyll biosynthesized by microalgae (*Haematococcus pluvialis*, *Chlorella zofingiensis*, and *Chlorococcum* sp), the yeast *Phaffia rhodozyma* and the bacterium *Agrobacterium aurantiacum*. Animals (zooplankton, crustaceans, fish) incorporate it through the diet [193]. In general, the major dietary source for humans is salmon. Commercially, this carotenoid, which can be used as feed additive or human dietary supplement, is largely obtained by synthesis or biotechnologically from *H. pluvialis* [194]. There is evidence that astaxanthin could provide benefits at the level of skin, such as protection against erythema or reduced wrinkling [194].

8.4.2. Canthaxanthin

Canthaxanthin, which is not one of the major dietary carotenoids but is approved as a food additive in many countries, has also proven useful to treat erythropoietic protoporphyria, although its accumulation in the retina over extended use raised concern about use of this carotenoid in general [175,195].

8.4.3. Beta-Carotene

Beta-carotene is a widely distributed carotenoid found in many foods. Some important sources are carrots, palm oil, mango, sweet potato, apricot, and green vegetables [15,72]. Beta-carotene has been long known to be beneficial for the treatment of erythropoietic protoporphyria, a rare inborn haematological disease that leads to increased levels of protoporphyrins in plasma, red blood cells, skin, and faeces. Protoporphyrin is an endogenous photosensitizer. This compound, upon exposure to UVR, becomes excited, and may eventually pass on the excitation energy to O_2 in the ground state, thus generating singlet oxygen, which is a ROS that can interact with different molecules (DNA, proteins, lipids), causing cellular damage and leading to clinical symptoms of photosensitivity. Specifically, the patients experience itching, burning and pain in the skin exposed to sunlight after even only minutes of exposure, followed by edema, erythema and purpura [11,39–41,54]. The photoprotective effect of β-carotene has been the subject of several original research articles and reviews. Altogether, they indicate that it protects against erythema caused by UVR and that such protection requires daily dosages of about 10 mg for ~10 weeks [38,54,196–199]. On the other hand, a (9Z)-β-carotene-rich algal powder from *Dunaliella bardawil* has been shown to reduce the severity of psoriasis in adult patients with mild, chronic, plaque-type psoriasis as assessed by changes in Psoriasis Area and Severity Index (PASI) [200].

8.4.4. Lutein

Lutein is a widely distributed dietary carotenoid present in all green vegetables, a wide variety of fruits, and egg yolk [72,75,201]. A recent placebo-controlled, double-blinded, randomized, crossover study has shown that an intervention with lutein capsules containing free lutein stabilized by 10% of the antioxidant carnosic acid, can protect against photodamage by decreasing the expression of UVR-modulated genes, including heme-oxygenase 1, intercellular adhesion molecule 1, and matrix metallopeptidase 1 genes [192].

8.4.5. Lycopene

Lycopene is an acyclic carotenoid found in foods including some varieties of tomatoes, watermelons, guava, papaya, apricots, and grapefruits, together with other carotenoids, including the colourless phytoene and phytofluene [23,72,110,202].

Having been shown to be a quencher of singlet oxygen in vitro [203], several studies indicate that lycopene may provide photoprotection, although most of the in vivo studies have used products containing lycopene extracts (e.g., tomato paste in olive oil, diverse tomato extracts, or even a tomato-containing carrot juice) that also include other accompanying compounds (e.g., vitamin E or the colourless carotenoids phytoene and phytofluene) [204]. Being precursors of carotenoids and very close to lycopene in the biosynthetic path of carotenoids, phytoene and phytofluene are always found together with lycopene in the main sources of the latter, and also occur in other foods where lycopene is not found, such as carrots, citrus and others [23]. In this sense, the possible contribution of such components must be considered, in addition to the possibilities of interactions such as synergisms [50]. Indeed, some reviews indicate that there is little evidence of the health benefits of lycopene alone, since in most cases tomato extracts also containing other carotenoids are used [116,117]. Concerning photoprotection, this is well illustrated in an elegant study in which human volunteers received synthetic lycopene, a tomato extract or a tomato-based drink (all of them supplying virtually the same lycopene amount) for 12 weeks. The results indicated that the intervention resulted in the prevention of the UV-induced erythema formation in all groups, although the effect was more intense in the volunteers receiving tomato based products than in the group receiving synthetic lycopene alone, suggesting that phytofluene and phytoene may have contributed to the effect [113]. Recently, evidence became available that a lycopene-rich tomato product also containing phytoene and phytofluene, tocopherols, and phytosterols can provide photoprotection by inhibiting UVR-induced upregulation of heme-oxygenase 1, intercellular adhesion molecule 1 and matrix metallopeptidase 1 genes [192]

Lastly it has been recently shown in SKH-1 hairless and immunocompetent mice that male mice that received diets containing lycopene, phytoene and phytofluene and other constituents from tomatoes developed fewer UVB-induced skin tumours relative to controls [205].

8.4.6. Other Carotenoid-Containing Products

Recently, paprika oleoresin has been shown to be effective in humans in increasing MED and reducing UV-induced skin darkening. Paprika is a carotenoid-rich product obtained from red peppers containing red xanthophylls (capsanthin or capsorubin), as well as other xanthophylls (zeaxanthin and β-cryptoxanthin, among others) and carotenes (β-carotene, phytoene, and phytofluene) [72,110]. In a randomized, placebo-controlled, parallel-group comparative clinical study, daily oral supplementation with a red paprika product led to a significant enhancement of the MED and reduction of skin tanning in skin exposed to UV on the back, allegedly through antioxidant and anti-inflammatory mechanisms. At the end of the four-week study the treatment did not lead to statistically significant changes in a* (redness), transepidermal water loss (TEWL) or stratum corneum hydration (SCH) in the back area exposed to UVR, although the change in skin lightness was statistically significant, indicating that the intervention effects a change in skin colour after UV irradiation. To evaluate the effect of paprika xanthophylls on non-UV-irradiated skin, facial skin colour (L*, a*, b*), TEWL and SCH values were determined, although no significant differences were observed [206].

8.5. UV Light-Absorbing Colourless-Carotenoids (Phytoene and Phytofluene) and Photoprotection in Humans

One of the first studies pointing to the beneficial role of carotenoids in skin health concluded that injected doses of phytoene provided protection against UVR-induced erythema in guinea pigs [207]. The pioneer Mathews-Roth [208] described that the prolonged administration of phytoene to mice reduced the appearance of UV-B light-induced skin tumours and their multiplicity. Another major finding of this study was that no anticarcinogenic activity was noticed when the tumours were induced chemically.

Regarding humans, aside from studies in which products containing lycopene plus colourless carotenoids were tested, there is further evidence that they exert photoprotection. Thus, a proprietary oral food supplement in the form of a tomato powder rich in PT and PTF (Israeli Biotechnology Research Ltd., Yavne, Israel) provided to women resulted in an mean increase of 10% in the minimum erythemal dose (MED), with 2/3 of the volunteers having a 20% increase at the end of the 12-week study [209].

Possible Mechanisms

Evidence is accumulating in relation to the beneficial effects of colourless carotenoids in terms of skin photoprotection, although the mechanistic aspects are still unclear. However, there is evidence of varying nature about actions that merit further investigation.

As already commented, phytoene absorbs maximally in the UVB region (280–320) and phytofluene in the UVA region (320–400 nm), unlike virtually all other carotenoids (Table 2). Taking this into consideration, it is expected that these colourless carotenoids could provide photoprotection through the absorption of UVR [23].

Additionally, it has been reported that phytoene and phytofluene could protect against erythema and DNA damage caused by UVR and hydroxyl radicals and that they could have anti-inflammatory effects, as observed in human peripheral blood lymphocytes and in vivo in a mouse ear edema model [210]. Finally, in an in vitro study, human neonatal dermal fibroblast cell cultures were either subjected to UVR or exposed to interleukin-1 and then treated with coenzyme Q10, phytoene+phytofluene or combinations of the coenzyme and the carotenoids. The latter treatment was shown to lead to an enhanced anti-inflamatory response [122].

9. Carotenoids and Cosmetic Benefits

9.1. Carotenoids and Colour Signalling in Animals

The importance of the colour of the skin of animals or associated structures, e.g., feathers in birds, from several points of view (biological, social) is beyond doubt. Thus, carotenoid-based signals in animals advertise information about health/disease or nutritional status, genetic quality, aggressiveness, fertility, and so on [211]. For example, it is thought that male birds devoting higher levels of carotenoids to sexual-related colouration are communicating their better health [212]. Thus, according to the carotenoid trade-off hypothesis, using carotenoids for colouration prevents their use as antioxidants, such that the trade-off leads to a correlation between external colouration and health as healthy individuals can afford to use more carotenoids for colour. Contrastingly, according to the carotenoid protection hypothesis, carotenoid-based external colouration in animals could be a sign of the occurrence of other antioxidants that prevent carotenoids from being degraded by oxidation, with concomitant colour loss [59].

9.2. Carotenoids as Cosmetics

9.2.1. From Cleopatra to Tanning Pills

Curiously, humans already used carotenoids topically with cosmetic purposes long before these compounds were "officially" discovered. Thus, it is reported that Cleopatra, the famous Pharaoh of Egypt, used saffron profusely for cosmetic purposes. Saffron is a product derived from the stigmas of *Crocus sativus* that exhibits a vivid orangish colour due to the presence of high levels of the apocarotenoid crocetin associated to sugar moieties. Similarly, indigenous people from South and Central America used to paint their faces with carotenoid-rich products, like annatto. This is obtained from the seeds of *Bixa orellana*, a small tree that bears in its scientific name the surname of the Spanish adventurer Francisco de Orellana, who is thought to have "discovered" it during his travels in the Amazonian region [213].

In modern times, carotenoids in supplements have been used since the 1970s as tanning agents, especially in Northern Europe. However, the use of canthaxanthin supplements raised concerns as it was observed that, in some cases, their continuous intake at high doses (from 30 mg/day) could lead to the formation of crystals of this carotenoid in the eye—though these could disappear when the intake of the product was discontinued [16,175]. Currently, EFSA recommends lower doses, specifically the Panel on Food Additives and Nutrient Sources added to Food (ANS) established an acceptable daily intake (ADI) of 0.03 mg/kg bw/day, which is in agreement with earlier recommendations made by the Joint FAO/WHO Expert Committee on Food Additives (JECFA) and the Scientific Committee on Food (SCF) [195].

9.2.2. New Trends

Evidence that the intake of carotenoids from fruits and vegetables leads to perceived cosmetic benefits is accumulating in the last years. More specifically, the association between skin carotenoid-based colour and facial appeal has drawn attention only in the last years [59].

Dietary interventions with carotenoid-containing products leads to perceived changes in skin colour. Whitehead et al. [163] informed that self-reported increases in the dietary intakes of fruits and vegetables for 6 weeks led to increases of the CIELAB colour parameters a* and b* (regarded as estimations of redness and yellowness contributions to overall colour, respectively) in the skin. More recently, Pezdirc et al. [55] clearly demonstrated that the consumption of a diet high in fruits and vegetables by young women led to significant increases in the readings of the b* parameter in skin, consistent with increased yellowness.

In a very interesting paper, data on the contribution of melanin and carotenoids to the colouration of skin and the healthy appearance of human faces were evaluated [214]. It was concluded that the skin colour attributed to carotenoids is associated to the quality of the diet and health status and that such "carotenoid skin colouration" can be a valid cue of importance for the choice of mate [214], a situation similar to that described for other animals [211,212] Furthermore, the effect of facial skin carotenoid and melanin colouration on the perceived health was investigated. For this purpose, Caucasian participants were allowed to manipulate the skin colour of computer-generated facial images from the same racial group along carotenoid and melanin colour axes that were empirically measured. They were asked to "make the face as healthy as possible". In this survey, it was concluded that the participants chose to enhance derived "carotenoid colouration" more than "melanin colouration" to maximize apparent facial health. This, according to the authors, indicated that the colouration imparted by carotenoids had more impact on the perceived human facial health than that attributable to melanin [214].

Evidence that skin colour linked to carotenoids is preferred over that attributable to melanin in certain populations is accumulating. Thus, in a recent report Lefevre et al. [215], provides more interesting information in this respect. The authors used controlled facial images manipulated to be high or low on carotenoid or melanin colouration to evaluate not only that aspect, but also whether both kinds of pigments had an impact on the perceived appeal and if the results were dependent on the gender of the face. The results of the study indicated that, under the experimental conditions, carotenoid colouration was consistently preferred over melanin with more marked preferences for carotenoids in female compared to male faces, regardless of the sex of the judging observer [215]. More recently, it has been concluded that young Australian adults see the skin colour of the face linked with carotenoids (derived from the consumption of fruit and vegetables) and melanin (owed to sunlight exposure) as conveying a healthy appearance in young adults, although carotenoid colouration was more important to health perception [216].

9.3. The Colourless UV-Absorbing Carotenoids Phytoene and Phytofluene in Cosmetics

Given their unique characteristics as colourless UV-absorbing carotenoids, phytoene and phytofluene offer distinctive possibilities relative to other carotenoids to provide cosmetic benefits at different levels.

9.3.1. Skin Whitening by Phytoene and Phytofluene-Rich Products

An increase of the deposition of melanin in certain areas of the skin to produce dark spots and freckles is related to exposure to sun, skin disorders, aging or hormonal disorders. The importance of dark spots goes beyond aesthetic preferences since they may lead to cancer in some cases, hence the interest of using whitening agents [210]. The use of whitening agents for cosmetic and other purposes (psychological sociological, political or economic reasons) has been common in African and Asian societies, having been traced back to the 16th century in some Asian countries (India, China, Japan, or Korea). Currently, some commonly used whitening agents (corticosteroids, hydroquinone, monobenzyl hydroquinone, tretinoin, or mercury salts) raise concerns and are even forbidden in some countries due to associated side effects [217]. For example, hydroquinone at low levels (2%) has been the whitening treatment of choice for dyspigmentation, for decades, due to its ability of inhibit the activity of tyrosinase, the key enzyme for melanogenesis. However, the safety of its use raises controversies as it may cause irritation and has been associated to the possible development of malignancies [10]. In this context, the use of phytoene and phytofluene-containing products for skin whitening offers obvious advantages, including their safety, which may be assumed from their constant consumption in the human diet worldwide [29]. The use of these carotenoids for this purpose may also result in additional cosmetic and health benefits, due to their distinctive strong UV radiation absorbing properties and various attributed effects (antioxidant, antiinflammatory, anticarcinogenic [22–24].

Previous experiments with phytoene and phytofluene-rich topical formulations (IBR, Israeli Biotechnology Research Ltd., Yavne, Israel) result in skin lightening effects and beneficial effects like anti-ageing and anti-wrinkling effects [218,219]. More specifically, in a 12-week clinical study the skin whitening effect of a dietary supplementation with capsules providing 5 mg of phytoene and phytofluene per day) was evaluated in women with Fitzpatrick skin phototype IV (Table 1). In this study it was reported that a lightening effect, as assessed from increases in L* values and ITA, was observed in up to 82% of the volunteers [219]. L* is a measurement of the relative lightness of the skin, and places a given skin colour on the grey scale, between black (L* = 0) and white (L* = 100) [220], whereas ITA° is a parameter that helps assess the degree of skin pigmentation and is inversely related to skin lightness [209].

The study by von Oppen-Bezalel et al. [209] showed that, contrarily to the perceived change of skin colouration produced by other carotenoid-rich products [55,163], a tomato powder rich in colourless carotenoids (Israeli Biotechnology Research Ltd., Yavne, Israel) administered orally to women for 12 weeks at dietary achievable doses (~5 mg of PT plus PTF per day) increased MED but did not lead to statistically significant changes in the colour parameters L*, a*, and b* nor the individual typological angle (ITA°) Indeed, although the aim of the study was not to measure skin whitening (for example, women qualifying as skin phototype II were enrolled; see Table 1 for characteristics of this light phototype), the results obtained from the instrumental measurements carried out with a spectrocolourimeter revealed clear, albeit non-statistically significant, changes in L* [209]

The results of these studies using phytoene and phytofluene-rich products open the doors to the oral use of these carotenoids in nutricosmetics as whitening agents [192], for the treatment of dark spots or to cater for the preferences of certain populations (like East Asians or Afro-Americans) for lighter skin colours.

9.3.2. Effect on Other Skin Aesthetical Parameters

The photoprotective effects of the intervention described in the study by von Oppen-Bezalel et al. [209] was accompanied by perceptible improvements in skin radiance, suppleness, evenness, smoothness, moisturization, elasticity, visible skin health, visible skin youthfulness, and overall skin beauty at the end of the 12-week study. Interestingly some enhancements were already noticed after 6 weeks. Notably, the improvements in the parameters were perceived both clinically and by the human volunteers [192,209]. Evidence of skin evening and anti-wrinkling effects derived from the use of topical formulations containing phytoene and phytofluene have also been reported [218,219].

Finally, the fact that phytofluene is fluorescent may have cosmetic implications and be harnessed for the development of innovative products.

9.4. Carotenoids and Aesthetic Benefits: Public Health Implications

It is well-known that the skin tone of certain ethnicities (for instance, Caucasians) is linked to the healthiness of the diet [8,214,221]. Overall, the results of some of the studies commented in previous sections, point to the fact that individuals, including young adults, from different geographical locations show preference for skin colouration linked to carotenoids (that is, to higher intakes of fruit and vegetables, their main dietary sources) over skin colouration associated with melanin (derived from sunlight exposure), which may be harnessed to increase fruits and vegetables intakes, especially in sectors with low intakes, like young adults [214–216]. Beyond skin tone, the intake of colourless carotenoid-containing products seem to have other aesthetical benefits at the level of the skin, resulting in the self-perception of the skin as more beautiful, healthier and younger [192,209]. On the other hand, a study involving young college women indicated that nutrition educators and health practitioners should be aware that such population groups (and probably many more similar groups) are less aware of and probably less interested in the health benefits derived from increasing fruits and vegetables intakes compared with older adults. Within this context, it seems sensible that such professionals revise their strategies and focus on aspects like showing to young men and women the relationship of fruit and vegetable intake with satiety, weight and appearance [222]. In this scenario, it is not surprising that the relationships between perceived attractiveness, skin pigmentation and the intake of carotenoid-rich fruits and vegetables could be used to boost the consumption of such products as a measure to tackle unhealthy dietary patterns leading to higher risks of several diseases, as envisaged by Whitehead et al. [223,224] who argued that this new paradigm based on an "appeal to vanity" in relation to carotenoid pigmentation can be an alternative to health-based messages. One example of this would be the recommendation of increasing the consumption of fruit and vegetables to reduce the risk of developing chronic diseases [225] which, according to Whitehead et al. needs alternatives, like interventions appealing to vanity, some of which have already proven promising [224].

Whitehead et al. [223] concluded that the majority of interventions targeting appearance stressed noncompliance-derived negative effects in attractiveness. For instance, exposure to young adults of UV photographs and photoaging information (for instance effect on wrinkles and age spots) appears promising as a brief and cheap strategy to increase young adults' sun protection intentions and attitudes, which may in turn reduce their chances of developing skin cancer [226]. A new paradigm encouraging the intake of fruits and vegetables as a means to improve appearance seems promising, since showing individuals images of how their faces improve because of the dietary change is motivating. For this strategy to be viable, more studies providing empirical data about how the diet impacts the appearance are neede. For instance investigations comparing the current appearance of the individual and that achievable through better or worse dietary patterns. As already discussed, some studies indicate that individuals from different ethnicities are expected to prefer facial skin colouration attributable to increased fruit and vegetable intakes [214,221].

10. Conclusions

The protection of skin is important in the context of health as a means of preventing disorders that eventually lead to harmful conditions. Additionally, the appearance of the skin, notably the face, is an attribute of great relevance in signalling, since it conveys information with impacts at the socioeconomic level.

The role of nutrition in skin health and appearance is undeniable and long-known, hence the efforts of the industry to innovate in cosmetics, cosmeceuticals, nutricosmetics, functional foods, or nutraceuticals.

Carotenoids are natural dietary products that have been shown to intervene in health-promoting actions and whose value in the context of nutricosmetics continues to grow. From the literature it can be inferred that a diet rich in carotenoid-containing products and the avoidance of stress factors have a beneficial impact on skin health and appearance, with other likely beneficial systemic effects.

Excellent recent original studies and reviews point to the fact that the positive perceivable effects that dietary carotenoids cause in the skin may be harnessed in the context of public health. For instance, they can be used to promote healthy dietary patterns rich in carotenoid containing products as a strategy to reduce the risk of developing serious diseases, including cancer, cardiovascular disease, eye disorders, osteoporosis, or metabolic diseases.

Among dietary carotenoids, the UVR-absorbing colourless carotenes phytoene and phytofluene have been largely overlooked, probably due to their lack of colour, which made their detection more challenging in the past compared to other carotenoids. Hence, the considerable lack of abundant data about their presence in foods and tissues, in contrast with the other major dietary carotenoids found in humans. However, it is well-established that they are major dietary carotenoids (found in products frequently consumed as tomatoes, carrots, citrus, and derivatives), present in plasma, human milk, skin, and other tissues, and involved in several health-promoting actions, as revealed by studies of different nature. Notably, evidence is accumulating that they could be involved in the health benefits traditionally associated to lycopene, since the latter seems to always occur along with the colourless carotenoids in foods. Being the unique major dietary carotenoids absorbing maximally in the UV region and possessing other distinctive characteristics within the carotenoid family, research and applications in the use of these carotenoids in the promotion of health and cosmetics is a timely and expanding area recently featuring in the carotenoid field.

Future studies should devote attention to generating more data about phytoene and phytofluene skin levels in order to provide accurate information about skin carotenoid status, since mainly coloured carotenoids are currently being considered. Additionally, mechanistic studies about the beneficial effects of colourless carotenoids in the skin (whitening, improvement of aging signs, etc.) are needed.

Acknowledgments: Research on colourless carotenoids by A.J.M.M.'s team has been funded by the Andalusian Council of Economy, Innovation, Science and Employment (ref. CAROTINCO-P12-AGR-1287), the Spanish State Secretariat of Research, Development and Innovation (Ministry of Economy and Competitiveness, project ref. AGL2012-37610, co-funded by FEDER, Carotenoid Network: from microbia and plants to food and health, CaRed, BIO2015-71703-REDT), CaRed: Spanish carotenoid network (BIO2017-90877-REDT) and IBR—Israeli Biotechnology Research, Ltd. The publication costs were covered by IBR—Israeli Biotechnology Research, Ltd.

References

1. Lai-Cheong, J.E.; McGrath, J.A. Structure and function of skin, hair and nails. *Medicine (Baltimore).* **2017**, *45*, 347–351. [CrossRef]
2. Rittie, L.; Fisher, G.J.; Rittié, L.; Fisher, G.J. Natural and sun-induced aging of human skin. *Cold Spring Harb. Perspect. Med.* **2015**, *5*, a015370. [CrossRef] [PubMed]
3. Presland, R.B.; Dale, B.A. Epithelial Structural Proteins of the Skin and Oral Cavity: Function in Health and Disease. *Crit. Rev. Oral Biol. Med.* **2000**, *11*, 383–408. [CrossRef] [PubMed]
4. Dąbrowska, A.K.; Spano, F.; Derler, S.; Adlhart, C.; Spencer, N.D.; Rossi, R.M. The relationship between skin function, barrier properties, and body-dependent factors. *Ski. Res. Technol.* **2018**, *24*, 165–174. [CrossRef]
5. Pérez-Sánchez, A.; Barrajón-Catalán, E.; Herranz-López, M.; Micol, V. Nutraceuticals for skin care: A comprehensive review of human clinical studies. *Nutrients* **2018**, *10*, 403. [CrossRef]
6. Fink, B.; Grammer, K.; Matts, P.J. Visible skin color distribution plays a role in the perception of age, attractiveness, and health in female faces. *Evol. Hum. Behav.* **2006**, *27*, 433–442. [CrossRef]
7. Matts, P.J.; Fink, B.; Grammer, K.; Burquest, M. Color homogeneity and visual perception of age, health, and attractiveness of female facial skin. *J. Am. Acad. Dermatol.* **2007**, *57*, 977–984. [CrossRef]
8. Little, A.C.; Jones, B.C.; Debruine, L.M. Facial attractiveness: Evolutionary based research. *Philos. Trans. R. Soc. B Biol. Sci.* **2011**, *366*, 1638–1659. [CrossRef] [PubMed]
9. Samson, N.; Fink, B.; Matts, P.J. Visible skin condition and perception of human facial appearance. *Int. J. Cosmet. Sci.* **2010**, *32*, 167–184. [CrossRef]
10. Lee, C.-M. Fifty years of research and development of cosmeceuticals: A contemporary review. *J. Cosmet. Dermatol.* **2016**, *15*, 527–539. [CrossRef] [PubMed]
11. Goralczyk, R.; Wertz, K. Skin Photoprotection by Carotenoids. In *Carotenoids. Volume 5. Nutrition and Health*; Britton, G., Liaaen-Jensen, S., Pfander, H., Eds.; Birkhäuser: Basel, Switzerland, 2009; pp. 335–362, ISBN 978-3-7643-7501-0.
12. Draelos, Z.D. Nutrition and enhancing youthful-appearing skin. *Clin. Dermatol.* **2010**, *28*, 400–408. [CrossRef]
13. Anunciato, T.P.; da Rocha Filho, P.A. Carotenoids and polyphenols in nutricosmetics, nutraceuticals, and cosmeceuticals. *J. Cosmet. Dermatol.* **2012**, *11*, 51–54. [CrossRef]
14. Madhere, S.; Simpson, P. A market overview of nutricosmetics. *Cosmet. Dermatology* **2010**, *23*, 268–274.
15. Britton, G.; Khachik, F. Carotenoids in Food. In *Carotenoids. Volume 5: Nutrition and Health*; Britton, G., Liaaen-Jensen, S., Pfander, H., Eds.; Birkhäuser: Basel, Switzerland, 2009; pp. 45–66, ISBN 978-3-7643-7501-0.
16. Mortensen, A. Supplements. In *Carotenoids: Volume 5: Nutrition and Health*; Britton, G., Pfander, H., Liaaen-Jensen, S., Eds.; Birkhäuser: Basel, Switzerland, 2009; pp. 67–82, ISBN 978-3-7643-7501-0.
17. Meléndez-Martínez, A.J.; Pérez-Gálvez, A.; Roca, M.; Estévez Santiago, R.; Olmedilla Alonso, B.; Mercadante, A.Z.; Jesús Ornelas-Paz, J.D. Biodisponibilidad de carotenoides, factores que la determinan y métodos de estimación. In *Carotenoides en Agroalimentación y Salud*; Meléndez-Martínez, A.J., Ed.; Editorial Terracota: Ciudad de México, México, 2017; pp. 574–608, ISBN 978-84-15413-35-6.

18. Britton, G.; Liaaen-Jensen, S.; Pfander, H. *Carotenoids. Volume 5: Nutrition and Health*; Birkhäuser: Basel, Switzerland, 2009; ISBN 978-3-7643-7501-0.
19. Krinsky, N.I.; Johnson, E.J. Carotenoid actions and their relation to health and disease. *Mol. Aspects Med.* **2005**, *26*, 459–516. [CrossRef] [PubMed]
20. Krinsky, N.; Mayne, S.T.; Sies, H. *Carotenoids in Health and Disease*; Marcel Dekker: New York, NY, USA, 2004.
21. Rodriguez-Concepcion, M.; Avalos, J.; Bonet, M.L.; Boronat, A.; Gomez-Gomez, L.; Hornero-Mendez, D.; Limon, M.C.; Meléndez-Martínez, A.J.; Olmedilla-Alonso, B.; Palou, A.; et al. A global perspective on carotenoids: Metabolism, biotechnology, and benefits for nutrition and health. *Prog. Lipid Res.* **2018**, *70*, 62–93. [CrossRef]
22. Engelmann, N.J.; Clinton, S.K.; Erdman, J.W. Nutritional aspects of phytoene and phytofluene, carotenoid precursors to lycopene. *Adv. Nutr.* **2011**, *2*, 51–61. [CrossRef]
23. Meléndez-Martínez, A.J.; Mapelli-Brahm, P.; Benítez-González, A.; Stinco, C.M. A comprehensive review on the colorless carotenoids phytoene and phytofluene. *Arch. Biochem. Biophys.* **2015**, *572*, 188–200. [CrossRef] [PubMed]
24. Meléndez-Martínez, A.J.; Mapelli-Brahm, P.; Stinco, C.M. The colourless carotenoids phytoene and phytofluene: From dietary sources to their usefulness for the functional foods and nutricosmetics industries. *J. Food Compos. Anal.* **2018**, *67*, 91–103. [CrossRef]
25. De Spirt, S.; Lutter, K.; Stahl, W. Carotenoids in Photooxidative Stress. *Curr. Nutr. Food Sci.* **2010**, *6*, 36–43. [CrossRef]
26. Brenner, M.; Hearing, V.J.V.J. The protective role of melanin against UV damage in human skin. *Photochem. Photobiol.* **2008**, *84*, 539–549. [CrossRef]
27. Darvin, M.E.; Fluhr, J.W.; Schanzer, S.; Richter, H.; Patzelt, A.; Meinke, M.C.; Zastrow, L.; Golz, K.; Doucet, O. Dermal carotenoid level and kinetics after topical and systemic administration of antioxidants: Enrichment strategies in a controlled in vivo study. *J. Dermatol. Sci.* **2011**, *64*, 53–58. [CrossRef]
28. Beckenbach, L.; Baron, J.M.; Merk, H.F.; Amann, P.M. Retinoid treatment of skin diseases. *Eur J Dermatol* **2015**, *25*, 384–391. [CrossRef]
29. Havas, F.; Krispin, S.; Meléndez-Martínez, A.J.; von Oppen-Bezalel, L. Preliminary data on the safety of phytoene and phytofluene-rich products for human use including topical application. *J. Toxicol.* **2018**, *2018*, 5475784. [CrossRef]
30. Sorg, O.; Antille, C.; Kaya, G.; Saurat, J.-H. Retinoids in cosmeceuticals. *Dermatol. Ther.* **2006**, *19*, 289–296. [CrossRef]
31. Bear, M.; Connors, B.W.; Paradiso, M.A. The somatic sensory system. In *Neuroscience. Exploring the Brain*; Lippincott Williams & Wilkins: Philadelphia, PA, USA, 2007; pp. 387–423.
32. Chu, D.H.; Haake, A.R.; Holbrook, K.; Loomis, C.A. Nerves and receptors of the skin in Chapter 6: The structure and development of skin. In *Fitzpatrick's Dermatology General Medicine*; Freedberg, I.M., Eisen, A.Z., Wolff, K., Austen, K.F., Goldsmith, L.A., Katz, S.I., Eds.; McGraw-Hill: New York, NY, USA, 2003; pp. 89–115.
33. Kandel, E.R.; Schwartz, J.H.; Jessell, T.M.; Siegelbaum, S.A.; Hudspeth, A.J. Touch. In *Principles of Neural Science*; McGraw-Hill: New York, NY, USA, 2013.
34. Bikle, D.D. Vitamin D and the skin: Physiology and pathophysiology. *Rev. Endocr. Metab. Disord.* **2012**, *13*, 3–19. [CrossRef]
35. Fitzpatrick, T.B. The validity and practicality of sun-reactive skin types I through VI. *Arch. Dermatol.* **1988**, *124*, 869. [CrossRef] [PubMed]
36. Halliwell, B. Reactive species and antioxidants. Redox biology is a fundamental theme of aerobic life. *Plant Physiol.* **2006**, *141*, 312–322. [CrossRef]
37. Sies, H.; Stahl, W. Nutritional protection against skin damage from sunlight. *Annu. Rev. Nutr.* **2004**, *24*, 173–200. [CrossRef]
38. Stahl, W.; Sies, H. Photoprotection by dietary carotenoids: Concept, mechanisms, evidence and future development. *Mol. Nutr. Food Res.* **2012**, *56*, 287–295. [CrossRef]
39. Mathews-Roth, M.M. Carotenoids in Erythropoietic Protoporphyria and Other Photosensitivity Diseases. *Ann. N. Y. Acad. Sci.* **1993**, *691*, 127–138. [CrossRef]
40. Von Laar, J.; Stahl, W.; Bolsen, K.; Goerz, G.; Sies, H. β-Carotene serum levels in patients with erythropoietic protoporphyria on treatment with the synthetic all-trans isomer or a natural isomeric mixture of β-carotene. *J. Photochem. Photobiol. B Biol.* **1996**, *33*, 157–162. [CrossRef]

41. Kou, J.; Dou, D.; Yang, L. Porphyrin photosensitizers in photodynamic therapy and its applications. *Oncotarget* **2017**, *8*, 81591–81603. [CrossRef] [PubMed]
42. Fitzpatrick, T.B. Soleil et peau. *J Med Esthet.* **1975**, *2*, 33–34.
43. Fitzpatrick, T.B. Ultraviolet-induced pigmentary changes: Benefits and hazards. *Curr. Probl. Dermatol.* **1986**, *15*, 25–38.
44. Pathak, M.A. Sunlight and melanin pigmentation. In *Photochemical and Photobiological Reviews*; Smith, K.C., Ed.; Plenum Press: New York, NY, USA, 1976; pp. 211–239.
45. Schagen, S.K.; Zampeli, V.A.; Makrantonaki, E.; Zouboulis, C.C. Discovering the link between nutrition and skin aging. *Dermatoendocrinol.* **2012**, *4*, 298–307. [CrossRef]
46. Terao, J.; Minami, Y.; Bando, N. Singlet molecular oxygen quenching activity of carotenoids: Relevance to protection of the skin from photoaging. *J. Clin. Biochem. Nutr.* **2011**, *48*, 57–62. [CrossRef]
47. Kochevar, I.E.; Pathak, M.A.; Parrish, J.A. Photophysics, photochemistry, and phobiology. In *Fitzpatrick's Dermatology General Medicine*; Freedberg, I., Eisen, A.Z., Wolff, K., Al, E., Eds.; McGraw-Hill: New York, NY, USA, 1999; pp. 220–229.
48. Akhalaya, M.Y.; Maksimov, G.V.; Rubin, A.B.; Lademann, J.; Darvin, M.E. Molecular action mechanisms of solar infrared radiation and heat on human skin. *Ageing Res. Rev.* **2014**, *16*, 1–11. [CrossRef]
49. Freitas, J.V.; Junqueira, H.C.; Martins, W.K.; Baptista, M.S.; Gaspar, L. Antioxidant role on the protection of melanocytes against visible light-induced photodamage. *Free Radic. Biol. Med.* **2019**, *131*, 399–407. [CrossRef]
50. Ascenso, A.; Ribeiro, H.; Marques, H.C.; Oliveira, H.; Santos, C.; Simões, S. Chemoprevention of photocarcinogenesis by lycopene. *Exp. Dermatol.* **2014**, *23*, 874–878. [CrossRef] [PubMed]
51. Pullar, J.; Carr, A.; Vissers, M. The Roles of Vitamin C in Skin Health. *Nutrients* **2017**, *9*, 866. [CrossRef]
52. Reich, P.; Shwachman, H.; Craig, J.M. Lycopenemia. *N. Engl. J. Med.* **1960**, *262*, 263–269. [CrossRef]
53. Maharshak, N.; Shapiro, J.; Trau, H. Carotenoderma - a review of the current literature. *Int. J. Dermatol.* **2003**, *42*, 178–181. [CrossRef]
54. Stahl, W.; Sies, H. β-Carotene and other carotenoids in protection from sunlight. *Am. J. Clin. Nutr.* **2012**, *96*, 1179–1184. [CrossRef]
55. Pezdirc, K.; Hutchesson, M.J.; Williams, R.L.; Rollo, M.E.; Burrows, T.L.; Wood, L.G.; Oldmeadow, C.; Collins, C.E. Consuming High-Carotenoid Fruit and Vegetables Influences Skin Yellowness and Plasma Carotenoids in Young Women: A Single-Blind Randomized Crossover Trial. *J. Acad. Nutr. Diet.* **2016**, *116*, 1257–1265. [CrossRef] [PubMed]
56. Darvin, M.E.; Sterry, W.; Lademann, J.; Vergou, T. The Role of Carotenoids in Human Skin. *Molecules* **2011**, *16*, 10491–10506. [CrossRef]
57. Darvin, M.E.; Fluhr, J.W.; Caspers, P.; van der Pool, A.; Richter, H.; Patzelt, A.; Sterry, W.; Lademann, J. In vivo distribution of carotenoids in different anatomical locations of human skin: Comparative assessment with two different Raman spectroscopy methods. *Exp. Dermatol.* **2009**, *18*, 1060–1063. [CrossRef] [PubMed]
58. Niu, C.; Aisa, H.A. Upregulation of Melanogenesis and Tyrosinase Activity: Potential Agents for Vitiligo. *Molecules* **2017**, *22*, 1303. [CrossRef] [PubMed]
59. Foo, Y.Z.; Simmons, L.W.; Rhodes, G. Predictors of facial attractiveness and health in humans. *Sci. Rep.* **2017**, *7*, 1–12. [CrossRef]
60. Hunter, M.L. If You're Light You're Alright: Light Skin Color as Social Capital for Women of Color. *Gend. Soc.* **2002**, *16*, 175–193. [CrossRef]
61. Hill, M.E. Skin color and the perception of attractiveness among African Americans: Does gender make a difference? *Soc. Psychol. Q.* **2002**, *65*, 77–91. [CrossRef]
62. Awad, G.H.; Norwood, C.; Taylor, D.S.; Martinez, M.; McClain, S.; Jones, B.; Holman, A.; Chapman-Hilliard, C. Beauty and Body Image Concerns Among African American College Women. *J Black Psychol. 2015* **2015**, *41*, 1–20. [CrossRef]
63. Coley, M.K.; Alexis, A.F. Cosmetic concerns in skin of color, part 1. *Cosmet. Dermatology* **2009**, *22*, 360–370.
64. Tranggono, R.I. Adityarini Cosmeceuticals for Asians who are living in the tropics. *J. Appl. Cosmetol.* **2010**, *28*, 71–86.
65. Howlett, J. *Functional foods from science To health and claims*; ILSI Press: Brussels, Belgium, 2008; ISBN 0849313724.
66. DeFelice, S.L. The nutraceutical revolution: Its impact on food industry. *Trends Food Sci. Technol.* **1995**, *6*, 59–61. [CrossRef]

67. Santini, A.; Cammarata, S.M.; Capone, G.; Ianaro, A.; Tenore, G.C.; Pani, L.; Novellino, E. Nutraceuticals: Opening the debate for a regulatory framework. *Br. J. Clin. Pharmacol.* **2018**, *84*, 659–672. [CrossRef]
68. The European Parliament and the Council of the European Union (institution) Regulation (EC) no 1223/2009 of The European Parliament and of the Council of 30 November 2009 on cosmetic products. *Off. J. Eur. Union* **2009**, *342*, 59–209.
69. FDA. *Federal Food, Drug, and Cosmetic Act*; 2019. Available online: https://www.fda.gov/cosmetics/guidanceregulation/lawsregulations/ucm074201.htm (accessed on 14 May 2019).
70. Saint-Leger, D. 'Cosmeceuticals'. Of men, science and laws .... *Int. J. Cosmet. Sci.* **2012**, *34*, 396–401. [CrossRef]
71. Meléndez-Martínez, A.J. Carotenoides: Estructura, propiedades y funciones. In *Carotenoides en agroalimentación y salud*; Meléndez-Martínez, A., Ed.; Editorial Terracota: Ciudad de México, México, 2017; ISBN 978-84-15413-35-6.
72. Dias, M.G.; Olmedilla-Alonso, B.; Hornero-Méndez, D.; Mercadante, A.Z.; Osorio, C.; Vargas-Murga, L.; Meléndez-Martínez, A.J. Comprehensive Database of Carotenoid Contents in Ibero-American Foods. A Valuable Tool in the Context of Functional Foods and the Establishment of Recommended Intakes of Bioactives. *J. Agric. Food Chem.* **2018**, *66*, 5055–5107. [CrossRef]
73. Singh, J.; Fan, D.; Banskota, A.H.; Stefanova, R.; Khan, W.; Hafting, J.; Craigie, J.; Critchley, A.T.; Prithiviraj, B. Bioactive components of the edible strain of red alga, Chondrus crispus, enhance oxidative stress tolerance in Caenorhabditis elegans. *J. Funct. Foods* **2013**, *5*, 1180–1190. [CrossRef]
74. Zarekarizi, A.; Hoffmann, L.; Burritt, D. Approaches for the sustainable production of fucoxanthin, a xanthophyll with potential health benefits. *J. Appl. Phycol.* **2018**, 1–19. [CrossRef]
75. Rasmussen, H.M.; Muzhingi, T.; Eggert, E.M.R.; Johnson, E. Lutein, zeaxanthin, meso-zeaxanthin content in egg yolk and their absence in fish and seafood. *J. Food Compos. Anal.* **2012**, *27*, 139–144. [CrossRef]
76. Schlatterer, J.; Breithaupt, D.E. Xanthophylls in commercial egg yolks: Quantification and identification by HPLC and LC-(APCI)MS using a C30 phase. *J. Agric. Food Chem.* **2006**, *54*, 2267–2273. [CrossRef]
77. Álvarez, R.; Meléndez-Martínez, A.J.; Vicario, I.M.; Alcalde, M.J. Carotenoid and Vitamin A Contents in Biological Fluids and Tissues of Animals as an Effect of the Diet: A Review. *Food Rev. Int.* **2015**, *31*, 319–340. [CrossRef]
78. Maoka, T. Carotenoids in Marine Animals. *Mar. Drugs* **2011**, *9*, 278–293. [CrossRef] [PubMed]
79. Shahidi, F.; Metusalach; Brown, J.A.; Taylor, P. Carotenoid pigments in seafoods and aquaculture. *Crit. Rev. Food Sci. Nutr.* **1998**, *38*, 1–67. [CrossRef]
80. Lehto, S.; Buchweitz, M.; Klimm, A.; Straßburger, R.; Bechtold, C.; Ulberth, F. Comparison of food colour regulations in the EU and the US: A review of current provisions. *Food Addit. Contam. Part A Chem. Anal. Control. Expo. Risk Assess.* **2017**, *34*, 335–355. [CrossRef]
81. Martins, N.; Roriz, C.L.; Morales, P.; Barros, L.; Ferreira, I.C.F.R. Food colorants: Challenges, opportunities and current desires of agro-industries to ensure consumer expectations and regulatory practices. *Trends Food Sci. Technol.* **2016**, *52*, 1–15. [CrossRef]
82. Phelan, D.; Prado-Cabrero, A.; Nolan, J.M. Stability of Commercially Available Macular Carotenoid Supplements in Oil and Powder Formulations. *Nutrients* **2017**, *9*, 1. [CrossRef]
83. Khachik, F. Analysis of carotenoids in nutritional studies. In *Carotenoids. Volume 5: Nutrition and Health*; Britton, G., Liaaen-Jensen, S., Pfander, H., Eds.; Birkhäuser: Basel, Switzerland, 2009; pp. 7–44, ISBN 978-3-7643-7501-0.
84. Canene-Adams, K.; Erdman, J.W., Jr. Absorption, Transport, Distribution in Tissues and Bioavailability. In *Carotenoids. Volume 5. Nutrition and Health*; Britton, G., Liaaen-Jensen, S., Pfander, H., Eds.; Birkhäuser: Basel, Switzerland, 2009; pp. 115–148, ISBN 978-3-7643-7501-0.
85. Meléndez-Martínez, A.; Stinco, C.M.; Liu, C.; Wang, X.-D. A simple HPLC method for the comprehensive analysis of cis/trans (Z/E) geometrical isomers of carotenoids for nutritional studies. *Food Chem.* **2013**, *138*, 1341–1350. [CrossRef]
86. Burrows, T.; Rollo, M.; Williams, R.; Wood, L.; Garg, M.; Jensen, M.; Collins, C. A Systematic Review of Technology-Based Dietary Intake Assessment Validation Studies That Include Carotenoid Biomarkers. *Nutrients* **2017**, *9*, 140. [CrossRef]
87. Britton, G. Vitamin A and Vitamin A Deficiency. In *Carotenoids. Volume 5. Nutrition and Health*; Britton, G., Liaaen-Jensen, S., Pfander, H., Eds.; Birkhäuser: Basel, Switzerland, 2009; pp. 173–190, ISBN 978-3-7643-7501-0.

88. Giuliano, G. Provitamin A biofortification of crop plants: A gold rush with many miners. *Curr. Opin. Biotechnol.* **2017**, *44*, 169–180. [CrossRef]
89. Van Hoang, D.; Pham, N.; Lee, A.; Tran, D.; Binns, C. Dietary Carotenoid Intakes and Prostate Cancer Risk: A Case-Control Study from Vietnam. *Nutrients* **2018**, *10*, 70. [CrossRef]
90. Yamaguchi, M. β-Cryptoxanthin and bone metabolism: The preventive role in osteoporosis. *J. Heal. Sci.* **2008**, *54*, 356–369. [CrossRef]
91. Böhm, V. Lycopene and heart health. *Mol. Nutr. Food Res.* **2012**, *56*, 296–303. [CrossRef]
92. Nishino, H.; Murakoshi, M.; Tokuda, H.; Satomi, Y. Cancer prevention by carotenoids. *Arch. Biochem. Biophys.* **2009**, *483*, 165–168. [CrossRef]
93. Mares, J. Lutein and Zeaxanthin Isomers in Eye Health and Disease. *Annu. Rev. Nutr.* **2016**, *36*, 571–602. [CrossRef]
94. Johnson, E.J. Role of lutein and zeaxanthin in visual and cognitive function throughout the lifespan. *Nutr. Rev.* **2014**, *72*, 605–612. [CrossRef]
95. Bonet, M.; Canas, J.A.; Ribot, J.; Palou, A. Carotenoids and their conversion products in the control of adipocyte function, adiposity and obesity. *Arch. Biochem. Biophys.* **2015**, *572*, 112–125. [CrossRef]
96. Coyne, T.; Ibiebele, T.I.; Baade, P.D.; McClintock, C.S.; Shaw, J.E. Metabolic syndrome and serum carotenoids: Findings of a cross-sectional study in Queensland, Australia. *Br. J. Nutr.* **2009**, *102*, 1668–1677. [CrossRef] [PubMed]
97. Than, A.; Bramley, P.M.; Davies, B.H.; Rees, A.F. Stereochemistry of phytoene. *Phytochemistry* **1972**, *11*, 3187–3192. [CrossRef]
98. Britton, G. Structure and properties of carotenoids in relation to function. *FASEB J.* **1995**, *9*, 1551–1558. [CrossRef] [PubMed]
99. Meléndez-Martínez, A.J.; Britton, G.; Vicario, I.M.; Heredia, F.J. Relationship between the colour and the chemical structure of carotenoid pigments. *Food Chem.* **2007**, *101*, 1145–1150. [CrossRef]
100. Rodriguez-Amaya, D. *A Guide to Carotenoid Analysis in Foods*; ILSI Press: Washington, DC, USA, 2001; ISBN 1578810728.
101. Davies, B.H. Carotenoids. In *Chemistry and Biochemistry of Plant Pigments*; Goodwin, T.W., Ed.; Academic Press: London, UK, 1976; pp. 38–165.
102. Britton, G.; Liaaen-Jensen, S.; Pfander, H. *Carotenoids. Handbook*; Birkhäuser: Basel, Switzerland, 2004.
103. Martínez, A.; Stinco, C.M.; Meléndez-Martínez, A.J. Free radical scavenging properties of phytofluene and phytoene isomers as compared to lycopene: A combined experimental and theoretical study. *J. Phys. Chem. B* **2014**, *118*, 9819–9825. [CrossRef] [PubMed]
104. Cooperstone, J.L.; Francis, D.M.; Schwartz, S.J. Thermal processing differentially affects lycopene and other carotenoids in cis-lycopene containing, tangerine tomatoes. *Food Chem.* **2016**, *210*, 466–472. [CrossRef]
105. Meléndez-Martínez, A.J.; Paulino, M.; Stinco, C.M.; Mapelli-Brahm, P.; Wang, X.-D. Study of the Time-Course of cis/trans (Z/E) Isomerization of Lycopene, Phytoene, and Phytofluene from Tomato. *J. Agric. Food Chem.* **2014**, *62*, 12399–12406. [CrossRef] [PubMed]
106. Desmarchelier, C.; Borel, P. Overview of carotenoid bioavailability determinants: From dietary factors to host genetic variations. *Trends Food Sci. Technol.* **2017**, *69*, 270–280. [CrossRef]
107. Mapelli-Brahm, P.; Corte-Real, J.; Meléndez-Martínez, A.J.A.J.; Bohn, T. Bioaccessibility of phytoene and phytofluene is superior to other carotenoids from selected fruit and vegetable juices. *Food Chem.* **2017**, *229*, 304–311. [CrossRef]
108. Mapelli-Brahm, P.; Stinco, C.M.; Rodrigo, M.J.; Zacarías, L.; Meléndez-Martínez, A.J. Impact of thermal treatments on the bioaccessibility of phytoene and phytofluene in relation to changes in the microstructure and size of orange juice particles. *J. Funct. Foods* **2018**, *46*, 38–47. [CrossRef]
109. Mapelli-Brahm, P.; Desmarchelier, C.; Margier, M.; Reboul, E.; Meléndez Martínez, A.J.; Borel, P. Phytoene and Phytofluene Isolated from a Tomato Extract are Readily Incorporated in Mixed Micelles and Absorbed by Caco-2 Cells, as Compared to Lycopene, and SR-BI is Involved in their Cellular Uptake. *Mol. Nutr. Food Res.* **2018**, 1800703. [CrossRef]
110. Biehler, E.; Alkerwi, A.; Hoffmann, L.; Krause, E.; Guillaume, M.; Lair, M.L.; Bohn, T. Contribution of violaxanthin, neoxanthin, phytoene and phytofluene to total carotenoid intake: Assessment in Luxembourg. *J. Food Compos. Anal.* **2012**, *25*, 56–65. [CrossRef]

111. Paetau, I.; Khachik, F.; Brown, E.D.; Beecher, G.R.; Kramer, T.R.; Chittams, J.; Clevidence, B.A. Chronic ingestion of lycopene-rich tomato juice or lycopene supplements significantly increases plasma concentrations of lycopene and related tomato carotenoids in humans. *Int. J. Cancer* **1998**, *68*, 1187–1195. [CrossRef]
112. Müller, H.; Bub, A.; Watzl, B.; Rechkemmer, G.; Contribution, O. Plasma concentrations of carotenoids in healthy volunteers after intervention with carotenoid-rich foods. *Eur. J. Nutr.* **1999**, *38*, 35–44. [CrossRef]
113. Aust, O.; Stahl, W.; Sies, H.; Tronnier, H.; Heinrich, U. Supplementation with tomato- based products increase lycopene, phytofluene, and phytoene levels in human serum and protects against UV-light-induced erythema. *Int. J. Vitam. Nutr. Res.* **2005**, *75*, 54–60. [CrossRef] [PubMed]
114. Khachik, F.; Spangler, C.J.; Smith, J.C., Jr.; Canfield, L.M.; Steck, A.; Pfander, H. Identification, quantification, and relative Concentrations of carotenoids and their metabolites in Human Milk and Serum. *Anal. Chem.* **1997**, *69*, 1873–1881. [CrossRef]
115. Khachik, F.; Carvalho, L.; Bernstein, P.S.; Muir, G.J.; Zhao, D.-Y.; Katz, N.B. Chemistry, distribution, and metabolism of tomato carotenoids and their impact on human health. *Exp. Biol. Med. (Maywood).* **2002**, *227*, 845–851. [CrossRef]
116. Basu, A.; Imrhan, V. Tomatoes versus lycopene in oxidative stress and carcinogenesis: Conclusions from clinical trials. *Eur. J. Clin. Nutr.* **2007**, *61*, 295–303. [CrossRef] [PubMed]
117. Jacques, P.F.; Lyass, A.; Massaro, J.M.; Vasan, R.S.; D'Agostino Sr, R.B. Relationship of lycopene intake and consumption of tomato products to incident CVD. *Br. J. Nutr.* **2013**, *110*, 545–551. [CrossRef]
118. Ben-dor, A.; Steiner, M.; Gheber, L.; Danilenko, M.; Dubi, N.; Linnewiel, K.; Zick, A.; Sharoni, Y.; Levy, J. Carotenoids activate the antioxidant response element transcription system Carotenoids activate the antioxidant response element transcription system. *Mol. Cancer Ther.* **2005**, *4*, 177–186.
119. Shaish, A.; Harari, A.; Kamari, Y.; Soudant, E.; Harats, D.; Ben-Amotz, A. A carotenoid algal preparation containing phytoene and phytofluene inhibited LDL oxidation in vitro. *Plant Foods Hum. Nutr.* **2008**, *63*, 83–86. [CrossRef] [PubMed]
120. Porrini, M.; Riso, P.; Brusamolino, A.; Berti, C.; Guarnieri, S.; Visioli, F. Daily intake of a formulated tomato drink affects carotenoid plasma and lymphocyte concentrations and improves cellular antioxidant protection. *Br. J. Nutr.* **2005**, *93*, 93. [CrossRef]
121. Simmons, D.L.; Botting, R.M.; Hla, T. Cyclooxygenase isozymes: The biology of prostaglandin synthesis and inhibition. *Pharmacol. Rev.* **2004**, *56*, 387–437. [CrossRef] [PubMed]
122. Fuller, B.; Smith, D.; Howerton, A.; Kern, D. Anti-inflammatory effects of CoQ10 and colorless carotenoids. *J. Cosmet. Dermatol.* **2006**, *5*, 30–38. [CrossRef]
123. Meléndez-Martínez, A.J.; Nascimento, A.F.; Wang, Y.; Liu, C.; Mao, Y.; Wang, X.-D. Effect of tomato extract supplementation against high-fat diet-induced hepatic lesions. *Hepatobiliary Surg. Nutr.* **2013**, *2*, 198–208. [CrossRef]
124. Kotake-Nara, E.; Kushiro, M.; Zhang, H.; Sugawara, T.; Miyashita, K.; Nagao, A. Carotenoids affect proliferation of human prostate cancer cells. *J. Nutr.* **2001**, *131*, 3303–3306. [CrossRef]
125. Nara, E.; Hayashi, H.; Kotake, M.; Miyashita, K.; Nagao, A. Acyclic Carotenoids and Their Oxidation Mixtures Inhibit the Growth of HL-60 Human Promyelocytic Leukemia Cells Acyclic Carotenoids and Their Oxidation Mixtures Inhibit the Growth of HL-60 Human Promyelocytic Leukemia Cells. *Nutr. Cancer* **2009**, *39*, 37–41. [CrossRef]
126. Hirsch, K.; Atzmon, A.; Danilenko, M.; Levy, J.; Sharoni, Y. Lycopene and other carotenoids inhibit estrogenic activity of 17-β-estradiol and genistein in cancer cells. *Breast Cancer Res. Treat.* **2007**, *104*, 221–230. [CrossRef]
127. Boileau, T.W.-M.; Liao, Z.; Kim, S.; Lemeshow, S.; Erdman, J.; Clinton, S.K. Prostate Carcinogenesis in N-methyl-N-nitrosourea (NMU)-Testosterone-Treated Rats Fed Tomato Powder, Lycopene, or Energy-Restricted Diets. *J. Natl. Cancer Inst.* **2003**, *95*, 1578–1586. [CrossRef] [PubMed]
128. Campbell, J.K.; Stroud, C.K.; Nakamura, M.T.; Lila, M.A.; Erdman, J.W. Serum testosterone is reduced following short-term phytofluene, lycopene, or tomato powder consumption in F344 rats. *J. Nutr.* **2006**, *136*, 2813–2819. [CrossRef] [PubMed]
129. FDA. *GRAS Notice 163*; 2005. Available online: https://www.accessdata.fda.gov/scripts/fdcc/index.cfm?set=GRASNotices&id=163 (accessed on 12 August 2018).
130. FDA. *GRAS Notice 185*; 2006. Available online: https://www.accessdata.fda.gov/scripts/fdcc/index.cfm?set=GRASNotices&id=185 (accessed on 12 August 2018).
131. EFSA Safety of Lycopene oleoresin from tomatoes. *EFSA J.* **2008**, *675*, 1–22. [CrossRef]

132. Darvin, M.E.; Patzelt, A.; Knorr, F.; Blume-Peytavi, U.; Sterry, W.; Lademann, J. One-year study on the variation of carotenoid antioxidant substances in living human skin: Influence of dietary supplementation and stress factors. *J. Biomed. Opt.* **2008**, *13*, 044028-1–044028-9. [CrossRef]
133. Mayne, S.T.; Cartmel, B.; Scarmo, S.; Lin, H.; Leffell, D.J.; Welch, E.; Ermakov, I.; Bhosale, P.; Bernstein, P.S.; Gellermann, W. Noninvasive assessment of dermal carotenoids as a biomarker of fruit and vegetable intake. *Am. J. Clin. Nutr.* **2010**, *92*, 794–800. [CrossRef] [PubMed]
134. Ermakov, I.V.; Gellermann, W. Validation model for Raman based skin carotenoid detection. *Arch. Biochem. Biophys.* **2010**, *504*, 40–49. [CrossRef]
135. Ermakov, I.V.; Ermakova, M.; Sharifzadeh, M.; Gorusupudi, A.; Farnsworth, K.; Bernstein, P.S.; Stookey, J.; Evans, J.; Arana, T.; Tao-Lew, L.; et al. Optical assessment of skin carotenoid status as a biomarker of vegetable and fruit intake. *Arch. Biochem. Biophys.* **2018**, *646*, 46–54. [CrossRef] [PubMed]
136. Stahl, W.; Heinrich, U.; Jungmann, H.; von Laar, J.; Schietzel, M.; Sies, H.; Tronnier, H. Increased Dermal Carotenoid Levels Assessed by Noninvasive Reflection Spectrophotometry Correlate with Serum Levels in Women Ingesting Betatene. *J. Nutr.* **1998**, *128*, 903–907. [CrossRef] [PubMed]
137. Stahl, W.; Heinrich, U.; Jungmann, H.; Tronnier, H.; Sies, H. Carotenoids in human skin: Noninvasive measurement and identification of dermal carotenoids and carotenol esters. *Methods Enzymol.* **2000**, *319*, 494–502. [CrossRef] [PubMed]
138. Lademann, J.; Meinke, M.C.; Sterry, W.; Darvin, M.E. Carotenoids in human skin. *Exp. Dermatol.* **2011**, *20*, 377–382. [CrossRef]
139. Ermakov, I.V.; Gellermann, W. Optical detection methods for carotenoids in human skin. *Arch. Biochem. Biophys.* **2015**, *572*, 101–111. [CrossRef]
140. Meinke, M.C.; Lohan, S.B.; Köcher, W.; Magnussen, B.; Darvin, M.E.; Lademann, J. Multiple spatially resolved reflection spectroscopy to monitor cutaneous carotenoids during supplementation of fruit and vegetable extracts in vivo. *Ski. Res. Technol.* **2017**, *23*, 459–462. [CrossRef]
141. Jilcott Pitts, S.B.; Jahns, L.; Wu, Q.; Moran, N.E.; Bell, R.A.; Truesdale, K.P.; Laska, M.N. A non-invasive assessment of skin carotenoid status through reflection spectroscopy is a feasible, reliable and potentially valid measure of fruit and vegetable consumption in a diverse community sample. *Public Health Nutr.* **2018**, *21*, 1664–1670. [CrossRef]
142. Ashton, L.M.; Pezdirc, K.B.; Hutchesson, M.J.; Rollo, M.E.; Collins, C.E. Is skin coloration measured by reflectance spectroscopy related to intake of nutrient-dense foods? A cross-sectional evaluation in Australian young adults. *Nutrients* **2018**, *10*, 11. [CrossRef] [PubMed]
143. Coyle, D.H.; Pezdirc, K.; Hutchesson, M.J.; Collins, C.E. Intake of specific types of fruit and vegetables is associated with higher levels of skin yellowness in young women: A cross-sectional study. *Nutr. Res.* **2018**, *56*, 23–31. [CrossRef]
144. Stinco, C.M.; Rodríguez-Pulido, F.J.; Escudero-Gilete, M.L.; Gordillo, B.; Vicario, I.M.; Meléndez-Martínez, A.J. Lycopene isomers in fresh and processed tomato products: Correlations with instrumental color measurements by digital image analysis and spectroradiometry. *Food Res. Int.* **2013**, *50*, 111–120. [CrossRef]
145. Meléndez-Martínez, A.J.; Gómez-Robledo, L.; Melgosa, M.; Vicario, I.M.; Heredia, F.J. Color of orange juices in relation to their carotenoid contents as assessed from different spectroscopic data. *J. Food Compos. Anal.* **2011**, *24*, 837–844. [CrossRef]
146. Meléndez-Martínez, A.J.; Vicario, I.M.; Heredia, F.J. Influence of white reference measurement and background on the colour specification of orange juices by means of diffuse reflectance spectrophotometry. *J. AOAC Int.* **2006**, *89*, 452–457.
147. Meléndez-Martínez, A.J.; Vicario, I.M.; Heredia, F.J. Instrumental measurement of orange juice colour: A review. *J. Sci. Food Agric.* **2005**, *85*, 894–901. [CrossRef]
148. Meléndez-Martínez, A.J.; Vicario, I.M.; Heredia, F.J. Rapid assessment of vitamin A activity through objective color measurements for the quality control of orange juices with diverse carotenoid profiles. *J. Agric. Food Chem.* **2007**, *55*, 2808–2815. [CrossRef] [PubMed]
149. Scarmo, S.; Cartmel, B.; Lin, H.; Leffell, D.J.; Ermakov, I.V.; Gellermann, W.; Bernstein, P.S.; Mayne, S.T. Single *v.* multiple measures of skin carotenoids by resonance Raman spectroscopy as a biomarker of usual carotenoid status. *Br. J. Nutr.* **2013**, *110*, 911–917. [CrossRef]
150. Aguilar, S.S.; Wengreen, H.J.; Lefevre, M.; Madden, G.J.; Gast, J. Skin Carotenoids: A Biomarker of Fruit and Vegetable Intake in Children. *J. Acad. Nutr. Diet.* **2014**, *114*, 1174–1180. [CrossRef] [PubMed]

151. Nguyen, L.M.; Scherr, R.E.; Linnell, J.D.; Ermakov, I.V.; Gellermann, W.; Jahns, L.; Keen, C.L.; Miyamoto, S.; Steinberg, F.M.; Young, H.M.; et al. Evaluating the relationship between plasma and skin carotenoids and reported dietary intake in elementary school children to assess fruit and vegetable intake. *Arch. Biochem. Biophys.* **2015**, *572*, 73–80. [CrossRef]
152. Holt, E.W.; Wei, E.K.; Bennett, N.; Zhang, L.M. Low skin carotenoid concentration measured by resonance Raman spectroscopy is associated with metabolic syndrome in adults. *Nutr. Res.* **2014**, *34*, 821–826. [CrossRef]
153. Stahl, W.; Heinrich, U.; Wiseman, S.; Eichler, O.; Sies, H.; Tronnier, H. Dietary Tomato Paste Protects against Ultraviolet Light–Induced Erythema in Humans. *J. Nutr.* **2001**, *131*, 1449–1451. [CrossRef]
154. Hata, T.R.; Scholz, T.A.; Ermakov, I.V.; McClane, R.W.; Khachik, F.; Gellermann, W.; Pershing, L.K. Non-invasive Raman spectroscopic detection of carotenoids in human skin. *J. Invest. Dermatol.* **2000**, *115*, 441–448. [CrossRef]
155. Wingerath, T.; Sies, H.; Stahl, W. Xanthophyll Esters in Human Skin. *Arch. Biochem. Biophys.* **1998**, *355*, 271–274. [CrossRef]
156. Wingerath, T.; Stahl, W.; Sies, H. β-Cryptoxanthin selectively increases in human chylomicrons upon ingestion of tangerine concentrate rich in beta-cryptoxanthin esters. *Arch. Biochem. Biophys.* **1995**, *324*, 385–390. [CrossRef]
157. Mercadante, A.Z.; Rodrigues, D.B.; Petry, F.C.; Mariutti, L.R.B. Carotenoid esters in foods—A review and practical directions on analysis and occurrence. *Food Res. Int.* **2017**, *99*, 830–850. [CrossRef]
158. Bohn, T.; McDougall, G.J.; Alegría, A.; Alminger, M.; Arrigoni, E.; Aura, A.-M.; Brito, C.; Cilla, A.; El, S.N.; Karakaya, S.; et al. Mind the gap-deficits in our knowledge of aspects impacting the bioavailability of phytochemicals and their metabolites-a position paper focusing on carotenoids and polyphenols. *Mol. Nutr. Food Res.* **2015**. [CrossRef] [PubMed]
159. Bohn, T.; Desmarchelier, C.; Dragsted, L.O.; Nielsen, C.S.; Stahl, W.; Rühl, R.; Keijer, J.; Borel, P. Host-related factors explaining interindividual variability of carotenoid bioavailability and tissue concentrations in humans. *Mol. Nutr. Food Res.* **2017**, *61*. [CrossRef]
160. Massenti, R.; Perrone, A.; Livrea, M.A.; Lo Bianco, R. Regular consumption of fresh orange juice increases human skin carotenoid content. *Int. J. Food Sci. Nutr.* **2015**, *66*, 718–721. [CrossRef]
161. Jahns, L.; Johnson, L.K.; Mayne, S.T.; Cartmel, B.; Sr, M.J.P.; Ermakov, I.V.; Gellermann, W.; Whigham, L.D.; Picklo, M.J.; Ermakov, I.V.; et al. Skin and plasma carotenoid response to a provided intervention diet high in vegetables and fruit: Uptake and depletion kinetics. *Am. J. Clin. Nutr.* **2014**, *100*, 930–937. [CrossRef] [PubMed]
162. Aguilar, S.S.; Wengreen, H.J.; Dew, J. Skin Carotenoid Response to a High-Carotenoid Juice in Children: A Randomized Clinical Trial. *J. Acad. Nutr. Diet.* **2015**, *115*, 1771–1778. [CrossRef]
163. Whitehead, R.D.; Re, D.; Xiao, D.; Ozakinci, G.; Perrett, D.I. You Are What You Eat: Within-Subject Increases in Fruit and Vegetable Consumption Confer Beneficial Skin-Color Changes. *PLoS ONE* **2012**, *7*, e32988. [CrossRef]
164. Sansone, R.A.; Sansone, L.A. Carrot Man: A Case of Excessive Beta-Carotene Ingestion. *Int. J. Eat. Disord.* **2012**, *45*, 816–818. [CrossRef]
165. Meinke, M.C.; Lauer, A.; Taskoparan, B.; Gersonde, I.; Lademann, J.; Darvin, M.E. Influence on the carotenoid levels of skin arising from age, gender, body mass index in smoking/non-smoking individuals. *Free Radicals Antioxidants* **2011**, *1*, 15–20. [CrossRef]
166. Biesalski, H.K.; Hemmes, C.; Hopfenmuller, W.; Schmid, C.; Gollnick, H.P. Effects of controlled exposure of sunlight on plasma and skin levels of beta-carotene. *Free Radic. Res.* **1996**, *24*, 215–224. [CrossRef]
167. Vandersee, S.; Beyer, M.; Lademann, J.; Darvin, M.E. Blue-violet light irradiation dose dependently decreases carotenoids in human skin, which indicates the generation of free radicals. *Oxid. Med. Cell. Longev.* **2015**, *2015*. [CrossRef]
168. Darvin, M.E.; Patzelt, A.; Meinke, M.; Sterry, W.; Lademann, J. Influence of two different IR radiators on the antioxidative potential of the human skin. *Laser Phys. Lett.* **2009**, *6*, 229–234. [CrossRef]
169. Darvin, M.E.; Fluhr, J.W.; Meinke, M.C.; Zastrow, L.; Sterry, W.; Lademann, J. Topical β-carotene protects against infra-red-light-induced free radicals. *Exp. Dermatol.* **2011**, *20*, 125–129. [CrossRef]
170. Lima, X.T.T.; Kimball, A.B.B. Skin carotenoid levels in adult patients with psoriasis. *J. Eur. Acad. Dermatol. Venereol.* **2011**, *25*, 945–949. [CrossRef] [PubMed]

171. Li, D.G.; LeCompte, G.; Golod, L.; Cecchi, G.; Irwin, D.; Harken, A.; Matecki, A. Dermal carotenoid measurement is inversely related to anxiety in patients with breast cancer. *J. Investig. Med.* **2018**, *66*, 329–333. [CrossRef] [PubMed]
172. Meinke, M.C.; Darvin, M.E.; Vollert, H.; Lademann, J. Bioavailability of natural carotenoids in human skin compared to blood. *Eur. J. Pharm. Biopharm.* **2010**, *76*, 269–274. [CrossRef]
173. Takaichi, S.; Mochimaru, M.; Sciences, M.L. Carotenoids and carotenogenesis in cyanobacteria: Unique ketocarotenoids and carotenoid glycosides. *Cell. Mol. Life Sci.* **2007**, *64*, 2607–2619. [CrossRef] [PubMed]
174. Britton, G. Functions of intact carotenoids. In *Carotenoids. Volume 4: Natural functions*; Britton, G., Liaaen-Jensen, S., Pfander, H., Eds.; Birkhäuser: Basel, Switzerland, 2008; pp. 189–212, ISBN 978-3-7643-7499-0.
175. Schalch, W.; Landrum, J.T.; Bone, R.A. The eye. In *Carotenoids. Volume 5: Nutrition and Health*; Britton, G., Liaaen-Jensen, S., Pfander, H., Eds.; Birkhäuser: Basel, Switzerland, 2009; pp. 301–334, ISBN 978-3-7643-7501-0.
176. Johnson, E.J.; Neuringer, M.; Russell, R.M.; Schalch, W.; Snodderly, D.M. Nutritional manipulation of primate retinas, III: Effects of lutein or zeaxanthin supplementation on adipose tissue and retina of xanthophyll-free monkeys. *Investig. Ophthalmol. Vis. Sci.* **2005**, *46*. [CrossRef]
177. Bhosale, P.; Larson, A.J.; Frederick, J.M.; Southwick, K.; Thulin, C.D.; Bernstein, P.S. Identification and characterization of a Pi isoform of glutathione S-transferase (GSTP1) as a zeaxanthin-binding protein in the macula of the human eye. *J. Biol. Chem.* **2004**, *279*, 49447–49454. [CrossRef]
178. Li, B.; Vachali, P.; Frederick, J.M.; Bernstein, P.S. Identification of StARD3 as a lutein-binding protein in the macula of the primate retina. *Biochemistry* **2011**, *50*, 2541–2549. [CrossRef]
179. Krinsky, N.I.; Landrum, J.T.; Bone, R. a Biologic mechanisms of the protective role of lutein and zeaxanthin in the eye. *Annu. Rev. Nutr.* **2003**, *23*, 171–201. [CrossRef]
180. Kopec, R.E.; Schick, J.; Tober, K.L.; Riedl, K.M.; Francis, D.M.; Young, G.S.; Schwartz, S.J.; Oberyszyn, T.M. Sex differences in skin carotenoid deposition and acute UVB-induced skin damage in SKH-1 hairless mice after consumption of tangerine tomatoes. *Mol. Nutr. Food Res.* **2015**, *59*, 2491–2501. [CrossRef]
181. Álvarez, R.; Vaz, B.; Gronemeyer, H.; ALera, Á.R.; Rosana, A.; Gronemeyer, H.; de Lera, A.R. Functions, therapeutic applications, and synthesis of retinoids and carotenoids. *Chem. Rev.* **2014**, *114*, 1–125. [CrossRef]
182. Niki, E. Lipid peroxidation: Physiological levels and dual biological effects. *Free Radic. Biol. Med.* **2009**, *47*, 469–484. [CrossRef] [PubMed]
183. Böhm, F.; Edge, R.; Truscott, G. Interactions of dietary carotenoids with activated (singlet) oxygen and free radicals: Potential effects for human health. *Mol. Nutr. Food Res.* **2012**, *56*, 205–216. [CrossRef] [PubMed]
184. Skibsted, L.H. Carotenoids in Antioxidant Networks. Colorants or Radical Scavengers. *J. Agric. Food Chem.* **2012**, *60*, 2409–2417. [CrossRef]
185. Meinke, M.C.; Friedrich, A.; Tscherch, K.; Haag, S.F.; Darvin, M.E.; Vollert, H.; Groth, N.; Lademann, J.; Rohn, S. Influence of dietary carotenoids on radical scavenging capacity of the skin and skin lipids. *Eur. J. Pharm. Biopharm.* **2013**, *84*, 365–373. [CrossRef]
186. Yeum, K.-J.; Aldini, G.; Russell, R.M.; Krinsky, N.I. Antioxidant/Pro-oxidant Actions of Carotenoids. In *Carotenoids. Volume 5. Nutrition and Health2*; Britton, G., Liaaen-Jensen, S., Pfander, H., Eds.; Birkhäuser: Basel, Switzerland, 2009; pp. 235–268.
187. Palozza, P. Prooxidant Actions of Carotenoids in Biologic Systems. *Nutr. Rev.* **2009**, *56*, 257–265. [CrossRef]
188. Ribeiro, D.; Freitas, M.; Silva, A.M.S.; Carvalho, F.; Fernandes, E. Antioxidant and pro-oxidant activities of carotenoids and their oxidation products. *Food Chem. Toxicol.* **2018**, *120*, 681–699. [CrossRef]
189. Grochot-Przeczek, A.; Dulak, J.; Jozkowicz, A. Haem oxygenase-1: Non-canonical roles in physiology and pathology. *Clin. Sci. (Lond).* **2012**, *122*, 93–103. [CrossRef]
190. Malemud, C. Matrix metalloproteinases (MMPs) in health and disease: An overview. *Front. Biosci.* **2006**, *11*, 1696–1701. [CrossRef] [PubMed]
191. Wertz, K.; Hunziker, P.B.; Seifert, N.; Riss, G.; Neeb, M.; Steiner, G.; Hunziker, W.; Goralczyk, R. beta-Carotene interferes with ultraviolet light A-induced gene expression by multiple pathways. *J. Invest. Dermatol.* **2005**, *124*, 428–434. [CrossRef]
192. Marini, A.; Jaenicke, T.; Stahl, W.; Krutmann, J.; Grether-Beck, S.; Marini, A.; Jaenicke, T.; Stahl, W.; Krutmann, J. Molecular evidence that oral supplementation with lycopene or lutein protects human skin against ultraviolet radiation: Results from a double-blinded, placebo-controlled, crossover study. *Br. J. Dermatol.* **2017**, *176*, 1231–1240. [CrossRef]

193. Yuan, J.P.; Peng, J.; Yin, K.; Wang, J.H. Potential health-promoting effects of astaxanthin: A high-value carotenoid mostly from microalgae. *Mol. Nutr. Food Res.* **2011**, *55*, 150–165. [CrossRef] [PubMed]
194. Davinelli, S.; Nielsen, M.; Scapagnini, G. Astaxanthin in Skin Health, Repair, and Disease: A Comprehensive Review. *Nutrients* **2018**, *10*, 522. [CrossRef]
195. EFSA Scientific Opinion on the re-evaluation of canthaxanthin (E 161 g) as a food additive. *EFSA J.* **2010**, *8*, 1852–1893. [CrossRef]
196. Heinrich, U.; Gärtner, C.; Wiebusch, M.; Eichler, O.; Sies, H.; Tronnier, H.; Stahl, W. Supplementation with beta-carotene or a similar amount of mixed carotenoids protects humans from UV-induced erythema. *J. Nutr.* **2003**, *133*, 98–101. [CrossRef] [PubMed]
197. Stahl, W.; Sies, H. Carotenoids and Protection against Solar UV Radiation. *Skin Pharmacol. Physiol.* **2002**, *15*, 291–296. [CrossRef]
198. Köpcke, W.; Krutmann, J. Protection from Sunburn with β-Carotene—A Meta-analysis. *Photochem. Photobiol.* **2008**, *84*, 284–288. [CrossRef]
199. Stahl, W.; Heinrich, U.; Jungmann, H.; Sies, H.; Tronnier, H. Carotenoids and carotenoids plus vitamin E protect against ultraviolet light-induced erythema in humans. *Am. Soc. Clin. Nutr.* **2000**, *71*, 795–798. [CrossRef]
200. Greenberger, S.; Harats, D.; Salameh, F.; Lubish, T.; Harari, A.; Trau, H.; Shaish, A. 9-cis-rich β-carotene powder of the alga Dunaliella reduces the severity of chronic plaque psoriasis: A randomized, double-blind, placebo-controlled clinical trial. *J. Am. Coll. Nutr.* **2012**, *31*, 320–326. [CrossRef]
201. Murillo, E.; Meléndez-Martínez, A.J.; Portugal, F. Screening of vegetables and fruits from Panama for rich sources of lutein and zeaxanthin. *Food Chem.* **2010**, *122*, 167–172. [CrossRef]
202. Rojas-Garbanzo, C.; Gleichenhagen, M.; Heller, A.; Esquivel, P.; Schulze-Kaysers, N.; Schieber, A. Carotenoid Profile, Antioxidant Capacity, and Chromoplasts of Pink Guava (Psidium guajava L. Cv. 'Criolla') during Fruit Ripening. *J. Agric. Food Chem.* **2017**, *65*. [CrossRef]
203. Beutner, S.; Bloedorn, B.; Frixel, S.; Blanco, I.H.; Hoffmann, T.; Martin, H.D.; Mayer, B.; Noack, P.; Ruck, C.; Schmidt, M.; et al. Quantitative assessment of antioxidant properties of natural colorants and phytochemicals: Carotenoids, flavonoids, phenols and indigoids. The role of β-carotene in antioxidant functions. *J. Sci. Food Agric.* **2001**, *81*, 559–568. [CrossRef]
204. Stahl, W.; Heinrich, U.; Aust, O.; Tronnier, H.; Sies, H. Lycopene-rich products and dietary photoprotection. *Photochem. Photobiol. Sci.* **2006**, *5*, 238–242. [CrossRef]
205. Cooperstone, J.L.; Tober, K.L.; Riedl, K.M.; Teegarden, M.D.; Cichon, M.J.; Francis, D.M.; Schwartz, S.J.; Oberyszyn, T.M. Tomatoes protect against development of UV-induced keratinocyte carcinoma via metabolomic alterations. *Sci. Rep.* **2017**, *7*, 1–9. [CrossRef]
206. Nishino, A.; Sugimoto, K.; Sambe, H.; Ichihara, T.; Takaha, T.; Kuriki, T. Effects of Dietary Paprika Xanthophylls on Ultraviolet Light-Induced Skin Damage: A Double-Blind Placebo-Controlled Study. *J. Oleo Sci.* **2018**, *67*, 863–869. [CrossRef] [PubMed]
207. Mathews Roth, M.M.; Pathak, M.A.; Mathews-Roth, M.M.; Pathak, M.A. Phytoene as a protective agent against sunburn (>280nm) radiation in guinea pigs. *Photochem. Photobiol.* **1975**, *21*, 261–263. [CrossRef] [PubMed]
208. Mathews-Roth, M.M. Antitumor activity of β-carotene, canthaxanthin and phytoene. *Oncology* **1982**, *39*, 33–37. [CrossRef]
209. Von Oppen-Bezalel, L.; Fishbein, D.; Havas, F.; Ben-Chitrit, O.; Khaiat, A. The photoprotective effects of a food supplement tomato powder rich in phytoene and phytofluene, the colorless carotenoids, a preliminary study. *Glob. Dermatol.* **2015**, *2*, 178–182.
210. Von Oppen-Bezalel, L.; Shaish, A. Application of the colorless carotenoids, phytoene, and phytofluene in cosmetics, wellness, nutrition, and therapeutics. In *The alga Dunaliella: Biodiversity, Physiology, Genomics & Biotechnology*; Ben-Amotz, A., Polle, J., Rao, S., Eds.; Science Publishers: Enfield, NH, USA, 2009; pp. 423–444, ISBN 978-1-5780-8545-3.
211. Blount, J.D.; McGraw, K.J. Signal functions of carotenoid colouration. In *Carotenoids. Volume 4: Natural functions*; Gritton, G., Liaaen-Jensen, S., Pfander, H., Eds.; Birkhäuser: Basel, Switzerland, 2008; pp. 213–236, ISBN 978-3-7643-7499-0.
212. Blount, J.D. Carotenoids and life-history evolution in animals. *Arch. Biochem. Biophys.* **2004**, *430*, 10–15. [CrossRef]

213. Britton, G.; Liaaen-Jensen, S.; Pfander, H. *Carotenoids: A Colourful History*; CaroteNature GmbH: Bern, Switzerland, 2017.
214. Stephen, I.D.; Coetzee, V.; Perrett, D.I. Carotenoid and melanin pigment coloration affect perceived. *Evol. Hum. Behav.* **2011**, *32*, 216–227. [CrossRef]
215. Lefevre, C.E.; Perrett, D.I.; Lefevre, C.E.; Perrett, D.I. Fruit over sunbed: Carotenoid skin colouration is found more attractive than melanin colouration. *Q. J. Exp. Psychol.* **2015**, *0218*, 1–10. [CrossRef]
216. Pezdirc, K.; Rollo, M.E.M.E.; Whitehead, R.; Hutchesson, M.J.M.J.; Ozakinci, G.; Perrett, D.; Collins, C.E.C.E. Perceptions of carotenoid and melanin colouration in faces among young Australian adults. *Aust. J. Psychol.* **2017**, *70*, 85–90. [CrossRef]
217. Desmedt, B.; Courselle, P.; De Beer, J.O.; Rogiers, V.; Grosber, M.; Deconinck, E.; De Paepe, K. Overview of skin whitening agents with an insight into the illegal cosmetic market in Europe. *J. Eur. Acad. Dermatol. Venereol.* **2016**, *30*, 943–950. [CrossRef]
218. Von Oppen-Bezalel, L. Colorless Carotenoids, phytoene and phytofluene for the skin: For prevention of aging/photo-aging from inside and out. *SOFW J.* **2007**, *133*, 1–3.
219. Von Oppen-Bezalel, L.; Havas, F.; Ramot, O.; Kalo, E.; Fishbein, D.; Ben-Chitrit, O. Phytoene and Phytofluene for (Photo) Protection, Anti Aging, Lightening and Evening of Skin Tone. *SOFW J.* **2014**, *140*, 8–12.
220. *CIE Recommendations on Uniform Color Spaces, Color-Difference Equations, Psychometric Color Terms*; CIE Publication No. 15 (E-1.3.1) 1971, Supplement 2; Bureau Central de la CIE: Vienna, Austria, 1978.
221. Stephen, I.D.; Law Smith, M.J.; Stirrat, M.R.; Perrett, D.I. Facial skin coloration affects perceived health of human faces. *Int. J. Primatol.* **2009**, *30*, 845–857. [CrossRef] [PubMed]
222. Chung, S.-J.; Hoerr, S.; Levine, R.; Coleman, G. Processes underlying young women's decisions to eat fruits and vegetables. *J. Hum. Nutr. Diet.* **2006**, *19*, 287–298. [CrossRef] [PubMed]
223. Whitehead, R.D.; Ozakinci, G.; Stephen, I.D.; Perrett, D.I. Appealing to Vanity: Could Potential Appearance Improvement Motivate Fruit and Vegetable Consumption? *Am. J. Public Health* **2012**, *102*, 207–211. [CrossRef] [PubMed]
224. Whitehead, R.D.; Ozakinci, G.; Perrett, D.I. Attractive skin coloration: Harnessing sexual selection to improve diet and health. *Evol. Psychol.* **2012**, *10*, 842–854. [CrossRef] [PubMed]
225. WHO. *Diet, Nutrition, and the Prevention of Chronic Diseases*; Report of the Joint WHO/FAO Expert Consultation WHO Technical Report Series, No. 916 (TRS 916); World Health Organization: Geneva, Switzerland, 2003.
226. Mahler, H.I.M.; Kulik, J.A.; Gerrard, M.; Gibbons, F.X. Long-term effects of appearance-based interventions on sun protection behaviors. *Heal. Psychol.* **2007**, *26*, 350–360. [CrossRef]

10

Mechanisms of Carotenoid Intestinal Absorption: Where Do We Stand?

Emmanuelle Reboul

Aix-Marseille University, INRA, INSERM, C2VN, 13005 Marseille, France; Emmanuelle.Reboul@univ-amu.fr;

Abstract: A growing literature is dedicated to the understanding of carotenoid beneficial health effects. However, the absorption process of this broad family of molecules is still poorly understood. These highly lipophilic plant metabolites are usually weakly absorbed. It was long believed that β-carotene absorption (the principal provitamin A carotenoid in the human diet), and thus all other carotenoid absorption, was driven by passive diffusion through the brush border of the enterocytes. The identification of transporters able to facilitate carotenoid uptake by the enterocytes has challenged established statements. After a brief overview of carotenoid metabolism in the human upper gastrointestinal tract, a focus will be put on the identified proteins participating in the transport and the metabolism of carotenoids in intestinal cells and the regulation of these processes. Further progress in the understanding of the molecular mechanisms regulating carotenoid intestinal absorption is still required to optimize their bioavailability and, thus, their health effects.

Keywords: carotenes; xanthophylls; bioavailability; intestine; membrane transporters

---

1. Introduction

Carotenoids are hydrophobic molecules synthesized by plants and by some microorganisms (bacteria, algae, or fungi). Carotenoid physicochemical properties determine their distribution in the cellular environment: carotenoids are associated with membrane lipid bilayers and cytosolic lipid droplets. More than 600 different carotenoids have been found in nature, but only 40 in the human diet and about 20 have been clearly identified in human blood and tissues [1,2].

Carotenoids are polymers of isopentenyl diphosphate with 40 carbon atoms. They derive chemically from a basic structure formed by the linear sequence of 8 isoprenic units, associated in two groups of four units head to tail. The first molecule of this biosynthesis pathway is phytoene, which presents 3 conjugated double bonds in the center of the molecule and 6 other unconjugated double bonds through the length of the molecule. Phytoene is then enzymatically desaturated to produce phytofluene and eventually lycopene, a linear basic structure (C40H56) with many conjugated double bonds showing a characteristic red color [3]. Other carotenes derive from lycopene by cyclization and dehydrogenation, and xanthophylls derive from carotenes by oxidation [4] (Table 1). Some xanthophyll carotenoids such as β-cryptoxanthin [5] or lutein [6] can be found in esterified forms. Additionally, each carotenoid double bond can take a *trans* or *cis* configuration. Most of natural carotenoids are *all-trans* molecules, but *cis*-isomers can be produced during heat treatments [7]. Finally, it is worth mentioning that small amounts of apocarotenoids, i.e., cleavage products of parent 40-C carotenoids, can be naturally found in foods and/or produced during food processing, but usually represent less than 5% of the parent carotenoid levels [8,9].

The main dietary sources of carotenoids are colored fruits and vegetables (Table 1).

Table 1. Main dietary carotenoids.

Carotenoids	Molecular Structure	Examples of Food Sources (mg/100 g) [10,11]
Phytoene	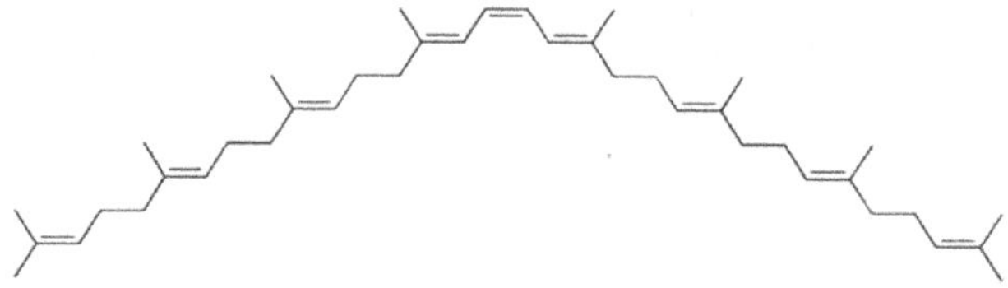	Tomato juice: 2.24 Carrot juice: 0.94
Phytofluene	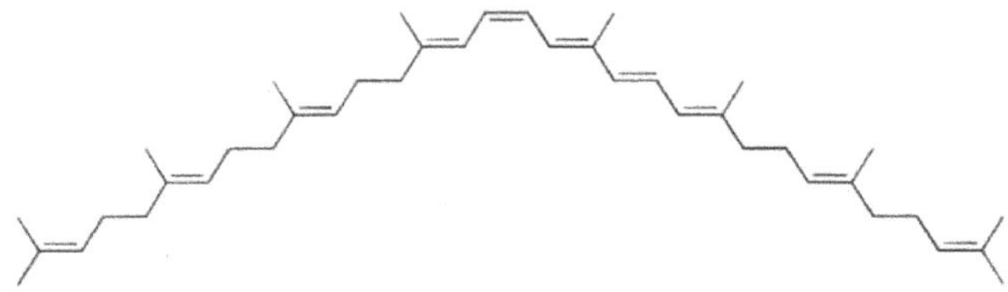	Tomato juice: 0.86 Carrot juice: 0.59
Lycopene	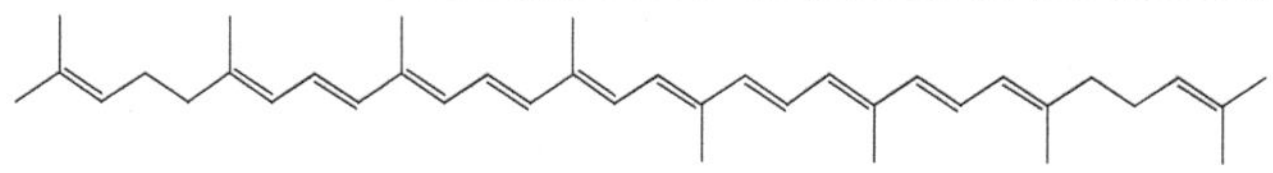	Tomato sauce: 15.92 Tomatoes: 3.03 Watermelon: 4.87
β-carotene	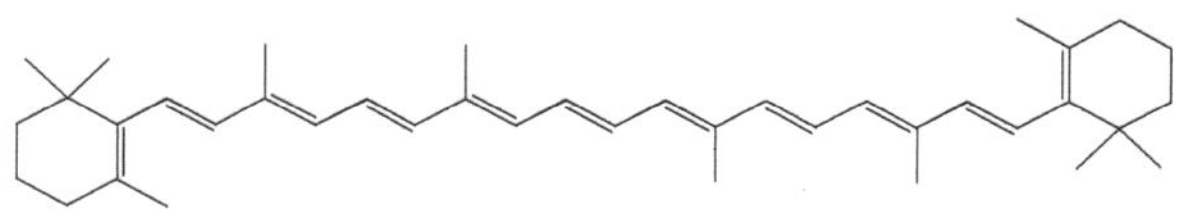	Raw carrot: 8.84 Canned carrot: 5.78 Cooked spinach: 5.24
α-carotene	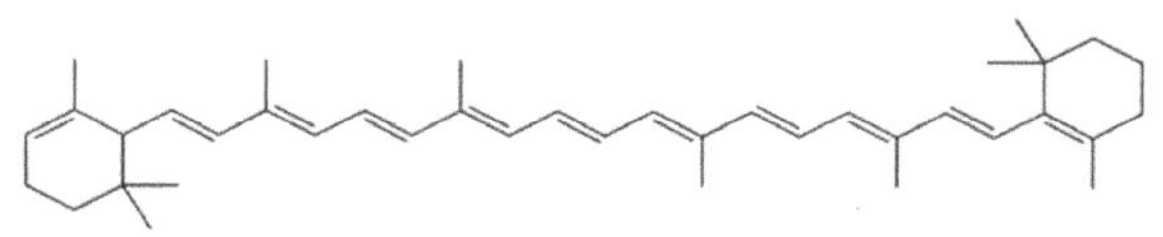	Carrot juice: 1.70
β-cryptoxanthin	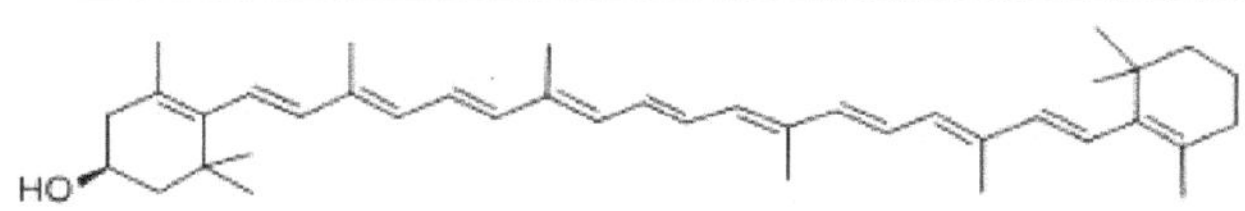	Sanguinello juice: 0.02
Lutein	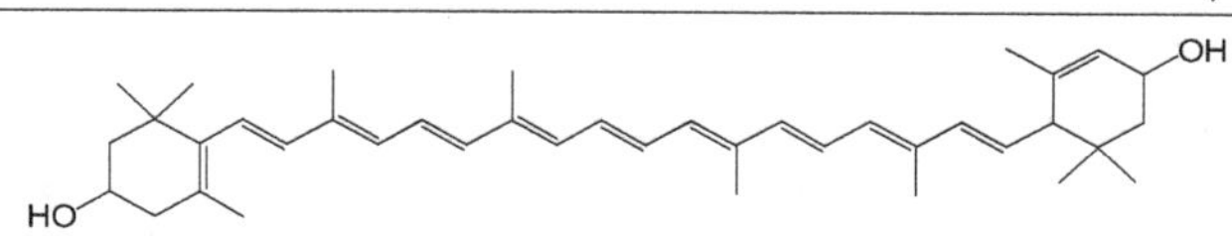	Cooked spinach: 7.04 Lettuce: 2.64

Carotenoid health properties were initially mainly accredited to their antioxidant properties as carotenoid are, at least in vitro, powerful radical quenchers [12]. Later, new investigations have highlighted the carotenoid ability to regulate intracellular signalling cascades, thus influencing both gene expression and protein translation in a broad number of metabolic pathways related to inflammatory and oxidative stress modulation [13]. However, the physiological relevance of these observations still needs to be fully established in humans. Interestingly, randomized placebo-controlled clinical trials have evidenced that supplementation with the xanthophylls lutein and zeaxanthin, which specifically accumulate into the human macula, was associated with improved visual function and decreased risk of progression to late age macular degeneration. These xanthophylls also display encouraging preventive and therapeutic effects on cataracts and retinopathies [14]. Finally, some carotenoids, such as α-carotene, β-carotene and β-cryptoxanthin, are vitamin A precursors. Indeed, they can be cleaved, mainly at the intestinal level, and metabolized into retinol (cf. Section 3.2).

After a short description of carotenoid fate in the human upper gastrointestinal lumen, a focus will be put on the identified proteins participating in carotenoid transport and metabolism in intestinal cells and on the regulation of these processes.

2. Digestion Process of Carotenoids

Fat-soluble micronutrients, including carotenoids, follow the fate of lipids in the human upper digestive tract. The first step of their digestion is thus their dissolution in the fat phase of the meal [15,16]. This phase is emulsified into lipid droplets in the stomach and duodenum.

The hypothesis that a carotenoid *cis*-isomerization could take place during gastric digestion was emitted [17], but finally refuted by a study in humans [16]. Recently, in vitro digestion experiments mimicking duodenal conditions showed that no significant isomerization of lycopene, β-carotene, or lutein occurred either [18].

It has been suggested that xanthophyll ester hydrolysis by lipases is indispensable prior to absorption. The cholesterol ester hydrolase (CEH) from pancreatic juice is likely responsible for the release of free xanthophyll from xanthophyll esters [5]. The remaining xanthophyll esters, if any, may either be cleaved at the brush border level or enter the enterocyte to be hydrolyzed in the cytosol [19].

During duodenal digestion, carotenoids are incorporated with other lipids (i.e., cholesterol, phospholipids) and lipid digestion products (i.e., free fatty acids, monoacylglycerols, lysophospholipids) into mixed micelles [20]. A fraction of carotenoids may also associate with proteins. For instance, the milk lipocalin β-lactoglobulin is able to bind β-carotene and does not alter its absorption compared to mixed micelles [21]. However, the mechanisms of carotenoid absorption may depend on carotenoid binding vehicles. Mixed micelles are likely isolated from the rest of the bolus in the unstirred water layer of the glycocalyx area and approach the brush border membrane [22] where carotenoids can be absorbed by passive diffusion and/or via a transporter-dependent process (see Section 3).

Carotenoid bioaccessibility (i.e., the fraction of carotenoids released form their food matrix and included in mixed micelles—which represents the fraction of carotenoids potentially able to be absorbed by the intestine) is highly variable. An in vitro digestion study highlighted that lycopene bioaccessibility was very limited (from 0.1% in raw tomatoes to 1.5% in tomato puree), β-carotene bioaccessibility was fairly low (from about 4% in carrot puree to 14% in carrot juice), while lutein bioaccessibility was the highest (from 37% in raw spinach leaves to 48% in boiled spinach). These values correlate with in vivo data and highlight the fact that the disruption of the food matrix by thermal treatment or processing can increase carotenoid bioaccessibility [10]. Xanthophylls were consistently shown to display a higher bioaccessibility than carotenes in different studies [10,11], probably because the presence of one or two hydroxylated group(s) increases their solubility into the micellar structures. Interestingly, phytoene and phytofluene also displayed a very high bioaccessibility. This may be linked to their more flexible molecular structure, compared to other carotenoids, which likely increase their incorporation into mixed micelles as well [11].

3. Carotenoid Absorption through the Enterocyte

Absorption efficiency of labelled β-carotene is widely variable among clinical studies, fluctuating from ≈3% to 80%, but usually ranging from 10% to 30% [23,24]. This can partly be due to the variable bioaccessibility of β-carotene (see above), but it may also reflect its moderate uptake and transport through the enterocyte. It should be mentioned that β-carotene absorption efficiency was usually measured following a single meal. However, the intestine can store β-carotene from a first meal to release it during subsequent postprandial phases in humans [25]. β-carotene absorption efficiency may, thus, be underestimated in some trials.

Studies using differentiated Caco-2 cell monolayers showed that phytofluene, β-carotene, and lutein uptakes were similar and significantly higher than that of phytoene, while lycopene uptake was the lowest [26,27]. In the same way as bioaccessibility, uptake efficiency thus seems to correlate with carotenoid polarity and flexibility. This may be explained by the fact that polar and flexible carotenoids present a better affinity for lipid transporters and/or for plasma membranes, which would lead to an increased absorption.

3.1. Apical Transport Across the Brush Border Membrane of the Enterocyte

Carotenoid uptake by the enterocytes has been considered to occur by passive diffusion for four decades, which was inconsistent with the high inter-individual variability in absorption observed in humans, as well as with the isomer selectivity and the competition for absorption between carotenoids and other fat-soluble micronutrients observed at the intestinal level (see [20] for review). Different teams started to re-explore carotenoid absorption mechanisms in the 2000s and several lipid transporters playing a role in carotenoid uptake by the intestinal cell have since been identified.

A first critical result was the identification of the gene ninaD encoding a class B scavenger receptor, essential for xanthophyll cellular distribution in *Drosophila* [28]. In 2005, we then identified the Scavenger Receptor class B type I: SR-BI as a key transporter of lutein in human intestinal Caco2 TC7 cells. This ubiquitous transmembrane glycoprotein found at the apical membrane of the enterocytes is expressed following a decreasing gradient from the duodenum to the colon [29]. Intestinal SR-BI was shown to facilitate the uptake of free cholesterol, but also of other lipids such as cholesterol esters, phospholipids, and triacylglycerol hydrolysis products, thus presenting a low substrate specificity [30,31]. The effective role of SR-BI in terms of cholesterol transport is still subject to debate [32] and SR-BI was recently presented as a cholesterol sensor [33], regulating chylomicron secretion [34]. Its involvement in the intestinal uptake of carotenoids has been extended to lycopene [35], provitamin A carotenoids [36], as well as to phytoene and phytofluene [27]. As SR-BI is also involved in the uptake of vitamin D [37], E [38], and K [39], in cultured cells and in mice, we suggest that another primary role of SR-BI in the gut is the transport of minor molecules, such as fat-soluble vitamins and carotenoids. However, we specifically showed, using both Caco2 cells and transfected HEK cells, that SR-BI was not involved in the uptake of micellar preformed vitamin A (retinol) [36].

Another pervasive scavenger receptor of interest is CD36 (CD 36 molecule). This membrane protein is highly expressed at the brush border level of the duodenum and the jejunum [40]. It is supposed to play a key role in the intestinal uptake of long-chain fatty acids [41], but also displays a broad substrate specificity [42,43]. Recently, CD36 has been described as a lipid sensor and its impact on chylomicron secretion has been established in many studies [44]. Besides, CD36 facilitates, directly or indirectly, fat-soluble vitamin uptake in the intestine [37,39,45]. CD36 was also shown to facilitate the uptake of lycopene, β-carotene, α-carotene, β-crypthoxanthine, and lutein, but not that of phytoene and phytofluene, in transfected Griptite cells and/or cultured adipocytes [27,36,46]. This result was confirmed ex vivo for β-carotene using brush-border membrane vesicles from CD36-deficient and wild-type mouse intestines [47].

A last candidate for carotenoid uptake is the NPC1-like transporter 1 (NPC1L1), which is a major sterol transporter in the intestine [37,48]. NPC1L1 was suggested to be involved in α-carotene, β-carotene, β-cryptoxanthin, and lutein intestinal uptake [49,50], but not in that of lycopene, phytoene, and phytofluene [27,35].

It is still possible that a fraction of carotenoid is absorption via a passive diffusion process, depending on the carotenoid concentration in the lumen. We previously showed in Caco-2 cells that vitamin D absorption is carrier-mediated at physiological concentrations and occurs by passive diffusion at pharmacological concentrations [37]. We suggest that a similar phenomenon occurs for carotenoids.

Recently, we showed that a fraction of phytoene and phytofluene taken up by the intestinal cells could be effluxed back to the lumen [27]. This phenomenon was previously acknowledged for fat-soluble vitamins such as vitamin D, E, and K and was shown to be, at least partly, SR-B-dependent [37–39]. This efflux may contribute to the limited absorption efficiency of carotenoids. Further research is needed to clearly identify the membrane transporters participating in this pathway. Besides SR-BI, ABCB1 (ATP binding cassette B1, also known as P-glycoprotein) and ABCG transporters, such as ABCG5, appear as good candidates. Indeed, a recent study combining in silico, cell culture, animal, and genetic approaches showed that ABCB1 was involved in vitamin D intestinal efflux [51]. Additionally, polymorphisms in the *ABCG5* gene tended to contribute to individual response to lutein supplementation in humans [52].

3.2. *Cytosolic Transport and Intracellular Metabolism*

No carotenoid carrier protein has clearly been identified in the human gut so far. However, the lutein-binding protein HR-LBP (Human Retinal Lutein-Binding Protein) present in the human retina cross-reacts with antibodies raised against a carotenoid-binding protein present in the *Bombyx mori* midgut [53], suggesting that it could be an intestinal intracellular transporter of xanthophylls [54]. As carotenoid membrane transporters SR-BI, CD36, and NPC1L1 can traffic in the enterocyte, especially after a fat load, we previously suggested that they may act as cytosolic carotenoid transporters [20]. However, this hypothesis still remains to be verified. Similarly, the association found between a genetic variant in the Intestinal Fatty-Acid Binding Protein (IFABP) and the fasting plasma lycopene concentrations in humans [55] still need to be challenged to assess whether IFABP is actually a carotenoid-carrier.

Up to 40% of absorbed carotenoids remain unmetabolized [56]. β-carotene can be cleaved into retinal by a cytosolic enzyme, BCO1 (β-carotene oxygenase 1), via a one-step process in the enterocyte [57]. β-Carotene "low-converter" phenotypes, which have been reported in several clinical studies [58], are likely due to genetic variation in *BCO1* gene. Other provitamin A carotenoids, such as β-crypthoxanthin, can be cleaved into retinal though a multi-step process involving both mitochondrial BCO2 (β-carotene oxygenase 2) and cytosolic BCO1 [59]. The produced retinal is subsequently converted into retinol and esterified into retinyl esters by the lecithin:retinol acyltransferase (LRAT) and probably by the diacylglycerol acyltransferase 1 (DGAT1) that displays an acyl-CoA:retinol acyltransferase activity [60,61]. Both provitamin A and nonprovitamin A carotenoids can also be cleaved asymmetrically in apocarotenoids by BCO2 [62]. However, a recent study showed that only traces of asymmetric [^{13}C]-β-apo-carotenals were found in plasma after [^{13}C]-β-carotene ingestion, suggesting a lack of significant postprandial intestinal BCO2 activity in healthy humans [63].

No *cis-trans* isomerization of β-carotene was measured in intestinal cultured cells [26]. As *cis*-isomerization does not occur in the gastrointestinal lumen (see above), the site of the 9-*cis* isomerization of β-carotene reported in vivo [64] remain undetermined. Conversely, lycopene isomerization in *cis*-isomers was identified to occur at the enterocyte level [65].

A summary of carotenoid transport pathways across the enterocyte is depicted in Figure 1.

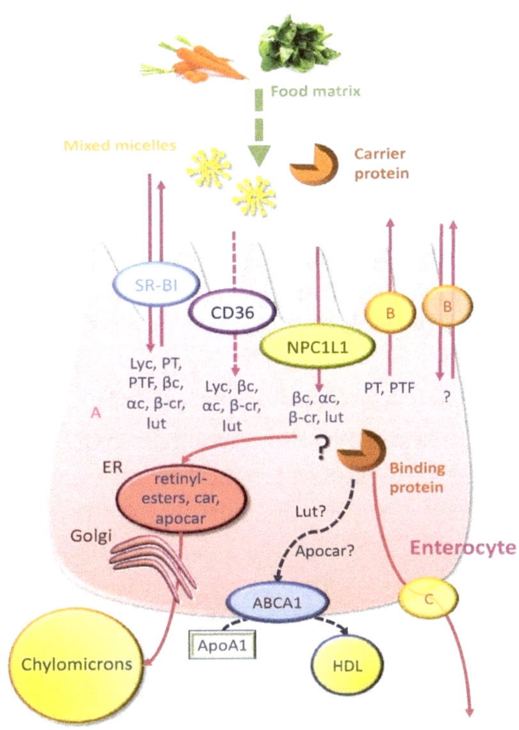

Figure 1. Uptake, transport, and secretion pathways of carotenoids across the enterocyte. PT = phytoene;

PTF = phytofluene; Lyc = lycopene; βC = β-carotene; αC = α-carotene; βCr = β-cryptoxanthine; Lut = lutein; Car = carotenoids; Apocar = apocarotenoids; A = passive diffusion; B = unidentified apical transporter; C = unidentified basolateral efflux transporter; ? = putative pathway, and ER = endoplasmic reticulum. Carotenoids are captured from mixed micelles and possibly from carrier proteins by apical membrane transporters SR-BI, CD36, and NPC1L1. A fraction of PT and PTF can then be effluxed back to the intestinal lumen via apical membrane transporters (likely SR-BI and possibly other transporters). Another fraction is transported to the site where they are incorporated into chylomicrons. Some proteins may be involved in intracellular transport of carotenoids, but none has been clearly identified. Provitamin A carotenoids are partly metabolized into retinyl-esters. Retinyl-esters and carotenoids are secreted in the lymph into chylomicrons, while a part of xanthophylls and a part of the more polar metabolites, such as some apocarotenoids, may be secreted via an HDL pathway.

3.3. Secretion Through the Basolateral Membrane of the Enterocyte

During the postprandial period, the major fraction of free carotenoids and retinyl esters originating from provitamin A carotenoid cleavage are packaged into chylomicrons (apoB-dependent pathway) that are secreted into the lymph to further join the bloodstream [20]. A non-apoB-dependent pathway (via high-density lipoproteins, HDL), mediated by the ABCA1 transporter, has been involved in vitamin E absorption [66] and possibly allows a part of free retinol absorption [20]. This HDL pathway may also exist for xanthophylls, such as lutein and zeaxanthin [67], but has not been proven to occur for other carotenoids. However, recent studies showed that several genetic variants in *ABCA1* gene were associated with lycopene [68], β-carotene [69], and lutein [70] postprandial responses in healthy subjects. Thus, further research is needed to fully understand the contribution of the intestinal HDL pathway to carotenoid absorption in humans.

4. Regulation of Carotenoid Transporter Expressions in the Enterocyte

Crucial factors modulating the expression and/or the activity of intestinal proteins involved in carotenoid absorption are provitamin A carotenoids, through a feedback regulation. Indeed, studies have pointed out that SR-BI activity is partly controlled by retinoids. Using both mouse models and human cell lines, it was specifically shown that retinoic acid produced from dietary precursors by BCO1 induced the expression of the intestinal transcription factor ISX that repressed the expression of both BCO1 [71] and SR-B1 [72], thus impacting both carotenoid conversion and uptake [73].

Additionally, many dietary factors other than retinoids were shown to regulate transporter expression in the intestine and may, thus, indirectly impact on carotenoid absorption.

Among these dietary factors, fat and fatty acids seem to play major roles. For instance, SR-BI expression in Caco-2 cells is increased by micellar oleic and ecosapentaenoic acids [74]. Conversely, CD36, NPC1L1, or ABCA1 expressions in rodent intestines are downregulated by dietary fat, including oleic acid [75,76] and cholesterol [77]. Such downregulation in NPC1L1 and ABCA1 expressions was also found after exposure of cultured intestinal FHs 74 or Caco-2 cells to phytosterols [78,79] and to long-chain polyunsaturated fatty acids [74,80].

In addition, dietary glucose increases SR-BI expression in both Caco-2 cells and mouse intestines [81] and decreases Caco2 cell ABCA1 expression [82].

Finally, some polyphenols were shown to decrease both SR-BI, NPCL1, and ABCA1 expressions in Caco-2 cells [83,84] and so did the cholesterol-lowering drug ezetimibe [49].

Host factors can also regulate carotenoid transporters. Among them, insulin resistance increases SR-BI intestinal expression in hamsters [85]. SR-BI post-transcriptional regulation also seems be dependent on bile secretion, with bile salts leading to a rise of intestinal SR-BI expression in rodents [86]. Finally, NPC1L1 expression was increased by estrogen [87] and cholecystokinin [88] in mouse intestines, while its expression was decreased by peptide YY in Caco-2 cells [89] (see [90] for review).

As the above results were exclusively obtained in cultured cells and animal studies, further investigations are deeply needed to address their relevance in humans.

5. Conclusions

To conclude, the understanding of carotenoid intestinal absorption by the intestine is far from being fully understood. Proteins including lipid membrane transporters (i.e., SR-BI, CD36, NPC1L1), the cleavage enzyme BCO1, and the transcription factor ISX have been showed to play important roles in carotenoid intestinal uptake and metabolism, but other proteins likely remain to be identified.

Genome-wide association studies (GWAS) and candidate gene association studies have identified correlations between single nucleotide polymorphisms in *SCARB1* (encoding SR-BI), *CD36*, *NPC1L1*, *BCO1*, and *ISX* and carotenoid blood concentrations. Interestingly, these studies also highlighted the impact of polymorphisms in genes encoding proteins likely indirectly linked to carotenoid metabolism (i.e., ELOVL fatty acid elongase 2). The involvement of such proteins in carotenoid intestinal metabolism still needs to be defined [91].

Carotenoid "low responder" or "high responder" phenotypes presumably correspond to individuals bearing associations of several "disadvantageous" or "advantageous" polymorphisms, respectively. In the future, it would thus be of major interest to take into account the carotenoid "low responder" or "high responder" phenotypes that are due to different transport and/or conversion efficiency, to propose tailored dietary recommendations to individuals and to thus optimize carotenoid health benefits.

Abbreviations

ABCA1	ATP binding cassette A1
ABCB1	ATB binding cassette B1
ABCG5	ATP binding cassette G5
BCO1	β-carotene-oxygenase 1
BCO2	β-carotene-oxygenase 2
CD36	CD36 molecule
CEH	cholesterol ester hydrolase
DGAT1	diacylglycerol acyltransferase 1
HR-LBP	human retinal lutein-binding protein
ISX	intestine-specific homebox
FABP	fatty-acid-binding protein
HDL	high-density lipoproteins
LRAT	lecithin retinol acyltransferase
NPC1L1	NPC1-like transporter 1
SR-BI	scavenger receptor class B type 1

References

1. Khachik, F.; Spangler, C.J.; Smith, J.C., Jr.; Canfield, L.M.; Steck, A.; Pfander, H. Identification, quantification, and relative concentrations of carotenoids and their metabolites in human milk and serum. *Anal. Chem.* **1997**, *69*, 1873–1881. [PubMed]
2. Tapiero, H.; Townsend, D.M.; Tew, K.D. The role of carotenoids in the prevention of human pathologies. *Biomed. Pharmacother.* **2004**, *58*, 100–110. [CrossRef]
3. Engelmann, N.J.; Clinton, S.K.; Erdman, J.W., Jr. Nutritional aspects of phytoene and phytofluene, carotenoid precursors to lycopene. *Adv. Nutr.* **2011**, *2*, 51–61. [PubMed]
4. Moise, A.R.; Al-Babili, S.; Wurtzel, E.T. Mechanistic aspects of carotenoid biosynthesis. *Chem. Rev.* **2014**, *114*, 164–193. [CrossRef] [PubMed]
5. Breithaupt, D.E.; Bamedi, A.; Wirt, U. Carotenol fatty acid esters: Easy substrates for digestive enzymes? *Comp. Biochem. Physiol. B Biochem. Mol. Biol.* **2002**, *132*, 721–728. [CrossRef]

6. Bowen, P.E.; Herbst-Espinosa, S.M.; Hussain, E.A.; Stacewicz-Sapuntzakis, M. Esterification does not impair lutein bioavailability in humans. *J. Nutr.* **2002**, *132*, 3668–3673. [CrossRef]
7. Shi, J.; Le Maguer, M. Lycopene in tomatoes: Chemical and physical properties affected by food processing. *Crit. Rev. Biotechnol.* **2000**, *20*, 293–334. [CrossRef]
8. Rodriguez, E.B.; Rodriguez-Amaya, D.B. Formation of apocarotenals and epoxycarotenoids from beta-carotene by chemical reactions and by autoxidation in model systems and processed foods. *Food Chem.* **2007**, *101*, 563–572. [CrossRef]
9. Kopec, R.E.; Riedl, K.M.; Harrison, E.H.; Curley, R.W., Jr.; Hruszkewycz, D.P.; Clinton, S.K.; Schwartz, S.J. Identification and quantification of apo-lycopenals in fruits, vegetables, and human plasma. *J. Agric. Food Chem.* **2010**, *58*, 3290–3296. [CrossRef]
10. Reboul, E.; Richelle, M.; Perrot, E.; Desmoulins-Malezet, C.; Pirisi, V.; Borel, P. Bioaccessibility of carotenoids and vitamin e from their main dietary sources. *J. Agric. Food Chem.* **2006**, *54*, 8749–8755. [CrossRef] [PubMed]
11. Mapelli-Brahm, P.; Corte-Real, J.; Melendez-Martinez, A.J.; Bohn, T. Bioaccessibility of phytoene and phytofluene is superior to other carotenoids from selected fruit and vegetable juices. *Food Chem.* **2017**, *229*, 304–311. [CrossRef] [PubMed]
12. Krinsky, N.I.; Yeum, K.J. Carotenoid-radical interactions. *Biochem. Biophys. Res. Commun.* **2003**, *305*, 754–760. [CrossRef]
13. Kaulmann, A.; Bohn, T. Carotenoids, inflammation, and oxidative stress—Implications of cellular signaling pathways and relation to chronic disease prevention. *Nutr. Res.* **2014**, *34*, 907–929. [CrossRef] [PubMed]
14. Scripsema, N.K.; Hu, D.N.; Rosen, R.B. Lutein, zeaxanthin, and meso-zeaxanthin in the clinical management of eye disease. *J. Ophthalmol.* **2015**, *2015*, 865179. [CrossRef]
15. Borel, P.; Grolier, P.; Armand, M.; Partier, A.; Lafont, H.; Lairon, D.; Azais-Braesco, V. Carotenoids in biological emulsions: Solubility, surface-to-core distribution, and release from lipid droplets. *J. Lipid Res.* **1996**, *37*, 250–261. [PubMed]
16. Tyssandier, V.; Reboul, E.; Dumas, J.F.; Bouteloup-Demange, C.; Armand, M.; Marcand, J.; Sallas, M.; Borel, P. Processing of vegetable-borne carotenoids in the human stomach and duodenum. *Am. J. Physiol. Gastrointest. Liver Physiol.* **2003**, *284*, G913–G923. [CrossRef] [PubMed]
17. Re, R.; Fraser, P.D.; Long, M.; Bramley, P.M.; Rice-Evans, C. Isomerization of lycopene in the gastric milieu. *Biochem. Biophys. Res. Commun.* **2001**, *281*, 576–581. [CrossRef]
18. Kopec, R.E.; Gleize, B.; Borel, P.; Desmarchelier, C.; Caris-Veyrat, C. Are lutein, lycopene, and beta-carotene lost through the digestive process? *Food Funct.* **2017**, *8*, 1494–1503. [CrossRef]
19. Dhuique-Mayer, C.; Borel, P.; Reboul, E.; Caporiccio, B.; Besancon, P.; Amiot, M.J. Beta-cryptoxanthin from citrus juices: Assessment of bioaccessibility using an in vitro digestion/caco-2 cell culture model. *Br. J. Nutr.* **2007**, *97*, 883–890. [CrossRef]
20. Reboul, E. Absorption of vitamin a and carotenoids by the enterocyte: Focus on transport proteins. *Nutrients* **2013**, *5*, 3563–3581. [CrossRef]
21. Mensi, A.; Borel, P.; Goncalves, A.; Nowicki, M.; Gleize, B.; Roi, S.; Chobert, J.M.; Haertle, T.; Reboul, E. Beta-lactoglobulin as a vector for beta-carotene food fortification. *J. Agric. Food Chem.* **2014**, *62*, 5916–5924. [CrossRef]
22. Phan, C.T.; Tso, P. Intestinal lipid absorption and transport. *Front. Biosci.* **2001**, *6*, D299–D319. [CrossRef] [PubMed]
23. van Lieshout, M.; West, C.E.; van Breemen, R.B. Isotopic tracer techniques for studying the bioavailability and bioefficacy of dietary carotenoids, particularly beta-carotene, in humans: A review. *Am. J. Clin. Nutr.* **2003**, *77*, 12–28. [CrossRef]
24. Van Loo-Bouwman, C.A.; Naber, T.H.; van Breemen, R.B.; Zhu, D.; Dicke, H.; Siebelink, E.; Hulshof, P.J.; Russel, F.G.; Schaafsma, G.; West, C.E. Vitamin a equivalency and apparent absorption of beta-carotene in ileostomy subjects using a dual-isotope dilution technique. *Br. J. Nutr.* **2010**, *103*, 1836–1843. [CrossRef]
25. Borel, P.; Grolier, P.; Mekki, N.; Boirie, Y.; Rochette, Y.; Le Roy, B.; Alexandre-Gouabau, M.C.; Lairon, D.; Azais-Braesco, V. Low and high responders to pharmacological doses of beta-carotene: Proportion in the population, mechanisms involved and consequences on beta-carotene metabolism. *J. Lipid Res.* **1998**, *39*, 2250–2260.
26. During, A.; Hussain, M.M.; Morel, D.W.; Harrison, E.H. Carotenoid uptake and secretion by caco-2 cells: Beta-carotene isomer selectivity and carotenoid interactions. *J. Lipid Res.* **2002**, *43*, 1086–1095. [CrossRef]

27. Mapelli-Brahm, P.; Desmarchelier, C.; Margier, M.; Reboul, E.; Melendez Martinez, A.J.; Borel, P. Phytoene and phytofluene isolated from a tomato extract are readily incorporated in mixed micelles and absorbed by caco-2 cells, as compared to lycopene, and sr-bi is involved in their cellular uptake. *Mol. Nutr. Food Res.* **2018**, *62*, e1800703. [CrossRef] [PubMed]
28. Kiefer, C.; Sumser, E.; Wernet, M.F.; Von Lintig, J. A class b scavenger receptor mediates the cellular uptake of carotenoids in drosophila. *Proc. Natl. Acad. Sci. USA* **2002**, *99*, 10581–10586. [CrossRef] [PubMed]
29. Reboul, E.; Soayfane, Z.; Goncalves, A.; Cantiello, M.; Bott, R.; Nauze, M.; Terce, F.; Collet, X.; Comera, C. Respective contributions of intestinal niemann-pick c1-like 1 and scavenger receptor class b type i to cholesterol and tocopherol uptake: In vivo v. In vitro studies. *Br. J. Nutr.* **2012**, *107*, 1296–1304. [CrossRef] [PubMed]
30. Hauser, H.; Dyer, J.H.; Nandy, A.; Vega, M.A.; Werder, M.; Bieliauskaite, E.; Weber, F.E.; Compassi, S.; Gemperli, A.; Boffelli, D.; et al. Identification of a receptor mediating absorption of dietary cholesterol in the intestine. *Biochemistry* **1998**, *37*, 17843–17850. [CrossRef] [PubMed]
31. Bietrix, F.; Yan, D.; Nauze, M.; Rolland, C.; Bertrand-Michel, J.; Comera, C.; Schaak, S.; Barbaras, R.; Groen, A.K.; Perret, B.; et al. Accelerated lipid absorption in mice overexpressing intestinal sr-bi. *J. Biol. Chem.* **2006**, *281*, 7214–7219. [CrossRef]
32. Nguyen, D.V.; Drover, V.A.; Knopfel, M.; Dhanasekaran, P.; Hauser, H.; Phillips, M.C. Influence of class b scavenger receptors on cholesterol flux across the brush border membrane and intestinal absorption. *J. Lipid Res.* **2009**, *50*, 2235–2244. [CrossRef]
33. Saddar, S.; Carriere, V.; Lee, W.R.; Tanigaki, K.; Yuhanna, I.S.; Parathath, S.; Morel, E.; Warrier, M.; Sawyer, J.K.; Gerard, R.D.; et al. Scavenger receptor class b type i is a plasma membrane cholesterol sensor. *Circ. Res.* **2013**, *112*, 140–151. [CrossRef] [PubMed]
34. Lino, M.; Farr, S.; Baker, C.; Fuller, M.; Trigatti, B.; Adeli, K. Intestinal scavenger receptor class b type i as a novel regulator of chylomicron production in healthy and diet-induced obese states. *Am. J. Physiol. Gastrointest. Liver Physiol.* **2015**, *309*, G350–G359. [CrossRef]
35. Moussa, M.; Landrier, J.F.; Reboul, E.; Ghiringhelli, O.; Comera, C.; Collet, X.; Frohlich, K.; Bohm, V.; Borel, P. Lycopene absorption in human intestinal cells and in mice involves scavenger receptor class b type i but not niemann-pick c1-like 1. *J. Nutr.* **2008**, *138*, 1432–1436. [CrossRef] [PubMed]
36. Borel, P.; Lietz, G.; Goncalves, A.; Szabo de Edelenyi, F.; Lecompte, S.; Curtis, P.; Goumidi, L.; Caslake, M.J.; Miles, E.A.; Packard, C.; et al. Cd36 and sr-bi are involved in cellular uptake of provitamin a carotenoids by caco-2 and hek cells, and some of their genetic variants are associated with plasma concentrations of these micronutrients in humans. *J. Nutr.* **2013**, *143*, 448–456. [CrossRef]
37. Reboul, E.; Goncalves, A.; Comera, C.; Bott, R.; Nowicki, M.; Landrier, J.F.; Jourdheuil-Rahmani, D.; Dufour, C.; Collet, X.; Borel, P. Vitamin d intestinal absorption is not a simple passive diffusion: Evidences for involvement of cholesterol transporters. *Mol. Nutr. Food Res.* **2011**, *55*, 691–702. [CrossRef]
38. Reboul, E.; Klein, A.; Bietrix, F.; Gleize, B.; Malezet-Desmoulins, C.; Schneider, M.; Margotat, A.; Lagrost, L.; Collet, X.; Borel, P. Scavenger receptor class b type i (sr-bi) is involved in vitamin e transport across the enterocyte. *J. Biol. Chem.* **2006**, *281*, 4739–4745. [CrossRef]
39. Goncalves, A.; Margier, M.; Roi, S.; Collet, X.; Niot, I.; Goupy, P.; Caris-Veyrat, C.; Reboul, E. Intestinal scavenger receptors are involved in vitamin k1 absorption. *J. Biol. Chem.* **2014**, *289*, 30743–30752. [CrossRef]
40. Terpstra, V.; van Amersfoort, E.S.; van Velzen, A.G.; Kuiper, J.; van Berkel, T.J. Hepatic and extrahepatic scavenger receptors: Function in relation to disease. *Arterioscler. Thromb. Vasc. Biol.* **2000**, *20*, 1860–1872. [CrossRef]
41. Drover, V.A.; Nguyen, D.V.; Bastie, C.C.; Darlington, Y.F.; Abumrad, N.A.; Pessin, J.E.; London, E.; Sahoo, D.; Phillips, M.C. Cd36 mediates both cellular uptake of very long chain fatty acids and their intestinal absorption in mice. *J. Biol. Chem.* **2008**, *283*, 13108–13115. [CrossRef] [PubMed]
42. Rigotti, A.; Acton, S.L.; Krieger, M. The class b scavenger receptors sr-bi and cd36 are receptors for anionic phospholipids. *J. Biol. Chem.* **1995**, *270*, 16221–16224. [CrossRef] [PubMed]
43. Endemann, G.; Stanton, L.W.; Madden, K.S.; Bryant, C.M.; White, R.T.; Protter, A.A. Cd36 is a receptor for oxidized low density lipoprotein. *J. Biol. Chem.* **1993**, *268*, 11811–11816. [PubMed]
44. Buttet, M.; Traynard, V.; Tran, T.T.; Besnard, P.; Poirier, H.; Niot, I. From fatty-acid sensing to chylomicron synthesis: Role of intestinal lipid-binding proteins. *Biochimie* **2014**, *96*, 37–47. [CrossRef] [PubMed]

45. Goncalves, A.; Roi, S.; Nowicki, M.; Niot, I.; Reboul, E. Cluster-determinant 36 (cd36) impacts on vitamin e postprandial response. *Mol. Nutr. Food Res.* **2014**, *58*, 2297–2306. [CrossRef] [PubMed]
46. Moussa, M.; Gouranton, E.; Gleize, B.; El Yazidi, C.; Niot, I.; Besnard, P.; Borel, P.; Landrier, J.F. Cd36 is involved in lycopene and lutein uptake by adipocytes and adipose tissue cultures. *Mol. Nutr. Food Res.* **2011**, *55*, 578–584. [CrossRef]
47. van Bennekum, A.; Werder, M.; Thuahnai, S.T.; Han, C.H.; Duong, P.; Williams, D.L.; Wettstein, P.; Schulthess, G.; Phillips, M.C.; Hauser, H. Class b scavenger receptor-mediated intestinal absorption of dietary beta-carotene and cholesterol. *Biochemistry* **2005**, *44*, 4517–4525. [CrossRef]
48. Davis, H.R., Jr.; Altmann, S.W. Niemann-pick c1 like 1 (npc1l1) an intestinal sterol transporter. *Biochim. Biophys. Acta* **2009**, *1791*, 679–683. [CrossRef]
49. During, A.; Dawson, H.D.; Harrison, E.H. Carotenoid transport is decreased and expression of the lipid transporters sr-bi, npc1l1, and abca1 is downregulated in caco-2 cells treated with ezetimibe. *J. Nutr.* **2005**, *135*, 2305–2312. [CrossRef] [PubMed]
50. Sato, Y.; Suzuki, R.; Kobayashi, M.; Itagaki, S.; Hirano, T.; Noda, T.; Mizuno, S.; Sugawara, M.; Iseki, K. Involvement of cholesterol membrane transporter niemann-pick c1-like 1 in the intestinal absorption of lutein. *J. Pharm. Pharm. Sci.* **2012**, *15*, 256–264. [CrossRef]
51. Margier, M.; Collet, X.; le May, C.; Desmarchelier, C.; Andre, F.; Lebrun, C.; Defoort, C.; Bluteau, A.; Borel, P.; Lespine, A.; et al. Abcb1 (p-glycoprotein) regulates vitamin d absorption and contributes to its transintestinal efflux. *FASEB J.* **2019**, *33*, 2084–2094. [CrossRef] [PubMed]
52. Herron, K.L.; McGrane, M.M.; Waters, D.; Lofgren, I.E.; Clark, R.M.; Ordovas, J.M.; Fernandez, M.L. The abcg5 polymorphism contributes to individual responses to dietary cholesterol and carotenoids in eggs. *J. Nutr.* **2006**, *136*, 1161–1165. [CrossRef] [PubMed]
53. Tabunoki, H.; Sugiyama, H.; Tanaka, Y.; Fujii, H.; Banno, Y.; Jouni, Z.E.; Kobayashi, M.; Sato, R.; Maekawa, H.; Tsuchida, K. Isolation, characterization, and cdna sequence of a carotenoid binding protein from the silk gland of bombyx mori larvae. *J. Biol. Chem.* **2002**, *277*, 32133–32140. [CrossRef] [PubMed]
54. Bhosale, P.; Li, B.; Sharifzadeh, M.; Gellermann, W.; Frederick, J.M.; Tsuchida, K.; Bernstein, P.S. Purification and partial characterization of a lutein-binding protein from human retina. *Biochemistry* **2009**, *48*, 4798–4807. [CrossRef] [PubMed]
55. Borel, P.; Moussa, M.; Reboul, E.; Lyan, B.; Defoort, C.; Vincent-Baudry, S.; Maillot, M.; Gastaldi, M.; Darmon, M.; Portugal, H.; et al. Human fasting plasma concentrations of vitamin e and carotenoids, and their association with genetic variants in apo c-iii, cholesteryl ester transfer protein, hepatic lipase, intestinal fatty acid binding protein and microsomal triacylglycerol transfer protein. *Br. J. Nutr.* **2009**, *101*, 680–687. [PubMed]
56. Castenmiller, J.J.M.; West, C.E. Bioavailability and bioconversion of carotenoids. *Annu. Rev. Nutr.* **1998**, *18*, 19–38. [CrossRef] [PubMed]
57. dela Sena, C.; Riedl, K.M.; Narayanasamy, S.; Curley, R.W., Jr.; Schwartz, S.J.; Harrison, E.H. The human enzyme that converts dietary provitamin a carotenoids to vitamin a is a dioxygenase. *J. Biol. Chem.* **2014**, *289*, 13661–13666. [CrossRef] [PubMed]
58. Lobo, G.P.; Amengual, J.; Palczewski, G.; Babino, D.; von Lintig, J. Mammalian carotenoid-oxygenases: Key players for carotenoid function and homeostasis. *Biochim. Biophys. Acta* **2012**, *1821*, 78–87. [CrossRef] [PubMed]
59. Amengual, J.; Widjaja-Adhi, M.A.; Rodriguez-Santiago, S.; Hessel, S.; Golczak, M.; Palczewski, K.; von Lintig, J. Two carotenoid oxygenases contribute to mammalian provitamin a metabolism. *J. Biol. Chem.* **2013**, *288*, 34081–34096. [CrossRef] [PubMed]
60. O'Byrne, S.M.; Wongsiriroj, N.; Libien, J.; Vogel, S.; Goldberg, I.J.; Baehr, W.; Palczewski, K.; Blaner, W.S. Retinoid absorption and storage is impaired in mice lacking lecithin:Retinol acyltransferase (lrat). *J. Biol. Chem.* **2005**, *280*, 35647–35657. [CrossRef]
61. Wongsiriroj, N.; Piantedosi, R.; Palczewski, K.; Goldberg, I.J.; Johnston, T.P.; Li, E.; Blaner, W.S. The molecular basis of retinoid absorption: A genetic dissection. *J. Biol. Chem.* **2008**, *283*, 13510–13519. [CrossRef]
62. Palczewski, G.; Amengual, J.; Hoppel, C.L.; von Lintig, J. Evidence for compartmentalization of mammalian carotenoid metabolism. *FASEB J.* **2014**, *28*, 4457–4469. [CrossRef]

63. Kopec, R.E.; Caris-Veyrat, C.; Nowicki, M.; Gleize, B.; Carail, M.; Borel, P. Production of asymmetric oxidative metabolites of [13c]-beta-carotene during digestion in the gastrointestinal lumen of healthy men. *Am. J. Clin. Nutr.* **2018**, *108*, 803–813. [CrossRef]
64. You, C.S.; Parker, R.S.; Goodman, K.J.; Swanson, J.E.; Corso, T.N. Evidence of cis-trans isomerization of 9-cis-beta-carotene during absorption in humans. *Am. J. Clin. Nutr.* **1996**, *64*, 177–183. [CrossRef]
65. Richelle, M.; Sanchez, B.; Tavazzi, I.; Lambelet, P.; Bortlik, K.; Williamson, G. Lycopene isomerisation takes place within enterocytes during absorption in human subjects. *Br. J. Nutr.* **2010**, *103*, 1800–1807. [CrossRef]
66. Reboul, E.; Trompier, D.; Moussa, M.; Klein, A.; Landrier, J.F.; Chimini, G.; Borel, P. Atp-binding cassette transporter a1 is significantly involved in the intestinal absorption of alpha- and gamma-tocopherol but not in that of retinyl palmitate in mice. *Am. J. Clin. Nutr.* **2009**, *89*, 177–184. [CrossRef]
67. Niesor, E.J.; Chaput, E.; Mary, J.L.; Staempfli, A.; Topp, A.; Stauffer, A.; Wang, H.; Durrwell, A. Effect of compounds affecting abca1 expression and cetp activity on the hdl pathway involved in intestinal absorption of lutein and zeaxanthin. *Lipids* **2014**, *49*, 1233–1243. [CrossRef]
68. Borel, P.; Desmarchelier, C.; Nowicki, M.; Bott, R. Lycopene bioavailability is associated with a combination of genetic variants. *Free Radic. Biol. Med.* **2015**, *83*, 238–244. [CrossRef]
69. Borel, P.; Desmarchelier, C.; Nowicki, M.; Bott, R. A combination of single-nucleotide polymorphisms is associated with interindividual variability in dietary beta-carotene bioavailability in healthy men. *J. Nutr.* **2015**, *145*, 1740–1747. [CrossRef]
70. Borel, P.; Desmarchelier, C.; Nowicki, M.; Bott, R.; Morange, S.; Lesavre, N. Interindividual variability of lutein bioavailability in healthy men: Characterization, genetic variants involved, and relation with fasting plasma lutein concentration. *Am. J. Clin. Nutr.* **2014**, *100*, 168–175. [CrossRef]
71. Seino, Y.; Miki, T.; Kiyonari, H.; Abe, T.; Fujimoto, W.; Kimura, K.; Takeuchi, A.; Takahashi, Y.; Oiso, Y.; Iwanaga, T.; et al. Isx participates in the maintenance of vitamin a metabolism by regulation of beta-carotene 15,15′-monooxygenase (bcmo1) expression. *J. Biol. Chem.* **2008**, *283*, 4905–4911. [CrossRef] [PubMed]
72. Choi, M.Y.; Romer, A.I.; Hu, M.; Lepourcelet, M.; Mechoor, A.; Yesilaltay, A.; Krieger, M.; Gray, P.A.; Shivdasani, R.A. A dynamic expression survey identifies transcription factors relevant in mouse digestive tract development. *Development* **2006**, *133*, 4119–4129. [CrossRef]
73. Lobo, G.P.; Hessel, S.; Eichinger, A.; Noy, N.; Moise, A.R.; Wyss, A.; Palczewski, K.; von Lintig, J. Isx is a retinoic acid-sensitive gatekeeper that controls intestinal beta,beta-carotene absorption and vitamin a production. *FASEB J.* **2010**, *24*, 1656–1666. [CrossRef] [PubMed]
74. Goncalves, A.; Gleize, B.; Roi, S.; Nowicki, M.; Dhaussy, A.; Huertas, A.; Amiot, M.J.; Reboul, E. Fatty acids affect micellar properties and modulate vitamin d uptake and basolateral efflux in caco-2 cells. *J. Nutr. Biochem.* **2013**, *24*, 1751–1757. [CrossRef] [PubMed]
75. de Vogel-van den Bosch, H.M.; de Wit, N.J.; Hooiveld, G.J.; Vermeulen, H.; van der Veen, J.N.; Houten, S.M.; Kuipers, F.; Muller, M.; van der Meer, R. A cholesterol-free, high-fat diet suppresses gene expression of cholesterol transporters in murine small intestine. *Am. J. Physiol. Gastrointest. Liver Physiol.* **2008**, *294*, G1171–G1180. [CrossRef] [PubMed]
76. Chen, M.; Yang, Y.; Braunstein, E.; Georgeson, K.E.; Harmon, C.M. Gut expression and regulation of fat/cd36: Possible role in fatty acid transport in rat enterocytes. *Am. J. Physiol. Endocrinol. Metab.* **2001**, *281*, E916–E923. [CrossRef] [PubMed]
77. Davis, H.R., Jr.; Zhu, L.J.; Hoos, L.M.; Tetzloff, G.; Maguire, M.; Liu, J.; Yao, X.; Iyer, S.P.; Lam, M.H.; Lund, E.G.; et al. Niemann-pick c1 like 1 (npc1l1) is the intestinal phytosterol and cholesterol transporter and a key modulator of whole-body cholesterol homeostasis. *J. Biol. Chem.* **2004**, *279*, 33586–33592. [CrossRef]
78. Jesch, E.D.; Seo, J.M.; Carr, T.P.; Lee, J.Y. Sitosterol reduces messenger rna and protein expression levels of niemann-pick c1-like 1 in fhs 74 int cells. *Nutr. Res.* **2009**, *29*, 859–866. [CrossRef]
79. Brauner, R.; Johannes, C.; Ploessl, F.; Bracher, F.; Lorenz, R.L. Phytosterols reduce cholesterol absorption by inhibition of 27-hydroxycholesterol generation, liver x receptor alpha activation, and expression of the basolateral sterol exporter atp-binding cassette a1 in caco-2 enterocytes. *J. Nutr.* **2012**, *142*, 981–989. [CrossRef] [PubMed]
80. Alvaro, A.; Rosales, R.; Masana, L.; Vallve, J.C. Polyunsaturated fatty acids down-regulate in vitro expression of the key intestinal cholesterol absorption protein npc1l1: No effect of monounsaturated nor saturated fatty acids. *J. Nutr. Biochem.* **2010**, *21*, 518–525. [CrossRef] [PubMed]

81. Malhotra, P.; Boddy, C.S.; Soni, V.; Saksena, S.; Dudeja, P.K.; Gill, R.K.; Alrefai, W.A. D-glucose modulates intestinal niemann-pick c1-like 1 (npc1l1) gene expression via transcriptional regulation. *Am. J. Physiol. Gastrointest. Liver Physiol.* **2013**, *304*, G203–G210. [CrossRef] [PubMed]
82. Boztepe, T.; Gulec, S. Investigation of the influence of high glucose on molecular and genetic responses: An in vitro study using a human intestine model. *Genes Nutr.* **2018**, *13*, 11. [CrossRef]
83. Kim, B.; Park, Y.; Wegner, C.J.; Bolling, B.W.; Lee, J. Polyphenol-rich black chokeberry (aronia melanocarpa) extract regulates the expression of genes critical for intestinal cholesterol flux in caco-2 cells. *J. Nutr. Biochem.* **2013**, *24*, 1564–1570. [CrossRef] [PubMed]
84. Feng, D.; Zou, J.; Zhang, S.; Li, X.; Lu, M. Hypocholesterolemic activity of curcumin is mediated by down-regulating the expression of niemann-pick c1-like 1 in hamsters. *J. Agric. Food Chem.* **2017**, *65*, 276–280. [CrossRef]
85. Hayashi, A.A.; Webb, J.; Choi, J.; Baker, C.; Lino, M.; Trigatti, B.; Trajcevski, K.E.; Hawke, T.J.; Adeli, K. Intestinal sr-bi is upregulated in insulin-resistant states and is associated with overproduction of intestinal apob48-containing lipoproteins. *Am. J. Physiol. Gastrointest. Liver Physiol.* **2011**, *301*, G326–G337. [CrossRef] [PubMed]
86. Voshol, P.J.; Schwarz, M.; Rigotti, A.; Krieger, M.; Groen, A.K.; Kuipers, F. Down-regulation of intestinal scavenger receptor class b, type i (sr-bi) expression in rodents under conditions of deficient bile delivery to the intestine. *Biochem. J.* **2001**, *356*, 317–325. [CrossRef]
87. Duan, L.P.; Wang, H.H.; Ohashi, A.; Wang, D.Q. Role of intestinal sterol transporters abcg5, abcg8, and npc1l1 in cholesterol absorption in mice: Gender and age effects. *Am. J. Physiol. Gastrointest. Liver Physiol.* **2006**, *290*, G269–G276. [CrossRef]
88. Zhou, L.; Yang, H.; Okoro, E.U.; Guo, Z. Up-regulation of cholesterol absorption is a mechanism for cholecystokinin-induced hypercholesterolemia. *J. Biol. Chem.* **2014**, *289*, 12989–12999. [CrossRef]
89. Grenier, E.; Garofalo, C.; Delvin, E.; Levy, E. Modulatory role of pyy in transport and metabolism of cholesterol in intestinal epithelial cells. *PLoS ONE* **2012**, *7*, e40992. [CrossRef]
90. Reboul, E. Vitamin e intestinal absorption: Regulation of membrane transport across the enterocyte. *IUBMB Life* **2019**, *71*, 416–423. [CrossRef]
91. Desmarchelier, C.; Landrier, J.F.; Borel, P. Genetic factors involved in the bioavailability of tomato carotenoids. *Curr. Opin. Clin. Nutr. Metab. Care* **2018**, *21*, 489–497. [CrossRef] [PubMed]

11

Effect of Tomato Nutrient Complex on Blood Pressure: A Double Blind, Randomized Dose–Response Study

Talia Wolak [1,†], Yoav Sharoni [2,*], Joseph Levy [2], Karin Linnewiel-Hermoni [3], David Stepensky [2] and Esther Paran [1]

1 Hypertension Unit, Soroka University Medical center and Ben-Gurion University of the Negev, Beer Sheva 84101, Israel; twolak@bgu.ac.il (T.W.); paran@bgu.ac.il (E.P.)
2 Department of Clinical Biochemistry and Pharmacology, Ben-Gurion University of the Negev, Beer Sheva 84105, Israel; lyossi@bgu.ac.il (J.L.); davidst@bgu.ac.il (D.S.)
3 Lycored Ltd., Secaucus, NJ 07094, USA; Karin.Hermoni@lycored.com
* Correspondence: yoav@bgu.ac.il;
† Present address: Internal medicine D, Shaare Zedek Medical Center, Jerusalem 9103102, Israel.

Abstract: Oxidative stress is implicated in the pathogenesis of essential hypertension, a risk factor for cardiovascular morbidity and mortality. Tomato carotenoids such as lycopene and the colorless carotenoids phytoene and phytofluene induce the antioxidant defense mechanism. This double-blind, randomized, placebo-controlled study aimed to find effective doses of Tomato Nutrient Complex (TNC) to maintain normal blood pressure in untreated hypertensive individuals. The effect of TNC treatment (5, 15 and 30 mg lycopene) was compared with 15 mg of synthetic lycopene and a placebo over eight weeks. Results indicate that only TNC treatment standardized for 15 or 30 mg of lycopene was associated with significant reductions in mean systolic blood pressure (SBP). Treatment with the lower dose standardized for 5 mg of lycopene or treatment with 15 mg of synthetic lycopene as a standalone had no significant effect. To test carotenoid bioavailability, volunteers were treated for four weeks with TNC providing 2, 5 or 15 mg lycopene. The increase in blood levels of lycopene, phytoene, and phytofluene was dose dependent. Results suggest that only carotenoid levels achieved by the TNC dose of 15 mg lycopene or higher correlate to a beneficial effect on SBP in hypertensive subjects while lower doses and lycopene alone do not.

Keywords: hypertension; carotenoids; tomato extract; lycopene; phytoene; phytofluene; bioavailability

---

1. Introduction

Hypertension (HT) is a major risk factor for cardiovascular morbidity and mortality. Prior studies provide strong evidence that oxidative stress and inflammatory processes correlate with the pathogenesis of HT. Although many drugs related to this chronic pathology are available, the high profile of side effects of anti-HT drugs warrant alternative and complementary treatment for blood pressure (BP) control [1,2]. This includes lifestyle modifications, especially dietary interventions such as consumption of more fruits and vegetables [3,4]. In line with these, the antioxidant lycopene has gained considerable attention in improving vascular function and regulating BP [5]. However, intervention trials investigating the role of lycopene supplementation or lycopene-containing foods in BP regulation have produced conflicting results. Several studies demonstrate that oral supplementation with tomato extract or tomato juice significantly decreases BP [5–9], while other studies show no relation [10] or no obvious association [11,12]. Interestingly one study even shows that lycopene can elevate BP [13].

In a meta-analysis, Ried et al. [14] reviewed four studies investigating the effect of lycopene-containing foods on BP and concluded that lycopene treatment could effectively decrease systolic BP (SBP), but had no statistically significant effect on diastolic BP (DBP). In an updated meta-analysis of intervention trials, Li et al. [15] similarly concluded a significant reduction in SBP by lycopene, but no significant effect on DBP. An important finding in this report is that lycopene treatment is more efficient in decreasing higher SBP (above 120 mmHg), but has no effect on normal BP.

Tomato products or extracts are used as the lycopene source in most of these studies. The extracts contain lycopene, β-carotene and the colorless carotenoids phytoene and phytofluene, in addition to a myriad of other active nutrients such as tocopherols and polyphenols. Many of these are strong antioxidants and known inducers of the antioxidant defense pathway, which is one of the mechanisms for the cardiovascular protective effect. The fact that these preparations are not pure lycopene has been frequently ignored, for example, in meta-analysis publications [14,15]. Thus, one of the major aims of the current work was to compare the effect on BP of a pure synthetic lycopene to a proprietary tomato extract. To complement our previous results showing the improvement of BP by natural antioxidants from tomato extract in pre-HT patients [6,9], we tested its BP-lowering effects in Stage 1 and 2 HT patients, attempting to establish a dose dependency and to show bioavailability of the major carotenoids present in tomato extract.

2. Materials and Methods

2.1. Study Population

The original sample size was 26 subjects in each study arm (see Section 2.5). However, following completion of treatment of the first 46 subjects (9–10 subjects in each treatment arm), an interim analysis was performed. Based on this, the study recruitment was stopped, and all study data were analyzed.

Sixty-one hypertensive individuals (according to the 2017 ACC guidelines) [16] without anti-HT treatment, aged 35–60 years, were recruited from primary-care clinics and through advertisements posted in local newspapers. The recruited patients had BP values in the range of $130 < SBP < 145$ mmHg or $80 < DBP < 95$ mmHg, measured as detailed in Section 2.3. Subjects treated for HT or dyslipidemia; who had any suspected allergy to tomato, carotenoids or α-tocopherol; or were taking vitamins or other food additives were excluded from the study. Smokers, persons with diabetes or cardiovascular, gastrointestinal, hepatic or malignant diseases were also excluded. All included subjects signed an informed consent form presented to them by the researchers after receiving an explanation regarding the course of the trial. The local Helsinki ethics committee approved the study protocol (approval No. 4594, 2008). The study was registered at ClinicalTrials.gov with the Identifier: NCT00637858.

2.2. Materials

Tomato Nutrient Complex, a proprietary tomato extract, was supplied by Lycored Ltd., Beer Sheva, Israel at doses corresponding to 5, 15 and 30 mg lycopene. Lycored also supplied identical-looking capsules with 15 mg synthetic lycopene (18–20% cis isomers) and placebo capsules containing soybean oil. The TNC 15-mg capsule contained the indicated amounts of the following tomato phytonutrients: lycopene (6%; 8–10% cis isomers), phytoene (1%), phytofluene (1%); β-carotene (0.15–0.2%), vitamin E (2%), and other fat-soluble phytonutrients naturally present in the tomato, suspended in tomato oleoresin oil.

2.3. Procedure

At the screening visit, held at the Hypertension Outpatient Clinic of the Soroka University Medical Center, a thorough physical examination was performed, and a comprehensive medical and dietary history was collected for each participant. Blood pressure, pulse rate, height and weight were measured, and body mass index (BMI) was calculated. BP was measured after 10 min of rest in a sitting position using a new and calibrated Omron HEM–705CP electronic semiautomatic sphygmomanometer (Tokyo, Japan), which was used only for this study. Recorded BP was calculated as the average of three serial measurements if the difference between them was <8 mmHg for SBP and <5 mmHg for DBP. A trained research nurse blinded to the study periods and treatment took all measurements. BP measurements were taken at the same hour of the morning after abstinence from food and caffeine for a minimum of 30 min.

Allocated participants started treatment with a four-week single-blind placebo run-in period, in which they were asked to consume one placebo capsule a day. This phase was used to confirm that participants indeed had HT. Only subjects with BP values of 130 < SBP < 145 mmHg or 80 < DBP < 95 mmHg were randomized for the double-blind placebo-controlled treatment phase. The study was performed under complete blind conditions (single-blind or double-blind, in accordance with the study phase). Knowledge of the randomization list was limited to the independent study statistician responsible for the creation of the list (Dr. Michael Friger, Department of Epidemiology, Ben-Gurion University) and the LycoRed designee responsible for preparation of the study medication. The subjects were allocated sequential subject numbers, and the investigator entered the subject randomization number into each subject's file. There were five treatment arms: TNC 5 mg, TNC 15 mg, TNC 30 mg, synthetic lycopene (15 mg) and a placebo administered once daily for eight weeks. Participants were blinded to the different study periods and were instructed to take the capsules with the main meal of the day to improve absorption of its ingredients. No other dietary supplements were allowed throughout the study, and participants were instructed to keep their usual dietary habits. Follow-up visits were held every two weeks and included a short clinical evaluation, and BP and pulse rate measurements. Study medications were dispensed, and compliance was verified by counting the remaining capsules and giving reinforcement at each visit.

Blood was drawn after an overnight fast at the end of the run-in phase and the end of the eight-week treatment phase. Blood analysis for safety included: complete blood count; plasma levels of glucose, urea, uric acid, sodium, potassium, creatinine, aspartate amino transferase (AST), alanine amino transferase (ALT), alkaline phosphatase (ALP), lactate dehydrogenase (LDH) and bilirubin; and blood lipid profile: cholesterol, high-density lipoprotein (HDL), low-density lipoprotein (LDL) and triglycerides. Additional plasma samples were stored at −70 °C. Stored samples were extracted with ethanol and hexane/dichloromethane, and then analyzed for lycopene using a high-performance liquid chromatography (HPLC)-based analytical method.

2.4. *Steady-State Bioavailability of Tomato Carotenoids TNC Dose–Response*

The study was performed with a different group of subjects from the ones participating in the BP study. It was conducted at the Endocrine Laboratory, Department of Clinical Biochemistry and Pharmacology of the Ben-Gurion University and the Soroka University Medical Center and was approved by the Helsinki Committee of the medical center (approval No. 0012-15-SOR). Twenty-five healthy volunteers, aged 20–40, were recruited from students of Ben-Gurion University through advertisements posted on the university electronic bulletin board. Written informed consent was obtained from all volunteers prior to entry into the double-blind, randomized, cross-over study. In each experiment, baseline blood samples were collected after overnight fasting, and treatment with TNC at 2, 5 or 15 mg of lycopene was begun for four weeks, followed by a four-week washout period between experiments without consumption of any supplement. The capsules with the different doses were identical in appearance, and the different doses were randomly distributed to about one-third of the volunteers in each experiment. Both the volunteers and the researchers were blinded to the received doses. Participants were instructed to consume one capsule per day with their main meal and to keep their usual dietary habits throughout the experimental and washout periods. Blood samples were taken after two, three and four weeks of treatment, after overnight fasting and 24 h after taking the last supplement. Compliance was verified by counting the remaining capsules and it was 90% or higher.

Carotenoid analysis was performed after ethanol and hexane/dichloromethane (4/1) extraction by dedicated HPLC method using a C30 reverse phase column, gradient elution and detection at multiple wavelengths using a photodiode array detector.

2.5. Statistical Methods

Sample size calculations were performed by using appropriate formulas based on 80% power and a two-sided $\alpha = 0.05$ with assumption of a standard deviation of DBP equal to 3.8 mmHg. A clinically significant difference in DBP was determined at 3.0 mmHg. For this determination, the sample size was 26 patients in each treatment arm—in all, 130 participants.

The paired t-test or non-parametric signed-rank test was applied for testing the differences of the continuous assessments between all visits to the baseline. An ANOVA model using the Duncan method was applied for testing the differences in blood pressure changes between all study groups. All tests applied were two-tailed, and a p-value of 5% or less was considered statistically significant. The data were analyzed using the SAS® version 9.1 for Windows (SAS Institute, Cary, North Carolina). The missing data for early withdrawals who were not replaced and who attended at least four weeks of the double-blind placebo-controlled phase of the study were handled as LOCFs (last observation carried forward).

For the bioavailability study, summary statistics were calculated using a GraphPad Prism 5.0 program. Paired t-tests were used to compare the carotenoid concentrations at different time points. A p-value of <0.05 was deemed statistically significant.

3. Results

3.1. Demographics and Baseline Characteristics

Sixty-one patients with BP values in the range of 130 < SBP < 145 mmHg or 80 < DBP < 95 mmHg were enrolled in the study and began treatment with a four-week single-blind placebo run-in phase. These patients were randomized for the double-blind placebo-controlled treatment phase. At enrollment, there were 12 subjects in each of the following arms: TNC 5 mg, TNC 15 mg, synthetic lycopene 15 mg and placebo, in addition to 13 subjects in the TNC 30-mg arm. Forty-six subjects completed the eight-week treatment period and 15 (3 in each arm) dropped out of the study prematurely. There were neither adverse effects reported during the entire study period nor any significant changes in glucose, urea, creatinine, uric acid, sodium, potassium, chloride, cholesterol, triglycerides, AST, ALT, ALP, LDH, HDL, LDL levels, or in the blood count parameters.

The treatment arms were comparable with respect to all demographic and baseline characteristics (Table 1). Baseline SBP and DBP measurements were not statistically significantly different (Table 1). The mean age was 52.4 ± 8.2 years, and 73.8% were male. The mean SBP and DBP were 135.2 ± 7.4 mmHg and 82.0 ± 11.7 mmHg, respectively. There were no statistically significant differences between the five arms in the baseline plasma lycopene concentrations; however, the mean concentration of the TNC 15-mg arm was somewhat higher than the other arms.

Table 1. Baseline characteristics of the study population.

Parameter	TNC 5 mg	TNC 15 mg	TNC 30 mg	Synthetic Lycopene 15 mg	Placebo	All
Age (years) [1]	53.5 ± 8.0 (12)	54.0 ± 8.6 (12)	51.0 ± 10.1 (13)	52.1 ± 8.4 (12)	51.8 ± 6.3 (12)	52.4 ± 8.2 (61)
Males (%)	66.7% (8)	75.0% (9)	69.2% (9)	66.7% (8)	83.3% (10)	72.1% (44)
Females (%)	33.3% (4)	25.0% (3)	30.8 (4)	33.3% (4)	16.7% (2)	27.9% (17)
SBP (mmHg) [1]	133.6 ± 7.8 (12)	137.4 ± 5.6 (12)	136.4 ± 7.8 (13)	132.8 ± 9.3 (12)	135.7 ± 6.0 (12)	135.2 ± 7.4 (61)
DBP (mmHg) [1]	82.9 ± 9.3 (12)	83.8 ± 6.3 (12)	77.5 ± 21 (13)	82.3 ± 6.1 (12)	83.7 ± 8.7 (12)	82.0 ± 11.7 (61)
Plasma lycopene (μM)	0.97 ± 0.49 (7)	1.55 ± 0.86 (7)	0.80 ± 0.74 (10)	0.91 ± 0.95 (8)	1.01 ± 1.24 (10)	0.93 ± 0.68 (42)
TG (mg/dL)	152.0 ± 70.4 (11)	164.3 ± 65.3 (10)	124.5 ± 75.3 (12)	115.1 ± 50.5 (10)	166.0 ± 103.1 (12)	
HDL chol (mg/dL)	52.0 ± 12.2 (10)	49.5 ± 10.1 (10)	54.4 ± 10.0 (12)	59.1 ± 18.2 (10)	52.1 ± 11.7 (11)	
LDL chol (mg/dL)	142.1 ± 34.6 (10)	107.4 ± 26.0 (9)	104.8 ± 31.1 (11)	134.2 ± 29.5 (10)	112.9 ± 30.1 (9)	

[1] Age, BP, lycopene, TG, HDL, and LDL values are mean ± SD (N).

3.2. Changes in BP Values during the 8-Week Double-Blind Placebo-Controlled Treatment Phase

The average SBP in the five treatment arms during eight weeks of treatment is presented in Table 2. The change in SBP in the treatment arms during this same period are presented in Figure 1. Treatment with TNC containing 15 or 30 mg lycopene was associated with statistically significant reductions in mean SBP at almost all time points from two to eight weeks. Similar effects were not observed following treatment with 5 mg of TNC, 15 mg of synthetic lycopene or the placebo. A comparison between treatment arms revealed that the reduction in SBP in the TNC 15-mg arm following eight weeks of treatment was statistically different from that of the TNC 5-mg arm, the placebo arm and the synthetic lycopene arm ($p = 0.0495$). Remarkably, the rate of reduction in SBP with time of treatment for the 15-mg and 30-mg arms is almost parallel (Figure 1), suggesting that TNC containing 15 mg lycopene is both necessary and sufficient to normalize SBP.

Table 2. SBP during eight weeks of treatment.

SBP [1] (mmHg)	TNC 5 mg	TNC 15 mg	TNC 30 mg	Synthetic Lycopene 15 mg	Placebo
Baseline	133.6 ± 7.8 (12)	137.4 ± 5.6 (12)	136.4 ± 7.8 (13)	132.8 ± 9.3 (12)	135.7 ± 6.0 (12)
Week 2	132.7 ± 8.9 (10)	133.7 ± 5.3 (12)	131.5 ± 8.0 (13)	133.2 ± 8.9 (11)	137.1 ± 10.3 (11)
Week 4	133.1 ± 9.2 (9)	130.7 ± 4.7 (10)	131.7 ± 10.5 (11)	133.4 ± 7.2 (9)	134.5 ± 8.7 (10)
Week 6	132.8 ± 9.2 (9)	130.2 ± 10.6 (9)	129.9 ± 13.9 (10)	130.1 ± 9.8 (9)	133.7 ± 9.9 (9)
Week 8	131.4 ± 7.7 (9)	127.2 ± 6.3 (9)	130.0 ± 13.0 (10)	132.6 ± 5.1 (9)	133.0 ± 6.7 (9)

[1] SBP values are mean ± SD (N).

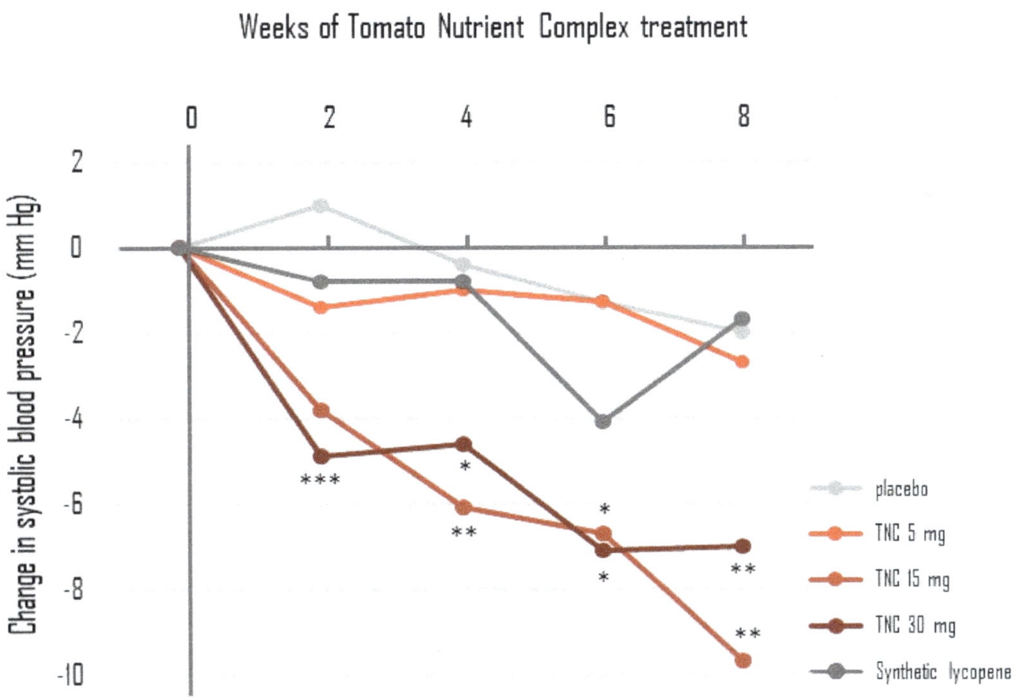

Figure 1. Tomato Nutrient Complex containing 15 mg and 30 mg lycopene reduces systolic blood pressure. Results are the mean of the individual changes from baseline to each time point from two to eight weeks. SDs are not shown for graph simplicity. N is the same as in Table 2. * $p < 0.05$; ** $p < 0.01$; *** $p < 0.001$ for changes to baseline within treatment arm.

The average DBP in the five treatment arms during the eight-week treatment is presented in Table 3. The changes in DBP in the five arms during this period are presented in Table 4. A significant reduction in DBP from baseline to eight weeks was observed only in the TNC 15-mg arm (−4.1 ± 5.0, $p = 0.038$, Table 4). There were no significant differences in DBP when treatment arms were compared.

Table 3. DBP during eight weeks of treatment.

DBP [1] (mmHg)	TNC 5 mg	TNC 15 mg	TNC 30 mg	Synthetic Lycopene 15 mg	Placebo
Baseline	82.9 ± 9.3 (12)	83.8 ± 6.3 (12)	77.5 ± 21 (13)	82.3 ± 6.1 (12)	83.7 ± 8.7 (12)
Week 2	81.4 ± 8.2 (10)	80.7 ± 7.1 (12)	80.5 ± 7.9 (13)	84.5 ± 6.1 (11)	84.2 ± 8.2 (11)
Week 4	82.8 ± 9.9 (9)	81.3 ± 3.9 (10)	82.6 ± 9.1 (11)	84.9 ± 6.6 (9)	83.0 ± 8.8 (10)
Week 6	82.6 ± 6.4 (9)	78.8 ± 7.5 (9)	72.3 ± 23 (10)	81.6 ± 6.0 (9)	83.2 ± 7.9 (9)
Week 8	81.7 ± 7.9 (9)	78.6 ± 7.9 (9)	74.4 ± 23 (10)	84.6 ± 5.0 (9)	85.3 ± 7.0 (9)

[1] DBP values are mean ± SD (*N*).

Table 4. Change in DBP from baseline during eight weeks of treatment.

DBP (mmHg)	TNC 5 mg	TNC 15 mg	TNC 30 mg	Synthetic Lycopene 15 mg	Placebo
	Mean ± SD (*p* [1])	Mean ± SD (*p*)	Mean ± SD (*p*)	Mean ± SD (*p*)	Mean ± SD (*p*)
Week 2	−2.9 ± 7.7 (0.265)	−3.2 ± 4.5 (0.032)	3.0 ± 4.9 (0.672)	0.9 ± 2.9 (0.331)	0.0 ± 5.0 (1.000)
Week 4	−0.9 ± 5.1 (0.613)	−1.9 ± 5.1 (0.268)	6.8 ± 7.0 (0.422)	1.2 ± 4.6 (0.449)	−0.4 ± 8.6 (0.887)
Week 6	−1.1 ± 5.8 (0.582)	−3.9 ± 6.5 (0.112)	−3.5 ± 5.9 (0.092)	−2.1 ± 4.5 (0.198)	−1.4 ± 9.8 (0.671)
Week 8	−2.0 ± 6.3 (0.371)	−4.1 ± 5.0 (0.038)	−1.4 ± 5.7 (0.454)	0.9 ± 5.6 (0.645)	0.7 ± 5.8 (0.740)

[1] *p*-value for changes to baseline within treatment arms. *N* is the same as in Table 3.

3.3. Changes in BP Values during the Single-Blind 16-Week Study Extension

Of the 46 subjects who completed the first phase of eight weeks of treatment, 31 agreed to continue for a single-blind four-month extension study with TNC containing 15 mg of lycopene. Four subjects ended this phase prematurely. The average SBP and DBP of the 27 subjects who completed the extension phase were compared to the average baseline values of the same subjects, measured at the randomization stage before the eight weeks of treatment. The results of SBP and DBP are presented in Table 5 and Figure 2. A statistically significant reduction in mean SBP was evident at all time points from one to four months. This result suggests that the SBP-reducing effect of TNC is long lasting. The changes in DBP from baseline to Month 4 were not significant.

Table 5. Mean SBP and DBP and changes from baseline in BP values during four-month study extension.

	SBP (mmHg) [1]	Change of SBP [1] from Baseline (mmHg)	*p*-Value for Change	DBP (mmHg) [1]	Change of DBP [1] from Baseline (mmHg)	*p*-Value for Change
Baseline	135.1 ± 8.76			85.1 ± 6.6		
Month 1	130.9 ± 8.6	−4.2 ± 6.5	0.0024	84.3 ± 6.2	−0.9 ± 5.7	0.422
Month 2	131.7 ± 10	−3.5 ± 7.4	0.0211	81.6 ± 15.5	−3.6 ± 15.8	0.252
Month 3	130.6 ± 8.8	−4.5 ± 7.0	0.0024	82.7 ± 7.7	−2.4 ± 6.3	0.056
Month 4	130.4 ± 10.9	−4.7 ±6.7	0.0012	83.9 ± 7.3	−1.4 ± 4.3	0.362

[1] BP values and changes in BP values are mean ± SD for the 27 subjects who completed the four-month extension phase.

3.4. Changes from Baseline of Plasma Levels of Lycopene

There was large variability in plasma lycopene baseline values (Table 6), and in the changes from baseline to eight weeks of treatment (Figure 3). Due to this variability and the small number of tested samples, there was no significant change in lycopene concentration in any of the arms, but the highest change was observed in the synthetic lycopene arm (Figure 3).

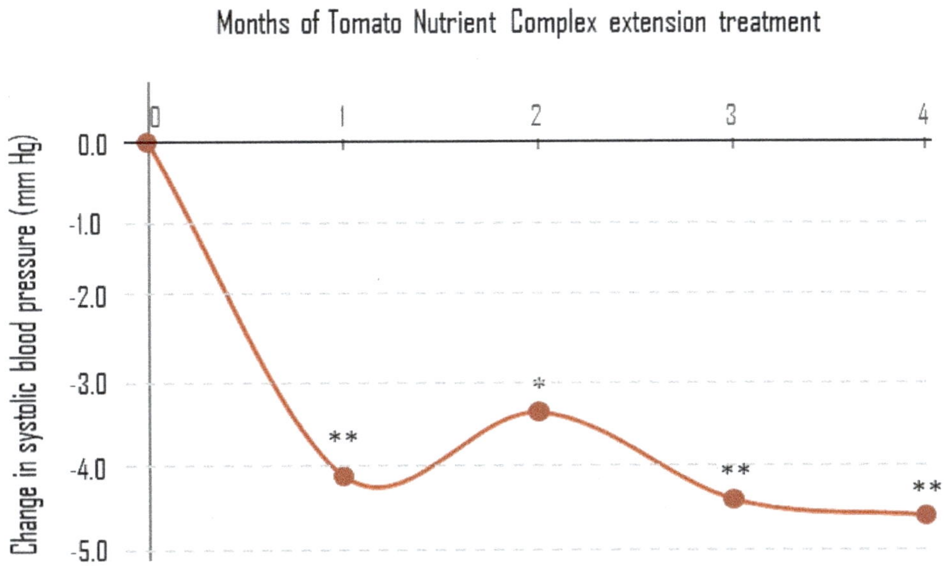

Figure 2. Changes in SBP values during the single-blind 16-week study extension. SBP values are the mean for the 27 subjects who completed this phase. * $p < 0.05$; ** $p < 0.01$ for changes to baseline within treatment arm.

Table 6. Plasma lycopene value at baseline and at eight weeks of treatment.

SBP [1] (mmHg)	TNC 5 mg	TNC 15 mg	TNC 30 mg	Synthetic Lycopene 15 mg	Placebo
Baseline	0.97 ± 0.49 (7)	1.55 ± 0.86 (7)	0.80 ± 0.74 (9)	0.91 ± 0.95 (7)	1.01 ± 1.24 (9)
Week 8	1.13 ± 0.97 (7)	1.89 ± 1.22 (7)	1.23 ±1.07 (9)	1.84 ± 1.14 (7)	0.72 ± 0.72 (9)

[1] Plasma lycopene values are mean ± SD (*N*).

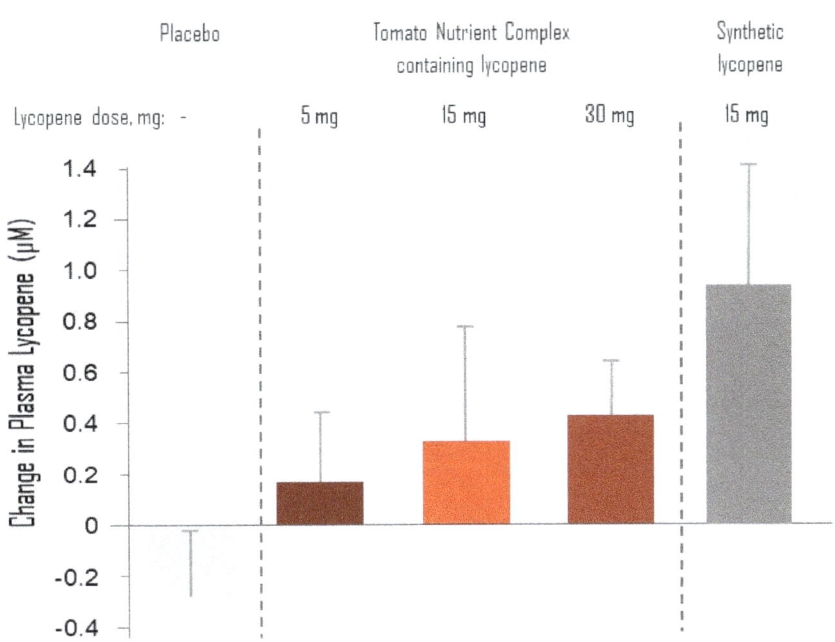

Figure 3. Changes of plasma levels of lycopene from baseline to eight weeks. Results are the mean ± SD of the changes from baseline to Week 8 within treatment arms. *N* was 9, 7, 7, 9, and 7 for the placebo, TNC 5 mg, TNC 15 mg, TNC 30 mg and synthetic lycopene arms, respectively.

3.5. Bioavailability of Tomato Carotenoids during 4 Weeks of Daily TNC Supplementation—A Dose–Response Study

Because of the large variability in the results of carotenoid plasma concentrations in the BP study patients (Section 3.4) and the low number of available samples, we conducted a separate bioavailability study of TNC with a different group of volunteers to evaluate the dose–response of steady-state carotenoid plasma concentrations during daily TNC treatment. A statistically significant increase in plasma lycopene was evident from Week 2 for the three supplemented doses (Table 7). For phytofluene, such an increase was not detected at all time points for the lowest dose (TNC 2 mg), but was evident at the highest dose (TNC 15 mg), and at Weeks 3 and 4 with TNC 5 mg. For phytoene, a significant increase was already detected for the two higher doses at Week 2 and at the lowest dose only at Week 4. No significant change was detected in the plasma concentrations of β-carotene, a control carotenoid that is found in very low amounts in the TNC preparations (e.g., 0.8 mg in the TNC 15 mg).

Table 7. Carotenoid plasma concentrations during 4-week treatment with TNC containing 2, 5 and 15 mg lycopene.

Carotenoid Plasma Concentration (μM)	Baseline Mean ± SD	Week 2 Mean ± SD (p) [1]	Week 3 Mean ± SD (p) [1]	Week 4 Mean ± SD (p) [1]
Lycopene				
TNC 2 mg [2]	1.021 ± 0.437	1.483 ± 0.481 (0.001)	1.354 ± 0.408 (0.009)	1.656 ± 0.537 (<0.000x)
TNC 5 mg [2]	1.149 ± 0.322	1.629 ± 0.444 (<0.000x)	1.677 ± 0.470 (<0.000x)	1.767 ± 0.473 (<0.000x)
TNC 15 mg [2]	1.036 ± 0.398	1.794 ± 0.453 (<0.000x)	1.754 ± 0.449 (<0.000x)	2.008 ± 0.627 (<0.000x)
Phytofluene				
TNC 2 mg [2]	0.310 ± 0.147	0.382 ± 0.211 (0.171)	0.300 ± 0.126 (0.805)	0.398 ± 0.242 (0.128)
TNC 5 mg [2]	0.354 ± 0.130	0.429 ± 0.190 (0.120)	0.456 ± 0.201 (0.046)	0.530 ± 0.263 (0.005)
TNC 15 mg [2]	0.270 ± 0.111	0.503 ± 0.235 (<0.000x)	0.536 ± 0.228 (<0.000x)	0.650 ± 0.275 (<0.000x)
Phytoene				
TNC 2 mg [2]	0.057 ± 0.040	0.073 ± 0.060 (0.300)	0.059 ± 0.037 (0.868)	0.091 ± 0.061 (0.028)
TNC 5 mg [2]	0.046 ± 0.032	0.096 ± 0.050 (<0.000x)	0.092 ± 0.057 (0.001)	0.124 ± 0.058 (<0.000x)
TNC 15 mg [2]	0.048 ± 0.031	0.133 ± 0.062 (<0.000x)	0.127 ± 0.068 (<0.000x)	0.158 ± 0.091 (<0.000x)
β-carotene				
TNC 2 mg [2]	0.842 ± 0.391	0.975 ± 0.484 (0.289)	0.872 ± 0.486 (0.811)	0.998 ± 0.502 (0.224)
TNC 5 mg [2]	0.947 ± 0.598	0.954 ± 0.580 (0.965)	0.919 ± 0.473 (0.866)	1.037 ± 0.533 (0.590)
TNC 15 mg [2]	0.885 ± 0.534	0.968 ± 0.609 (0.618)	0.970 ± 0.553 (0.587)	1.057 ± 0.631 (0.315)

[1] p-value for difference from baseline within the same dose arm. [2] N = 25 for TNC 2 mg and 15 mg. N = 24 for TNC 5 mg.

To calculate the average net increase in carotenoid concentrations, individual baseline concentrations were subtracted from values at other time points (Figure 4). The increase in plasma lycopene and phytofluene concentrations were significantly lower with TNC 5 mg and TNC 2 mg than with TNC 15 mg. This result suggests that the lower increase in these carotenoid concentrations for TNC 5 mg as compared to TNC 15 mg was not enough to drive the reduction in SBP in the HT subjects (Table 3). For phytoene, there was a significant difference between TNC 15 and TNC 2 mg, but not TNC 5 mg. When comparing the changes in carotenoid concentrations between TNC 5 mg and TNC 2 mg, a significantly higher increase was evident at the three time points only for phytoene concentrations, but not for lycopene and phytofluene.

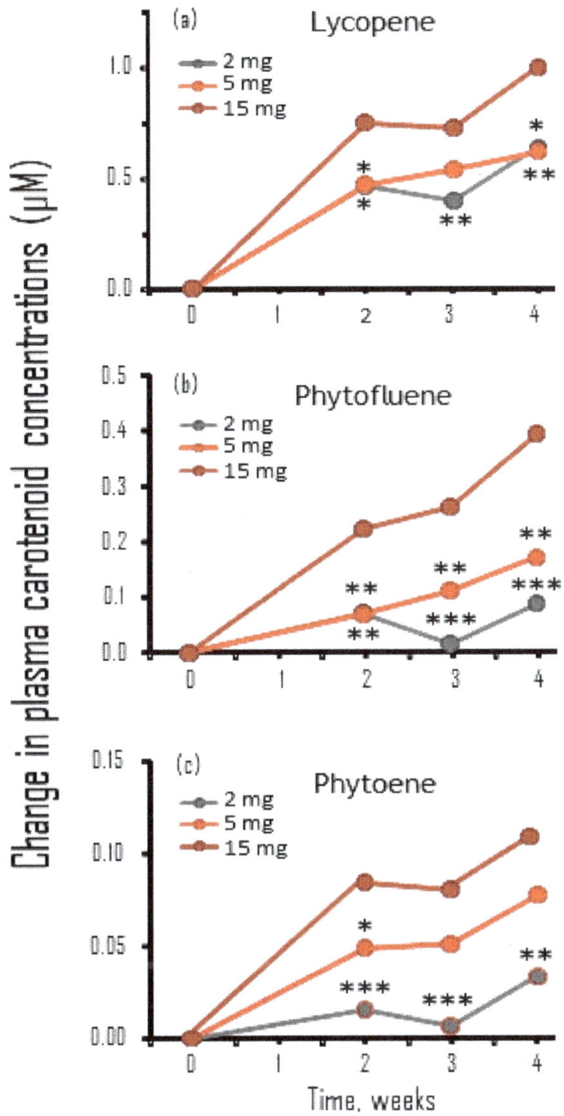

Figure 4. The increase in lycopene, phytofluene and phytoene concentrations after 2–4 weeks of treatment with TNC were significantly lower with TNC 5 mg and TNC 2 mg than with TNC 15 mg: (**a**) lycopene; (**b**) phytofluene; and (**c**) phytoene. Please note that the scale in the Y-axis is different for the three carotenoids. Results are the mean of individual changes in carotenoid concentrations of 25 subjects (TNC 2 mg and 15 mg) or 24 subjects (TNC 5 mg). SDs are not shown for graph simplicity. * $p < 0.05$; ** $p < 0.01$; *** $p < 0.001$ for the difference at each time point between TNC 15 mg to TNC 2 mg or TNC 5 mg.

A small continuous increase in the three carotenoid concentrations was observed from Week 2, to Weeks 3 and 4. However, there were no statistically significant differences between the concentrations at these time points, which suggests that steady-state concentrations were already attained after two weeks of TNC supplementation.

4. Discussion

The aims of the current study were to perform a dose–response analysis and uncover the optimal effective dose of a proprietary Tomato Nutrient Complex supplement in maintaining blood pressure within a normal range among untreated HT individuals and to compare the effect of TNC to that of synthetic lycopene. The bioavailability of the major tomato carotenoids was studied in a separate group of volunteers to gain insight into their relative contribution to the BP lowering effect of TNC.

Our study has several limitations. The minimum time between food and caffeine intake was determined to be 30 min. However, this time may be too short to prevent any effect of food intake on the BP measurement. In addition, the exact time and the type of food/beverages taken were not recorded; thus, it was not possible to estimate the effect of the food on BP analysis. The study lacks quantitative information on consumption of fruit and vegetables at baseline and at follow-up times. However, the lycopene plasma concentrations at baseline, which partially reflect this consumption, were not statistically different between study arms (Table 1), suggesting that this did not have a major effect on the study results. Although the participants were encouraged to maintain their dietary habits, there is no quantitative information on their food consumption during the study period to confirm that they did. In addition, there is no information on BMI or physical activity before and during the study, factors that may affect BP. These limitations should be considered in future studies, but it should be emphasized that, despite these limitations, the study resulted in showing significant effects of TNC on SBP.

Results of this double-blind, randomized, placebo-controlled study indicate that treatment with TNC standardized to contain 15 or 30 mg of lycopene was associated with statistically significant reductions in mean SBP. Treatment with the lower dose of TNC standardized for 5 mg of lycopene or treatment with 15 mg of synthetic lycopene did not produce a significant effect. DBP was not significantly different from the baseline with any treatment or control arm. Subjects from all treatment arms participated in an additional single-blind extension period for four months with TNC containing 15 mg lycopene, which resulted in a significant reduction of SBP that was persistent throughout the extension period. Thus, the reduction of SBP appears to be of a long-term nature. During the study and extension period, all treatments were safe and well tolerated, and no treatment-related adverse effects were reported.

The current results are in line with the recent meta-analysis of the effects of tomato products on BP [14,15] demonstrating a significant reduction of SBP, but no statistically significant effect on DBP. Subgroup analyses within the six studies [1,6–9,13], which met the inclusion criteria in the more recent study [15], demonstrated that higher dosage of tomato-derived supplements (containing more than 12 mg lycopene per day) could significantly lower SBP, whereas lower doses did not show a significant effect. This is similar to the results of the current study, which did not indicate a significant SBP reduction with TNC corresponding to 5 mg lycopene per day, but did show an effect at 15 and 30 mg. The low dose is probably the reason for the negative results in Paterson et al.'s study [13], which used only 4.5 mg/day lycopene, an amount close to the non-effective lycopene dose in the current study. Another important factor obtained in the meta-analysis was related to the baseline SBP. A significant reduction of SBP was observed if participants had higher baseline SBP (SBP $\geq$ 120 mmHg). Although this issue was not examined in the current study, it is important to note that the baseline SBP of all participants was above the threshold level (120 mmHg) suggested by the meta-analysis.

Remarkably, treatment with 15 mg of synthetic lycopene as a standalone did not cause a significant reduction in SBP. Apparently, this was not due to lower bioavailability of lycopene in the synthetic preparation. Actually, the mean increase in blood lycopene between the baseline and eight weeks was higher with the synthetic lycopene as compared to treatment with TNC containing 15 and 30 mg lycopene. Synthetic lycopene is different from tomato-derived lycopene in the ratio of cis:trans isomers—about 20% cis-isomers are in the synthetic lycopene and 10% in TNC. However, this difference cannot explain the better efficiency of TNC in lowering SBP, as we showed previously that the cis:trans ratio in supplemented lycopene does not affect the ratio in plasma and tissues [17]. The effects of purified lycopene was tested in another study on biomarkers of oxidative stress [18]. In that study, healthy volunteers were treated with 0, 6.5, 15 or 30 mg lycopene/day for eight weeks, which significantly increased plasma lycopene levels in agreement with our results. Interestingly, it was found that pure lycopene supplementation at all doses did not affect biomarkers of lipid peroxidation, whereas biomarkers of DNA damage were affected only at the highest dose of 30 mg/day of pure lycopene. This is similar to the lack of effect of 15 mg pure lycopene on BP in the current study.

One explanation for the lower efficacy of the synthetic lycopene is the presence of other active nutrients in the tomato extract preparation. Indeed, in a previous study [19], we found that the anti-cancer effects of carotenoids and other phytonutrients present in tomato extract (e.g., lycopene, phytoene and phytofluene) resides in their combined activity, which is synergistically higher than the activity of each compound alone. To assess the potential contribution of other tomato constituents to the BP-lowering effect, we analyzed the bioavailability of these carotenoids following treatment with different doses of TNC in a group of 25 healthy volunteers. Although the characteristics of these volunteers are different from those of the participants of the BP study, the information about the differences in the dose–response of the three major tomato carotenoids can shed light on the results of the BP study, as discussed below. The increase in blood levels of lycopene, phytoene and phytofluene was dose dependent, and was significantly higher with TNC 15 mg as compared to TNC 5 mg. A large increase in plasma concentrations of lycopene, phytofluene, and phytoene was already evident after two weeks of treatment. This correlates well with the reduction of SBP with TNC 15 mg, which was statistically significant after two weeks of treatment, suggesting that the increase in these tomato constituents was the reason and the driving force for the SBP reduction. It should be noted that the changes in phytofluene and phytoene plasma concentrations between the non-effective dose of TNC 5 mg and the effective TNC 15 mg was more pronounced than that of lycopene, which suggests that these carotenoids (and possibly other components of TNC) have an important role in reducing SBP. Such a role for phytofluene and phytoene can also explain the lower effect of pure synthetic lycopene, which does not contain these carotenoids or any other tomato component. This option is supported by a study showing that a reduction in UV-induced erythema by tomato extract enriched with phytofluene and phytoene was larger than that achieved with non-enriched tomato extract, whereas the lowest erythema reduction was found with synthetic lycopene [20].

An important question not addressed in the current study is what the mechanism might be by which the supplemented tomato carotenoids reduce BP. A possible answer is suggested by a study in endothelial cells [21], in which Di Tumo et al. found that lycopene and β-carotene reduce TNFα-induced inflammation in endothelial cells in culture. This effect was associated with reduced reactive oxygen species and nitrotyrosine [an index of interaction of NO with superoxide anion (O_2^-)] and an increase in NO and cGMP, which are known to cause vascular relaxation. The antioxidant effect of the carotenoids, which led to the observed effects in the endothelial cells, and possibly to lower SBP in the current human study, probably resulted from activation of the antioxidant response element and the Nrf2 transcription system that is induced by carotenoids, as we reported previously [22,23].

5. Conclusions

TNC containing 15 mg and 30 mg lycopene was well tolerated and showed efficacy in reducing SBP in the HT population, while lower doses and standalone pure lycopene were not sufficient to induce similar effects. The content of lycopene in raw tomatoes is 2.5–4 mg per 100 g [24]. Thus, reasonable consumption of tomatoes, e.g., 100–200 g per day, will supply 4–8 mg lycopene, but not enough to drive SBP reduction; therefore, inclusion in the daily diet of other lycopene-rich foods such as tomato products and supplements is recommended. It is not clear whether a supplement such as TNC can be used as a standalone treatment or in conjunction with other treatments. However, our previous study that used tomato extract in treated but uncontrolled hypertensive patients [9] suggests that patients treated with various antihypertensive drugs can benefit from the addition of TNC.

Author Contributions: Conceptualization, Y.S., J.L. and E.P.; Formal analysis, D.S. and E.P.; Funding acquisition, Y.S., J.L. and E.P.; Investigation, T.W., Y.S., J.L. and E.P.; Methodology, T.W., Y.S., J.L. and E.P.; Project administration, Y.S., J.L. and E.P.; Resources, Y.S., K.L.-H. and E.P.; Supervision, Y.S., J.L. and E.P.; Visualization, Y.S., J.L., K.L.-H. and D.S.; Writing—original draft, Y.S. and J.L.; and Writing—review and editing, T.W., Y.S., J.L., K.L.-H., D.S. and E.P.

Acknowledgments: We thank Arnon Aharon and Iris Alroy for initial analysis of the BP data, Michael Friger for the randomization process and for sample size calculation, Gil Harari, Medistat, Ltd. for the statistical analysis of the BP data, and Robin Miller for English editing.

References

1. Thies, F.; Masson, L.F.; Rudd, A.; Vaughan, N.; Tsang, C.; Brittenden, J.; Simpson, W.G.; Duthie, S.; Horgan, G.W.; Duthie, G. Effect of a tomato-rich diet on markers of cardiovascular disease risk in moderately overweight, disease-free, middle-aged adults: A randomized controlled trial. *Am. J. Clin. Nutr.* **2012**, *95*, 1013–1022. [CrossRef] [PubMed]
2. Yeh, G.Y.; Davis, R.B.; Phillips, R.S. Use of complementary therapies in patients with cardiovascular disease. *Am. J. Cardiol.* **2006**, *98*, 673–680. [CrossRef] [PubMed]
3. Chobanian, A.V.; Bakris, G.L.; Black, H.R.; Cushman, W.C.; Green, L.A.; Izzo, J.L., Jr.; Jones, D.W.; Materson, B.J.; Oparil, S.; Wright, J.T., Jr.; et al. The seventh report of the joint national committee on prevention, detection, evaluation, and treatment of high blood pressure: The jnc 7 report. *JAMA* **2003**, *289*, 2560–2572. [CrossRef]
4. Svetkey, L.P.; Simons-Morton, D.; Vollmer, W.M.; Appel, L.J.; Conlin, P.R.; Ryan, D.H.; Ard, J.; Kennedy, B.M. Effects of dietary patterns on blood pressure: Subgroup analysis of the dietary approaches to stop hypertension (dash) randomized clinical trial. *Arch. Intern. Med.* **1999**, *159*, 285–293. [CrossRef]
5. John, J.H.; Ziebland, S.; Yudkin, P.; Roe, L.S.; Neil, H.A.; Oxford, F.; Vegetable Study, G. Effects of fruit and vegetable consumption on plasma antioxidant concentrations and blood pressure: A randomised controlled trial. *Lancet* **2002**, *359*, 1969–1974. [CrossRef]
6. Engelhard, Y.N.; Gazer, B.; Paran, E. Natural antioxidants from tomato extract reduce blood pressure in patients with grade-1 hypertension: A double-blind, placebo-controlled pilot study. *Am. Heart J.* **2006**, *151*, 100. [CrossRef]
7. Kim, J.Y.; Paik, J.K.; Kim, O.Y.; Park, H.W.; Lee, J.H.; Jang, Y.; Lee, J.H. Effects of lycopene supplementation on oxidative stress and markers of endothelial function in healthy men. *Atherosclerosis* **2011**, *215*, 189–195. [CrossRef]
8. Ried, K.; Frank, O.R.; Stocks, N.P. Dark chocolate or tomato extract for prehypertension: A randomised controlled trial. *BMC Complement. Altern. Med.* **2009**, *9*, 22. [CrossRef] [PubMed]
9. Paran, E.; Novack, V.; Engelhard, Y.N.; Hazan-Halevy, I. The effects of natural antioxidants from tomato extract in treated but uncontrolled hypertensive patients. *Cardiovasc. Drugs Ther.* **2009**, *23*, 145–151. [CrossRef]
10. Hozawa, A.; Jacobs, D.R., Jr.; Steffes, M.W.; Gross, M.D.; Steffen, L.M.; Lee, D.H. Circulating carotenoid concentrations and incident hypertension: The coronary artery risk development in young adults (cardia) study. *J. Hypertens.* **2009**, *27*, 237–242. [CrossRef]
11. Itsiopoulos, C.; Brazionis, L.; Kaimakamis, M.; Cameron, M.; Best, J.D.; O'Dea, K.; Rowley, K. Can the mediterranean diet lower hba1c in type 2 diabetes? Results from a randomized cross-over study. *Nutr. Metab. Cardiovasc. Dis.* **2011**, *21*, 740–747. [CrossRef]
12. Upritchard, J.E.; Sutherland, W.H.; Mann, J.I. Effect of supplementation with tomato juice, vitamin e, and vitamin c on ldl oxidation and products of inflammatory activity in type 2 diabetes. *Diabetes Care* **2000**, *23*, 733–738. [CrossRef]
13. Paterson, E.; Gordon, M.H.; Niwat, C.; George, T.W.; Parr, L.; Waroonphan, S.; Lovegrove, J.A. Supplementation with fruit and vegetable soups and beverages increases plasma carotenoid concentrations but does not alter markers of oxidative stress or cardiovascular risk factors. *J. Nutr.* **2006**, *136*, 2849–2855. [CrossRef]
14. Ried, K.; Fakler, P. Protective effect of lycopene on serum cholesterol and blood pressure: Meta-analyses of intervention trials. *Maturitas* **2011**, *68*, 299–310. [CrossRef] [PubMed]
15. Li, X.; Xu, J. Lycopene supplement and blood pressure: An updated meta-analysis of intervention trials. *Nutrients* **2013**, *5*, 3696–3712. [CrossRef]
16. Whelton, P.K.; Carey, R.M.; Aronow, W.S.; Casey, D.E., Jr.; Collins, K.J.; Dennison Himmelfarb, C.; DePalma, S.M.; Gidding, S.; Jamerson, K.A.; Jones, D.W.; et al. 2017 acc/aha/aapa/abc/acpm/ags/apha/ash/aspc/nma/pcna guideline for the prevention, detection, evaluation, and management of high blood pressure

in adults: A report of the american college of cardiology/american heart association task force on clinical practice guidelines. *J. Am. Coll. Cardiol.* **2018**, *71*, e127–e248.

17. Walfisch, Y.; Walfisch, S.; Agbaria, R.; Levy, J.; Sharoni, Y. Lycopene in serum, skin and adipose tissues after tomato-oleoresin supplementation in patients undergoing haemorrhoidectomy or peri-anal fistulotomy. *Br. J. Nutr.* **2003**, *90*, 759–766. [CrossRef]
18. Devaraj, S.; Mathur, S.; Basu, A.; Aung, H.H.; Vasu, V.T.; Meyers, S.; Jialal, I. A dose-response study on the effects of purified lycopene supplementation on biomarkers of oxidative stress. *J. Am. Coll. Nutr.* **2008**, *27*, 267–273. [CrossRef]
19. Linnewiel-Hermoni, K.; Khanin, M.; Danilenko, M.; Zango, G.; Amosi, Y.; Levy, J.; Sharoni, Y. The anti-cancer effects of carotenoids and other phytonutrients resides in their combined activity. *Arch. Biochem. Biophys.* **2015**, *572*, 28–35. [CrossRef]
20. Aust, O.; Stahl, W.; Sies, H.; Tronnier, H.; Heinrich, U. Supplementation with tomato-based products increases lycopene, phytofluene, and phytoene levels in human serum and protects against uv-light-induced erythema. *Int. J. Vitam Nutr. Res.* **2005**, *75*, 54–60. [CrossRef]
21. Di Tomo, P.; Canali, R.; Ciavardelli, D.; Di Silvestre, S.; De Marco, A.; Giardinelli, A.; Pipino, C.; Di Pietro, N.; Virgili, F.; Pandolfi, A. Beta-carotene and lycopene affect endothelial response to tnf-alpha reducing nitro-oxidative stress and interaction with monocytes. *Mol. Nutr. Food Res.* **2012**, *56*, 217–227. [CrossRef] [PubMed]
22. Ben-Dor, A.; Steiner, M.; Gheber, L.; Danilenko, M.; Dubi, N.; Linnewiel, K.; Zick, A.; Sharoni, Y.; Levy, J. Carotenoids activate the antioxidant response element transcription system. *Mol. Cancer Ther.* **2005**, *4*, 177–186. [PubMed]
23. Linnewiel, K.; Ernst, H.; Caris-Veyrat, C.; Ben-Dor, A.; Kampf, A.; Salman, H.; Danilenko, M.; Levy, J.; Sharoni, Y. Structure activity relationship of carotenoid derivatives in activation of the electrophile/antioxidant response element transcription system. *Free Radic. Biol. Med.* **2009**, *47*, 659–667. [CrossRef] [PubMed]
24. Khachik, F.; Goli, M.B.; Beecher, G.R.; Holden, J.; Lusby, W.R.; Tenorio, M.D.; Barrera, M.R. Effect of food preparation on qualitative and quantitative distribution of major carotenoid constituents of tomatoes and several green vegetables. *J. Agric. Food Chem.* **1992**, *40*, 390–398. [CrossRef]

Low Serum Carotenoids are Associated with Self-Reported Cognitive Dysfunction and Inflammatory Markers in Breast Cancer Survivors

Krystle E. Zuniga [1,*] and Nancy E. Moran [2]

[1] Nutrition and Foods, Family and Consumer Sciences, Texas State University, 601 University Drive, San Marcos, TX 78666, USA

[2] United States Department of Agriculture/Agricultural Research Service Children's Nutrition Research Center, Department of Pediatrics, Baylor College of Medicine, Houston, TX 77030, USA; nancy.moran@bcm.edu

* Correspondence: k_z17@txstate.edu;

Abstract: Background: Dietary carotenoids may exert anti-inflammatory activities to reduce inflammation-driven cognitive impairments during cancer and cancer treatment. Our objective was to explore if cognitive function in breast cancer survivors (BCS) differs by serum carotenoid concentrations, and if blood carotenoids concentrations are associated with reduced systemic inflammation. **Methods:** Objective cognitive function and perceived cognitive impairment of 29 BCS and 38 controls were assessed cross-sectionally with the National Institutes of Health Toolbox Cognition Battery and The Functional Assessment of Cancer Therapy-Cognitive Function Questionnaire, respectively. Serum carotenoid and inflammatory marker (sTNF-RII, IL-6, IL-1ra, CRP) concentrations were measured. **Results:** Low-carotenoid BCS had more cognitive complaints compared to the low-carotenoid controls (Mdiff = −43.0, $p < 0.001$) and high-carotenoid controls (Mdiff = −44.5, $p < 0.001$). However, the cognitive complaints of high-carotenoid BCS were intermediate to and not different than the low-carotenoid BCS, or low- or high-carotenoid controls. BCS performed similarly to controls on all objective cognitive measures. Multiple linear regression, controlling for age and body mass index (BMI), demonstrated an inverse association between serum carotenoid concentrations and pro-inflammatory sTNFR-II ($\beta = 0.404$, $p = 0.005$) and IL-6 concentrations ($\beta = -0.35$, $p = 0.001$), but not IL-1ra or CRP. **Conclusions:** Higher serum carotenoid concentrations may convey cognitive and anti-inflammatory benefits in BCS. Future research should identify dietary components and patterns that support cognitive health in cancer survivors.

Keywords: cancer-related cognitive impairment; cognition; carotenoid; memory; inflammation

---

1. Introduction

With over 252,000 new breast cancer cases estimated in 2017 and a 90% five-year survival rate, the population of over 3.5 million U.S. breast cancer survivors (BCS) will continue to increase [1,2]. BCS live with many treatment-related side effects including cognitive dysfunction [3]. There is evidence that up to 75% of breast cancer patients experience cognitive decline during cancer treatment and that these impairments can persist up to twenty years following treatment completion [4,5]. However, there is marked variability in the incidence, duration, and severity of cancer-related cognitive impairments, suggesting that risk is modulated by treatment type, demographics, lifestyle, or genetics [4]. Recent advances in the field of nutritional neuroscience suggest that diet may play a role in preventing aging-associated cognitive decline; however, little to no research has focused on the mechanisms by which dietary factors reduce or prevent cancer-related cognitive decline.

Cancer-related cognitive impairments are hypothesized to arise as a result of cancer- and treatment-related inflammation. Cytokine elevation occurs in breast cancer patients before and during chemotherapy [6] and persists post-treatment [7–9]. These cytokines may be stimulated by the tumor, treatment, or psychological factors like fatigue or depression [10]. In breast cancer patients, elevated cytokines have been associated with reduced cognitive performance, changes in perceived cognitive function, and smaller hippocampal volume [10]. Oxidative stress and inflammation adversely affect neurogenesis and have a role in the pathogenesis of cognitive dysfunction [10], making these important target mechanisms to investigate with regard to the cognitive side effects of cancer treatment.

Nutrition has an important role in brain structure and function; for example, dietary components maintain neural tissue and membrane structure, provide substrates for signaling molecule synthesis, fuel metabolism, and some have antioxidant and anti-inflammatory actions [11]. Evidence suggests a correlation between fruit and vegetable intake and cognitive function [12,13], and fruits and vegetables are components of dietary patterns associated with reduced risks of cognitive impairment and neurodegenerative diseases [14–16]. In a prospective study of over 1000 breast cancer patients, both fruit and vegetable intake were associated with better verbal fluency scores post-diagnosis [17]. We previously discovered a positive relationship between fruit and vegetable intake and a measure of executive function (the ability to focus on relevant aspects of the environment) among BCS and age-matched controls [18]; however, the mechanisms underlying this relationship remain unknown. While fruits and vegetables contain an abundance of nutrients and bioactives, carotenoids, which are particularly concentrated in fruits and vegetables [19], have recently gained attention for potential cognitive benefits across the lifespan [20–22]. In addition to some carotenoids serving as vitamin A precursors, carotenoids confer many physiological activities, such as acting as anti-inflammatory or antioxidant agents, and may exert benefits for cognitive health, as some carotenoids may have potent activity in scavenging free radicals, protecting lipid membranes from peroxidation and reducing cellular inflammation [19,23,24]. A number of recent studies have suggested a particular benefit of dietary carotenoid intake for attenuating the symptoms of aging-related cognitive decline [25–28].

Some inflammatory and oxidative processes associated with cognitive decline in aging are believed to be similar to those that occur in cancer-related cognitive impairment; therefore, we hypothesize that potential anti-inflammatory and neuroprotective actions of carotenoids may elicit cognitive benefits in BCS. It is of interest to determine if the benefits of carotenoids to cognition and antioxidant status observed among a healthy population would be seen in other populations at risk of cognitive decline such as BCS. The objective of this research is to explore if cognitive function in BCS differs depending on their serum carotenoid concentrations and to explore reduction of inflammation as a potential mechanism by which carotenoids are associated with cognitive function in BCS.

2. Materials and Methods

Recruitment: Breast cancer survivors who completed primary treatment (chemotherapy, radiation therapy, or both) within the past 60 months and age-matched controls with no history of a cancer diagnosis were recruited from the Central Texas area. Potential participants were recruited via local oncology clinics, support groups, print media (flyers), social networking sites, websites, and listserv announcements. After expressing initial interest, individuals were contacted by phone and provided with a full study description and screened for eligibility. Inclusion criteria included: female; breast cancer survivor ≤60 months from last treatment, 30–70 years old; no history of stroke, heart attack, or transient ischemic attack; not currently pregnant; could speak, read, and write English; could attend all testing sessions; not blind or legally blind; nonsmoker. The exclusion criteria for this study included: current use of computer-based brain training games (e.g., Lumosity®, BrainHQ®). Eligible participants were scheduled for two testing appointments. Of the 83 total contacts, 70 consented and were eligible for testing (30 cancer survivors, 40 controls). Three women withdrew after consenting and did not complete testing owing to being no longer interested or no longer eligible (1 cancer, 2 control); thus, data are presented from sixty-seven women that consented and completed testing (38 control; 29 cancer). Participants were remunerated for their participation. All study procedures and recruitment materials were approved by the Texas State University Institutional Review Board and were performed in accordance with the ethical standards as laid down in the 1964 Declaration of Helsinki and its later amendments. Written informed consent was obtained from all subjects. This trial was registered at ClinicalTrials.gov as NCT02591316.

Demographics: Participants self-reported medical history, marital status, age, race, ethnicity, occupation, income, and education level. Additionally, BCS self-reported breast cancer specific diagnosis and treatment history. Height and weight were measured to calculate body mass index (BMI).

Dietary Intakes: Participants completed a modified version of the 2005 Block Food Frequency Questionnaire [29] reporting on intakes over the past 3 months delivered via NutritionQuest's online Data-on-Demand System. The questionnaire included 110 food items with details on portion sizes.

Neuropsychological assessment: The computer-based National Institutes of Health Toolbox Neurological and Behavioral Function Cognitive Function Battery (NIHTB-CB) was used to assess multiple domains of cognitive function. The NIHTB-CB has high reliability and validity and has been widely used in various research applications to assess cognitive performance [30]. Episodic memory and working memory were tested by the picture sequence and list sorting working memory tasks, respectively. Picture Vocabulary and Oral Reading Recognition tested language abilities. Fully-adjusted scores for each participant were provided by the NIHTB-CB and are normalized to reference groups by age, ethnicity, gender, and education.

Self-reported cognitive dysfunction: Perceived cognitive function was measured with the Functional Assessment of Cancer Therapy-Cognitive Function (FACT-Cog), a 37-item, 5-pt Likert scale questionnaire [31]. Possible scores range from 0–148, with higher FACT-Cog scores indicating fewer cognitive complaints. In this study, the Cronbach alpha was 0.98 for the total score, with subscale scores ranging from 0.91 to 0.96.

Inflammatory markers: Participants were instructed to fast for 10 h prior to blood collection. Fasted blood samples were collected via venipuncture into silica-coated BD Vacutainer serum collection tubes. Samples were allowed to clot for 30 min, centrifuged for 15 min at 2000× *g*, and the resultant serum was aliquoted and stored at −80 °C for subsequent analysis. Serum C-reactive protein (CRP), soluble tumor necrosis factor-alpha receptor type II (sTNF-RII), and interleukin-6 (IL-6) were quantified using their respective Quantikine ELISA Immunoassay kit (R&D Systems, Minneapolis, MN) per the manufacturer's instructions. Interleukin-1 receptor antagonist (IL-1ra) was analyzed with Biosource IL-1ra Cytoscreen kit (Biosource Europe S.A., Nivelles, Belgium) per the manufacturer's instructions.

Serum carotenoids: All sample analyses were performed under yellow lighting to protect carotenoids. Carotenoids were extracted from 300 uL thawed serum based on a previously described method with several modifications [32]. Apo-8′-carotenal (75 ng, #10810, Sigma-Aldrich, St. Louis, MO, USA) was added as an internal standard to duplicate samples from each subject. Dried extracts were reconstituted in 30 μL 80% methyl *tert*-butyl ether (MtBE): 20% methanol, held at 4 °C in a refrigerated autosampler, and 20 μL were injected onto an Ultimate 3000 UHPLC system coupled with a photodiode array detector (ThermoFisher, Waltham, MA, USA). Analytes were separated on a C30 Carotenoid Column (250 × 3 mm, 3 μm particle size) (ThermoFisher, Waltham, MA, USA) cooled to 18 °C, over 42 min at 0.4 mL/min by a gradient elution method, which was a modification of a previously published method [33]. The method utilized 3 HPLC-grade mobile phases: A: Methanol, B: MtBE, C: 1.5% Ammonium Acetate in water (*w/v*). The initial conditions were 98% A, 0% B, 2% C, which reached to 60% A, 38% B, 2% C at 12.5 min, then 48% A, 50% B, and 2% C at 20 min, then 38% A, 60% B, and 2% C at 30 min, which was held until 32 min, then returned to initial conditions (98% A, 0% B, 2% C) by 35 min and was held at initial conditions until 42 min. Analytes were detected by photodiode array detector at 472 nm (lycopene, beta-apo-8′-carotenal), 290 nm (phytoene), 450 nm (alpha- and beta-carotene, lutein & zeaxanthin, and beta-cryptoxanthin), and 330 nm (phytofluene). The data were analyzed using Chromeleon 7 software (ThermoFisher, Waltham, MA, USA). Analyte signals were quantitated by external calibration curves of authentic analytical standards for (*E/Z*)-phytoene, lycopene, beta-carotene, alpha-carotene, lutein, zeaxanthin, and beta-cryptoxanthin (Sigma-Aldrich, St. Louis, MO, USA), phytofluene (Carotenature, Lupsingen, Switzerland), and results were adjusted to the internal standard to correct for extraction efficiency. Total carotenoid concentration was the sum of all carotenoids analyzed.

Plasma Cholesterol: Samples were analyzed by commercial lab (LabCorp, Houston, TX, USA) using the lipid panel test (#303756) for frozen, EDTA-collected plasma. Triglycerides and total and HDL cholesterol were measured directly by enzymatic colorimetric assay on a clinical chemistry analyzer (COBAS 8000 c701, Roche Diagnostics International Ltd., Rotkreuz, Zug Switzerland) and VLDL and LDL cholesterol were calculated using standard clinical algorithms.

Statistical Analysis: The primary objective of this study was to determine if cognitive function in BCS differed by serum total carotenoid status. We also confirmed that serum carotenoid concentrations were positively associated with reported fruit and vegetable intake. As secondary outcomes, we explored whether serum carotenoids were associated with markers of inflammation. Characteristics of the BCS and controls were compared using independent t-tests for continuous variables and X^2-tests for categorical variables. Differences in serum carotenoids between groups were tested with the Mann–Whitney U-test. Univariate analysis of covariance (ANCOVA) was used to determine the difference in subjective cognitive function between BCS and controls after controlling for age. In order to compare cognitive function between BCS and controls with either low or high serum carotenoid concentrations, BCS and controls were each split into two groups: (1) BCS or control with serum carotenoid concentrations lower than, and including, the median; and (2) BCS or control with serum carotenoid concentrations above the median. Then, univariate ANCOVA, including age as a covariate, was used to compare cognitive function as a function of group (low carotenoid BCS, high carotenoid BCS, low carotenoid control, high carotenoid control), and post hoc analysis with *t*-tests was performed with a Bonferroni adjustment for the six comparisons, yielding an $\alpha = 0.008$. The significance level was set at $\alpha = 0.05$ for all other statistical analyses. Associations between serum carotenoids and inflammatory markers were determined using multiple linear regression, controlling for the a priori-identified covariates of age and BMI. All statistical analyses were performed in SPSS (v.24) (IBM, Armonk, NY, USA). When the assumption of normality was violated, values were log-transformed to the base 10 ($\log_{10}$) to provide increased normality.

3. Results

Participant Characteristics: There were no significant differences in age, education, race, ethnicity, socioeconomic status, or BMI between BCS and healthy controls (Table 1). Most BCS had early stage breast cancer at diagnosis (75.9% at stage II or lower) and were an average of 1.6 years post-completion of cancer treatment (M = 18.6 months, SD = 16.3). All had undergone surgery, 65.5% had received radiation therapy, 72.4% had received chemotherapy, and 65.5% were currently receiving hormonal therapy.

Table 1. Participant Characteristics.

	Breast Cancer Survivors	Controls	*p*
Age, y (Mean ± SD)	50.1 ± 10.1	50.8 ± 10.0	0.783
Income, *n* (%)			
≥$60,000	16 (61.5)	29 (78.4)	0.145
Race, *n* (%)			
White	20 (69.0)	33 (86.8)	0.075
Black	3 (10.3)	0 (0.0)	
Asian	2 (6.9)	1 (2.6)	
More than One Race	4 (13.8)	4 (10.5)	
Ethnicity, *n* (%)			
Hispanic or Latino	6 (20.7)	9 (23.7)	0.771
Education, *n* (%)			
≥ 4 year College Degree	20 (69.0)	32 (84.2)	0.138
Body Mass Index (BMI), kg/m^2 (Mean ± SD)	29.7 ± 6.3	27.3 ± 7.6	0.168
Stage at Diagnosis, *n* (%)			
Ductal Carcinoma in Situ (DCIS)	3 (10.3)	-	
Stage I	8 (27.6)	-	
Stage II	11 (37.9)	-	
Stage III	6 (20.7)	-	
Unknown	1 (3.4)	-	
Treatment, *n* (%)			
Chemotherapy Only	10 (34.5)	-	
Radiation Only	8 (27.6)	-	
Chemotherapy + Radiation	11 (37.9)	-	
Current Hormone Therapy	19 (65.5)	-	
Surgery	29 (100)	-	
Time since Treatment-Months (Mean ± SD)	18.6 ± 16.3	-	
Total Cholesterol (mg/dL) [1]	167 (130–189)	166 (146–189)	0.463
Serum Carotenoid Concentrations (nmol/L) [1]			
Alpha-carotene	41.1 (19.7–64.5)	53.3 (35.8–122.7)	0.121
Beta-carotene	163.0 (79.5–298.8)	217.5 (122.6–367.2)	0.260
Lycopene	298.1 (225.8–369.8)	312.4 (213.6–411.3)	0.968
Lutein & Zeaxanthin	163.2 (92.9–272.9)	214.7 (145.7–308.3)	0.199
Beta-cryptoxanthin	68.7 (45.3–115.8)	78.2 (49.6–154.9)	0.354
Phytofluene	65.2 (50.7–92.4)	62.1 (48.7–100.2)	0.958
Phytoene	68.6 (50.3–82.4)	53.6 (43.1–75.6)	0.083
Total Carotenoids	933.3 (663.2–1120.5)	1052.3 (782.2–1356.1)	0.314
Average Daily Intakes (Mean ± SD)			
Fruit (cups)	1.0 ± 0.8	1.1 ± 0.9	0.568
Vegetables (cups)	2.8 ± 1.7	2.6 ± 1.6	0.761
Total Carotenoid Intake (mg)	20.8 ± 13.5	18.7 ± 10.3	0.514

[1] median and interquartile range (25–75th percentile).

Dietary and serum carotenoids: Serum and dietary carotenoids were not significantly different between BCS and controls (Table 1). Fruit and vegetable intake were similar between BCS and age-matched controls (Table 1). After controlling for BMI and total cholesterol, reported fruit and vegetable intake (total servings per day) was positively correlated with total serum carotenoid concentrations ($r = 0.434$, $p < 0.001$) (data not shown).

Objective and Subjective Cognitive Function: BCS performed similarly to controls on all objective cognitive measures (Table 2). However, BCS reported significantly more cognitive complaints than controls (Table 3). After adjustment for age, there was a statistically significant difference in perceived cognitive function between the groups across all subscales and total score of the FACT-Cog, indicating more self-reported cognitive difficulties in BCS (Table 3).

Table 2. Objective Cognitive Function [1].

	Breast Cancer Survivors	Controls	*p*
List-Sorting Working Memory	108.8 (17.5)	105.3 (11.2)	0.353
Picture Vocabulary	108.2 (16.2)	115.2 (14.5)	0.072
Picture Sequence Memory	100.5 (18.9)	103.1 (14.7)	0.536
Oral Reading Recognition	117.4 (14.3)	116.7 (16.4)	0.864

Mean (SD).[1] fully-adjusted, standardized scores.

Table 3. Self-Reported Cognitive Dysfunction.

	Breast Cancer Survivors	Controls	*p*
Total FACT-Cog Score [1]	88.70 (5.27)	119.17 (4.60)	<0.001
Perceived Cognitive Impairments	45.43 (3.01)	61.66 (2.63)	<0.001
Impact of Perceived Cognitive Impairments on Quality of Life	10.06 (0.83)	13.60 (0.73)	0.002
Comments from Others	12.94 (0.53)	15.57 (0.46)	<0.001
Perceived Cognitive Abilities	20.28 (1.44)	28.34 (1.26)	<0.001

Data are adjusted mean (SE). ANCOVA with age as a covariate. [1] Functional Assessment of Cancer Therapy-Cognitive Function

Serum carotenoids and cognitive complaints: Serum carotenoid concentrations by group are described in Table 4. ANCOVA was used to determine the differences in FACT-Cog scores between serum carotenoid status groups. After adjustment for age, there was a statistically significant difference in FACT-Cog scores between the groups, $F(3, 60) = 9.498$, $p < 0.001$, partial $\eta 2 = 0.322$. The low-carotenoid BCS had significantly lower FACT-Cog scores (more cognitive complaints) compared to the low-carotenoid controls (Mdiff = −43.0, 95% CI [−68.8, −17.1], $p < 0.001$) and high-carotenoid controls (Mdiff = −44.54, 95% CI [−71.1, −18.0], $p < 0.001$) (Figure 1). However, FACT-Cog scores in high-carotenoid BCS were not significantly different than those of the low-carotenoid BCS, or low- or high-carotenoid controls.

Table 4. Serum Carotenoid Concentrations.

Serum Carotenoid Concentrations (nmol/L).	Low Carotenoid BCS	High Carotenoid BCS	Low Carotenoid Control	High Carotenoid Control
Alpha-carotene	27.3 (13.0)	153.8 (269.9)	43.3 (33.6)	90.3 (150.8)
Beta-carotene	103.9 (58.7) [a]	461.1 (427.4) [b]	140.7 (78.5) [a]	425.4 (215.7) [b]
Lycopene	275.0 (74.4) [a]	344.1 (99.4) [ab]	241.4 (80.8) [a]	417.3 (198.4) [b]
Lutein & Zeaxanthin	117.4 (44.5) [a]	366.3 (263.6) [b]	174.0 (79.5) [ac]	299.8 (121.7) [bc]
Beta-cryptoxanthin	54.4 (34.5) [a]	135.9 (133.5) [ab]	69.1 (58.1) [ab]	149.4 (105.3) [b]
Phytofluene	55.5 (34.6) [ab]	113.8 (91.8) [a]	53.9 (22.5) [b]	108.4 (63.4) [a]
Phytoene	56.5 (23.1) [ab]	87.5 (40.1) [a]	47.9 (9.9) [b]	79.7 (39.0) [a]
Total Carotenoids	689.9 (185.0) [a]	1662.4 (1065.7) [b]	770.3 (179.9) [a]	1619.6 (604.2) [b]

Mean (SD); Different letters indicate significant differences between groups ($p < 0.05$).

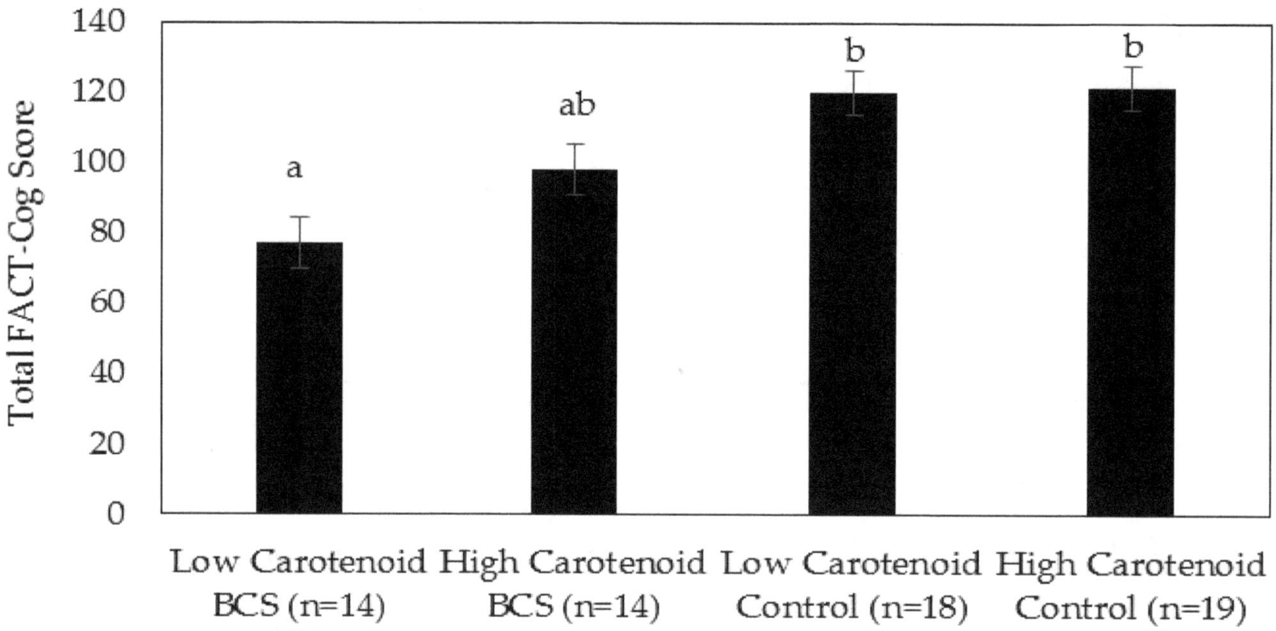

Figure 1. Perceived Cognitive Dysfunction by Group Carotenoid Status. Data are adjusted mean (standard error). ANCOVA with age as covariate. Different letters indicate significant differences between groups ($p < 0.05$).

Inflammatory Markers: Serum CRP, sTNF-RII, IL-6, and IL-1ra levels were not significantly different between BCS and controls (Table 5). In multiple linear regression models controlling for age and BMI, serum carotenoids were significant predictors of lower IL-6 ($\beta = -0.353$, $p = 0.001$) and sTNFR-II ($\beta = -0.404$, $p = 0.005$) concentrations, but not IL-1ra or CRP (Table 6).

Table 5. Inflammatory Markers.

	Breast Cancer Survivors	Controls	*p*
IL-6 (pg/mL)	2.0 (1.1)	1.8 (1.1)	0.431
IL-1ra (pg/mL)	476.8 (91.6)	513.1 (78.4)	0.766
sTNFRII (pg/mL)	3037.41 (128.0)	2717.3 (115.8)	0.073
CRP (ng/mL)	2156.8 (358.2)	3012.3 (296.3)	0.072

Data are mean adjusted (SE). ANCOVA with age, BMI, and moderate to vigorous physical activity as covariates.

Table 6. Regression analyses explaining variability in inflammatory markers.

	IL-6			sTNFR-II			CRP			IL-1ra		
	β	p	Model Adjusted R^2	β	p	Model Adjusted R^2	β	p	Model Adjusted R^2	β	p	Model Adjusted R^2
			0.483 **			0.175 *			0.142 *			0.032
Age	0.225	0.020		0.284	0.022		−0.064	0.622		0.264	0.046	
BMI	0.433	<0.001		0.036	0.790		0.337	0.024		−0.018	0.900	
Serum Carotenoids	−0.353	0.001		−0.404	0.005		−0.158	0.277		−0.162	0.267	

* $p < 0.01$, ** $p < 0.001$.

4. Discussion

Here we report, for the first time, that BCS with low blood carotenoid concentrations reported more cognitive complaints than healthy controls with no prior cancer diagnosis, and BCS with higher serum carotenoid concentrations reported cognitive complaints not different from both groups of controls. Furthermore, we found that several, but not all, serum markers of inflammation were significantly inversely associated with serum total carotenoid concentrations, suggesting a potential mechanism by which carotenoids may affect cognitive function.

In our sample, objectively assessed cognitive performance was similar between BCS and controls. Indeed, several meta-analyses have concluded that cognitive deficits in BCS are generally subtle [34–36], and may be more detectable by subjective report than by objective laboratory tests. Standard neuropsychological assessments likely command more focus than the tasks of everyday life and may not be representative of the routine cognitive challenges that BCS face [37,38]. Compared to age-matched controls, BCS reported significantly greater levels of perceived cognitive impairment. In non-cancer populations, memory complaints are a predictor of worse physical health and a higher degree of dependency for daily life activities [39,40]. In aging populations, self-reported, perceived memory impairments are associated with an increased risk of cognitive decline and impairment and all-cause dementia, suggesting that cognitive complaints may indicate neurodegenerative changes that precede significant changes in neuropsychological performance assessed with objective laboratory tests [41–43]. A minimal clinically important difference for FACT-Cog has been estimated to be 7–11 points [44] and has been demonstrated to be sensitive to interventions to improve cognitive function in cancer survivors including cognitive rehabilitation [45], physical activity [46,47], and meditation [48]. The low carotenoid BCS had an over 40 point difference on FACT-Cog scores compared to low and high carotenoid controls, which is clinically significant.

The neurotoxicity of cancer and treatment may be mediated, at least in part, through the action of cytokines crossing the blood-brain barrier to elicit oxidative stress and negatively impact neurogenesis [49]. Evidence suggests that several inflammatory markers are elevated in BCS including the cytokines IL-6, IL-8, and IL-10 [7–10]; however, BCS in our sample did not have significantly higher levels of inflammatory markers compared to controls. This may have been partially attributed to the heterogeneity in time since treatment in our small sample size, as it is suggested that some cytokine changes may be acute [8,50].

Carotenoids can accumulate in the brain and may function as reactive oxygen species scavengers, protecting lipid membranes from peroxidation and reducing cellular inflammation [23,51,52]. Evidence indicates an altered redox status in cancer patients [53,54], and other lines of evidence suggest oxidative stress in the brain can negatively affect neurogenesis and promote cognitive dysfunction [55,56]. However, the association between biomarkers of oxidative stress in cancer survivors and cancer-related cognitive dysfunction has not been thoroughly assessed, and future research is needed to determine which oxidative stress markers have clinical and prognostic utility in this sample. The current analyses focused on inflammatory markers that have consistently been identified to be both elevated and correlated with cognitive function in breast cancer patients and survivors. In this study, serum carotenoids were inversely associated with IL-6 and sTNFR-II, which is notable, as elevations in these markers of systemic inflammation have been associated with alterations in brain structure and function in breast cancer patients and survivors. sTNF-RII is a marker of the cytokine TNF-α's pro-inflammatory activity and can be reliably measured in circulation [57]. Higher sTNF-RII levels have been associated with greater memory complaints [50], worse memory performance [58], alterations in brain metabolism [50], and decreased gray matter volume in specific brain regions [59] of BCS. Additionally, a significant correlation between lower hippocampal volume and higher TNF-α has been observed among BCS [60]. In a longitudinal sample of BCS, elevated IL-6 levels were associated with more cognitive complaints [9], and in a sample of breast cancer patients, impaired memory function by radiation therapy was suggested to be partially mediated by elevated IL-6 [61]. The precise mechanism underlying how peripheral inflammatory cytokines impairs cognitive function in BCS is unknown. However, it is hypothesized that peripherally elevated levels of cytokines induce alterations among numerous neural substrates, including neurotransmitters and brain-derived neurotrophic factor [10]. It is mechanistically plausible that carotenoids have a direct effect on systemic inflammation, as carotenoids have been shown in model systems to reduce oxidative stress and downstream inflammatory signaling (reviewed in Reference [62]). In BCS, higher plasma carotenoid concentrations have previously shown to be associated with reduced oxidative stress [63,64]. Therefore, strategies to reduce inflammation, such as dietary changes to increase carotenoid intake, could provide cognitive benefits.

In addition to being bioactive compounds themselves, serum concentrations of carotenoids are a well-recognized biomarker of fruit and vegetable intake [65]. In our sample, serum carotenoid concentrations were positively associated with fruit and vegetable intake. Fruits and vegetables contain an array of antioxidants and anti-inflammatory nutrients and bioactives that may elicit neuroprotection by inhibiting neuroinflammation and neurodegeneration [66,67]. The carotenoids lutein and zeaxanthin have been more strongly associated with cognitive function than other individual carotenoids [22]. Further investigation is warranted to determine which specific compounds contribute to cognitive benefits observed with fruit and vegetable consumption, as many compounds likely interact to elicit cognitive benefits. The limited evidence of interventions with fruits and vegetables or carotenoids for improvement in cognitive function in aging populations does suggest a positive benefit [25–28,66,68,69]; thus, promotion of this dietary strategy may be useful for reducing the short- and/or long-term adverse cognitive effects of cancer treatment.

There are important limitations of this study including the cross-sectional design and small sample size which limits the interpretation of our findings. Our sample of BCS was heterogeneous in cancer stage, time since diagnosis, and treatment variables. The neuropsychological assessment was brief (~40 min), thus, a longer battery or field testing may have identified the subtle cognitive impairments common in BCS. There are several other inflammatory markers that were not assessed; however, CRP, IL-6, sTNF-RII, and IL-1ra were chosen because previous studies have demonstrated these markers to be elevated and correlated with cognitive decline in BCS [50,60,70]. While we cannot directly measure brain oxidative stress or inflammation, evidence indicates systemic inflammation is associated with lower white matter integrity, poorer cognitive performance, dementia, and cognitive decline in aging [71,72]. Future basic research can define the impact of carotenoids on other proposed mechanisms of cognitive dysfunction requiring model systems like oxidative stress, epigenetic changes, impaired neurogenesis, and treatment-induced hormonal alterations [4]. Despite these limitations, this is the first study, to our knowledge, to examine a potential mechanism by which food components could elicit cognitive benefits in cancer survivors. Although previous research has supported the hypothesis that dietary carotenoids have anti-inflammatory activity and may elicit cognitive benefits, these associations have never been explored in individuals with cancer-related cognitive impairment. Only two studies have examined the association between dietary intake and cognitive dysfunction in cancer survivors [17,18], and neither explored a potential mechanism of cognitive benefits from dietary components. Therefore, our findings are novel and provide much needed preliminary information to guide future dietary interventions.

Cancer survivorship research to date has primarily focused on improving survival and reducing risk of recurrence, yet strategies to support survivors' cognitive function are limited. Pharmacotherapies modestly alleviate cognitive deficits [73,74]; however, possible side effects and interactions highlight a need to explore modifiable lifestyle factors. While cognitive behavioral training and physical activity convey functional improvements in cancer survivors [75,76], there are no published dietary strategies. Nevertheless, survivors seek dietary changes to improve symptoms and reduce cancer risk [77]. Our findings suggest an association between serum carotenoids, perceived cognitive function, and markers of systemic inflammation. Future research should explore the mechanisms by which dietary patterns and corresponding food components can reduce memory complaints and support cognitive health in cancer survivors, providing evidence for future dietary interventions to improve BCS' quality of life.

Author Contributions: Conceptualization, K.E.Z. and N.E.M.; Methodology, K.E.Z.; Formal Analysis, K.E.Z.; Investigation, K.E.Z. and N.E.M.; Resources, K.E.Z. and N.E.M.; Data Curation, K.E.Z.; Writing – Original Draft Preparation, K.E.Z. and N.E.M.; Writing – Review & Editing, K.E.Z. and N.E.M.; Visualization, K.E.Z.; Supervision, K.E.Z.; Project Administration, K.E.Z.; Funding Acquisition, K.E.Z. and N.E.M.

References

1. Howlader, N.; Noone, A.M.; Krapcho, M.; Miller, D.; Bishop, K.; Kosary, C.L.; Yu, M.; Ruhl, J.; Tatalovich, Z.; Mariotto, A.; et al. SEER Cancer Statistics Review (CSR) 1975–2014. Available online: https://seer.cancer.gov/csr/1975_2015/ (accessed on 16 April 2018).
2. Miller, K.D.; Siegel, R.L.; Lin, C.C.; Mariotto, A.B.; Kramer, J.L.; Rowland, J.H.; Stein, K.D.; Alteri, R.; Jemal, A. Cancer treatment and survivorship statistics, 2016. *CA. Cancer J. Clin.* **2016**, *66*, 271–289. [CrossRef] [PubMed]
3. Palesh, O.; Scheiber, C.; Kesler, S.; Mustian, K.; Koopman, C.; Schapira, L. Management of side effects during and post-treatment in breast cancer survivors. *Breast J.* **2018**, *24*, 164–175. [CrossRef] [PubMed]
4. Janelsins, M.C.; Kesler, S.R.; Ahles, T.A.; Morrow, G.R. Prevalence, mechanisms, and management of cancer-related cognitive impairment. *Int. Rev. Psychiatry* **2014**, *26*, 102–113. [CrossRef] [PubMed]
5. Koppelmans, V.; Breteler, M.M.B.; Boogerd, W.; Seynaeve, C.; Gundy, C.; Schagen, S.B. Neuropsychological performance in survivors of breast cancer more than 20 years after adjuvant chemotherapy. *J. Clin. Oncol.* **2012**, *30*, 1080–1086. [CrossRef] [PubMed]
6. Janelsins, M.C.; Mustian, K.M.; Palesh, O.G.; Mohile, S.G.; Peppone, L.J.; Sprod, L.K.; Heckler, C.E.; Roscoe, J.A.; Katz, A.W.; Williams, J.P.; et al. Differential expression of cytokines in breast cancer patients receiving different chemotherapies: Implications for cognitive impairment research. *Support Care Cancer* **2012**, *20*, 831–839. [CrossRef] [PubMed]
7. Williams, A.M.; Shah, R.; Shayne, M.; Huston, A.J.; Krebs, M.; Murray, N.; Thompson, B.D.; Doyle, K.; Korotkin, J.; van Wijngaarden, E.; et al. Associations between inflammatory markers and cognitive function in breast cancer patients receiving chemotherapy. *J. Neuroimmunol.* **2018**, *314*, 17–23. [CrossRef] [PubMed]
8. Lyon, D.E.; Cohen, R.; Chen, H.; Kelly, D.L.; McCain, N.L.; Starkweather, A.; Ahn, H.; Sturgill, J.; Jackson-Cook, C.K. Relationship of systemic cytokine concentrations to cognitive function over two years in women with early stage breast cancer. *J. Neuroimmunol.* **2016**, *301*, 74–82. [CrossRef] [PubMed]
9. Cheung, Y.T.; Ng, T.; Shwe, M.; Ho, H.K.; Foo, K.M.; Cham, M.T.; Lee, J.A.; Fan, G.; Tan, Y.P.; Yong, W.S.; et al. Association of proinflammatory cytokines and chemotherapy-associated cognitive impairment in breast cancer patients: A multi-centered, prospective, cohort study. *Ann. Oncol.* **2015**, *26*, 1446–1451. [CrossRef] [PubMed]
10. Wang, X.M.; Walitt, B.; Saligan, L.; Tiwari, A.F.; Cheung, C.W.; Zhang, Z.J. Chemobrain: A critical review and causal hypothesis of link between cytokines and epigenetic reprogramming associated with chemotherapy. *Cytokine* **2015**, *72*, 86–96. [CrossRef] [PubMed]
11. Wahl, D.; Cogger, V.C.; Solon-Biet, S.M.; Waern, R.V.; Gokarn, R.; Pulpitel, T.; Cabo, R.; Mattson, M.P.; Raubenheimer, D.; Simpson, S.J.; et al. Nutritional strategies to optimise cognitive function in the aging brain. *Ageing Res. Rev.* **2016**, *31*, 80–92. [CrossRef] [PubMed]
12. Loef, M.; Walach, H. Fruit, vegetables and prevention of cognitive decline or dementia: A systematic review of cohort studies. *J. Nutr. Heal. Aging* **2012**, *16*, 626–630. [CrossRef]
13. Nurk, E.; Refsum, H.; Drevon, C.A.; Tell, G.S.; Nygaard, H.A.; Engedal, K.; Smith, A.D. Cognitive performance among the elderly in relation to the intake of plant foods. The Hordaland Health Study. *Br. J. Nutr.* **2010**, *104*, 1190–1201. [CrossRef] [PubMed]
14. Cheung, B.H.; Ho, I.C.; Chan, R.S.; Sea, M.M.; Woo, J. Current evidence on dietary pattern and cognitive function. *Adv. Food Nutr. Res.* **2014**, *71*, 137–163. [PubMed]
15. Morris, M.C.; Tangney, C.C.; Wang, Y.; Sacks, F.M.; Bennett, D.A.; Aggarwal, N.T. MIND diet associated with reduced incidence of Alzheimer's disease. *Alzheimers Dement.* **2015**, *11*, 1007–1014. [CrossRef] [PubMed]
16. Allès, B.; Samieri, C.; Féart, C.; Jutand, M.A.; Laurin, D.; Barberger-Gateau, P. Dietary patterns: A novel approach to examine the link between nutrition and cognitive function in older individuals. *Nutr. Res. Rev.* **2012**, *25*, 207–222. [CrossRef] [PubMed]
17. Huang, Z.; Shi, Y.; Bao, P.; Cai, H.; Hong, Z.; Ding, D.; Jackson, J.; Shu, X.-O.; Dai, Q. Associations of dietary

intake and supplement use with post-therapy cognitive recovery in breast cancer survivors. *Breast Cancer Res. Treat.* **2018**, 1–10. [CrossRef] [PubMed]

18. Zuniga, K.E.; Mackenzie, M.J.; Roberts, S.A.; Raine, L.B.; Hillman, C.H.; Kramer, A.F.; McAuley, E. Relationship between fruit and vegetable intake and interference control in breast cancer survivors. *Eur. J. Nutr.* **2016**, *55*, 1555–1562. [CrossRef] [PubMed]
19. Hammond, B.R., Jr.; Renzi, L.M. Nutrient Information: Carotenoids. *Adv. Nutr.* **2013**, *4*, 474–476. [CrossRef] [PubMed]
20. Akbaraly, N.T.; Faure, H.; Gourlet, V.; Favier, A.; Berr, C. Plasma carotenoid levels and cognitive performance in an elderly population: Results of the EVA study. *J. Gerontol. A Biol. Sci. Med. Sci.* **2007**, *62*, 308–316. [CrossRef] [PubMed]
21. Kesse-Guyot, E.; Andreeva, V.A.; Ducros, V.; Jeandel, C.; Julia, C.; Hercberg, S.; Galan, P. Carotenoid-rich dietary patterns during midlife and subsequent cognitive function. *Br. J. Nutr.* **2014**, *111*, 915–923. [CrossRef] [PubMed]
22. Johnson, E.J. Role of lutein and zeaxanthin in visual and cognitive function throughout the lifespan. *Nutr. Rev.* **2014**, *72*, 605–612. [CrossRef] [PubMed]
23. Mohn, E.S.; Erdman, J.W.; Kuchan, M.J.; Neuringer, M.; Johnson, E.J. Lutein accumulates in subcellular membranes of brain regions in adult rhesus macaques: Relationship to DHA oxidation products. *PLoS ONE* **2017**, *12*, e0186767. [CrossRef] [PubMed]
24. Ruxton, C.H.S.; Derbyshire, E.; Toribio-Mateas, M. Role of fatty acids and micronutrients in healthy ageing: A systematic review of randomised controlled trials set in the context of European dietary surveys of older adults. *J. Hum. Nutr. Diet.* **2016**, *29*, 308–324. [CrossRef] [PubMed]
25. Lindbergh, C.A.; Renzi-Hammond, L.M.; Hammond, B.R.; Terry, D.P.; Mewborn, C.M.; Puente, A.N.; Miller, L.S. Lutein and zeaxanthin influence brain function in older adults: A randomized controlled trial. *J. Int. Neuropsychol. Soc.* **2018**, *24*, 1–14. [CrossRef] [PubMed]
26. Hammond, B.R.; Miller, L.S.; Bello, M.O.; Lindbergh, C.A.; Mewborn, C.; Renzi-Hammond, L.M.; Renzi-Hammond, L.M. Effects of lutein/zeaxanthin supplementation on the cognitive function of community dwelling older adults: A randomized, double-masked, placebo-controlled trial. *Front. Aging Neurosci.* **2017**, *9*, 254. [CrossRef] [PubMed]
27. Power, R.; Coen, R.F.; Beatty, S.; Mulcahy, R.; Moran, R.; Stack, J.; Howard, A.N.; Nolan, J.M. Supplemental retinal carotenoids enhance memory in healthy individuals with Low levels of macular pigment in a randomized, double-blind, placebo-ontrolled clinical trial. *J. Alzheimers Dis.* **2018**, *61*, 947–961. [CrossRef] [PubMed]
28. Grodstein, F.; Kang, J.H.; Glynn, R.J.; Cook, N.R.; Gaziano, J.M. A randomized trial of beta carotene supplementation and cognitive function in men: The Physicians' Health Study II. *Arch. Intern. Med.* **2007**, *167*, 2184. [CrossRef] [PubMed]
29. Block, G.; Wakimoto, P.; Jensen, C.; Mandel, S.; Green, R.R. Validation of a food frequency questionnaire for Hispanics. *Prev. Chronic Dis.* **2006**, *3*, A77. [PubMed]
30. Heaton, R.K.; Akshoomoff, N.; Tulsky, D.; Mungas, D.; Weintraub, S.; Dikmen, S.; Beaumont, J.; Casaletto, K.B.; Conway, K.; Slotkin, J.; et al. Reliability and validity of composite scores from the NIH toolbox cognition battery in adults. *J. Int. Neuropsychol. Soc.* **2014**, *20*, 588–598. [CrossRef] [PubMed]
31. Cella, D.F.; Tulsky, D.S.; Gray, G.; Sarafian, B.; Linn, E.; Bonomi, A.; Silberman, M.; Yellen, S.B.; Winicour, P.; Brannon, J.; et al. The Functional Assessment of Cancer Therapy scale: Development and validation of the general measure. *J. Clin. Oncol.* **1993**, *11*, 570–579. [CrossRef] [PubMed]
32. Campbell, J.K.; Engelmann, N.J.; Lila, M.A.; Erdman, J.W. Phytoene, phytofluene, and lycopene from tomato powder differentially accumulate in tissues of male Fisher 344 rats. *Nutr. Res.* **2007**, *27*, 794–801. [CrossRef] [PubMed]
33. Lu, C.H.; Choi, J.H.; Engelmann Moran, N.; Jin, Y.S.; Erdman, J.W. Laboratory-scale production of 13C-labeled lycopene and phytoene by bioengineered Escherichia coli. *J. Agric. Food Chem.* **2011**, *59*, 9996–10005. [CrossRef] [PubMed]
34. Jim, H.S.; Phillips, K.M.; Chait, S.; Faul, L.A.; Popa, M.A.; Lee, Y.H.; Hussin, M.G.; Jacobsen, P.B.; Small, B.J. Meta-analysis of cognitive functioning in breast cancer survivors previously treated with standard-dose chemotherapy. *J. Clin. Oncol.* **2012**, *30*, 3578–3587. [CrossRef] [PubMed]
35. Ono, M.; Ogilvie, J.M.; Wilson, J.S.; Green, H.J.; Chambers, S.K.; Ownsworth, T.; Shum, D.H.K. A

meta-analysis of cognitive impairment and decline associated with adjuvant chemotherapy in women with breast cancer. *Front. Oncol.* **2015**, *5*, 59. [CrossRef] [PubMed]

36. Bernstein, L.J.; McCreath, G.A.; Komeylian, Z.; Rich, J.B. Cognitive impairment in breast cancer survivors treated with chemotherapy depends on control group type and cognitive domains assessed: A multilevel meta-analysis. *Neurosci. Biobehav. Rev.* **2017**, *83*, 417–428. [CrossRef] [PubMed]
37. Hutchinson, A.D.; Hosking, J.R.; Kichenadasse, G.; Mattiske, J.K.; Wilson, C. Objective and subjective cognitive impairment following chemotherapy for cancer: A systematic review. *Cancer Treat. Rev.* **2012**, *38*, 926–934. [CrossRef] [PubMed]
38. Pullens, M.J.; De Vries, J.; Roukema, J.A. Subjective cognitive dysfunction in breast cancer patients: A systematic review. *Psychooncology* **2010**, *19*, 1127–1138. [CrossRef] [PubMed]
39. Clarnette, R.M.; Almeida, O.P.; Forstl, H.; Paton, A.; Martins, R.N. Clinical characteristics of individuals with subjective memory loss in Western Australia: Results from a cross-sectional survey. *Int. J. Geriatr. Psychiatry* **2001**, *16*, 168–174. [CrossRef]
40. Montejo, P.; Montenegro, M.; Fernandez, M.A.; Maestu, F. Subjective memory complaints in the elderly: Prevalence and influence of temporal orientation, depression and quality of life in a population-based study in the city of Madrid. *Aging Ment. Health* **2011**, *15*, 85–96. [CrossRef] [PubMed]
41. Reid, L.; MacLullich, A.M. Subjective memory complaints and cognitive impairment in older people. *Dement. Geriatr. Cogn. Disord.* **2006**, *22*, 471–485. [CrossRef] [PubMed]
42. Wang, L.; van Belle, G.; Crane, P.K.; Kukull, W.A.; Bowen, J.D.; McCormick, W.C.; Larson, E.B. Subjective memory deterioration and future dementia in people aged 65 and older. *J. Am. Geriatr. Soc.* **2004**, *52*, 2045–2051. [CrossRef] [PubMed]
43. Saykin, A.J.; Wishart, H.A.; Rabin, L.A.; Santulli, R.B.; Flashman, L.A.; West, J.D.; McHugh, T.L.; Mamourian, A.C. Older adults with cognitive complaints show brain atrophy similar to that of amnestic MCI. *Neurology* **2006**, *67*, 834–842. [CrossRef] [PubMed]
44. Cheung, Y.T.; Foo, Y.L.; Shwe, M.; Tan, Y.P.; Fan, G.; Yong, W.S.; Madhukumar, P.; Ooi, W.S.; Chay, W.Y.; Dent, R.A.; et al. Minimal clinically important difference (MCID) for the functional assessment of cancer therapy: Cognitive function (FACT-Cog) in breast cancer patients. *J. Clin. Epidemiol.* **2014**, *67*, 811–820. [CrossRef] [PubMed]
45. Bray, V.J.; Dhillon, H.M.; Bell, M.L.; Kabourakis, M.; Fiero, M.H.; Yip, D.; Boyle, F.; Price, M.A.; Vardy, J.L. Evaluation of a web-based cognitive rehabilitation program in cancer survivors reporting cognitive symptoms after chemotherapy. *J. Clin. Oncol.* **2017**, *35*, 217–225. [CrossRef] [PubMed]
46. Hartman, S.J.; Nelson, S.H.; Myers, E.; Natarajan, L.; Sears, D.D.; Palmer, B.W.; Weiner, L.S.; Parker, B.A.; Patterson, R.E. Randomized controlled trial of increasing physical activity on objectively measured and self-reported cognitive functioning among breast cancer survivors: The memory and motion study. *Cancer* **2018**, *124*, 192–202. [CrossRef] [PubMed]
47. Derry, H.M.; Jaremka, L.M.; Bennett, J.M.; Peng, J.; Andridge, R.; Shapiro, C.; Malarkey, W.B.; Emery, C.F.; Layman, R.; Mrozek, E.; et al. Yoga and self-reported cognitive problems in breast cancer survivors: A randomized controlled trial. *Psychooncology* **2015**, *24*, 958–966. [CrossRef] [PubMed]
48. Milbury, K.; Chaoul, A.; Biegler, K.; Wangyal, T.; Spelman, A.; Meyers, C.A.; Arun, B.; Palmer, J.L.; Taylor, J.; Cohen, L. Tibetan sound meditation for cognitive dysfunction: Results of a randomized controlled pilot trial. *Psychooncology* **2013**, *22*, 2354–2363. [CrossRef] [PubMed]
49. Lacourt, T.E.; Heijnen, J.C. Mechanisms of neurotoxic symptoms as a result of breast cancer and its treatment: Considerations on the contribution of stress, inflammation, and cellular bioenergetics. *Curr. Breast Cancer Rep.* **2017**, *9*, 70–81. [CrossRef] [PubMed]
50. Ganz, P.A.; Bower, J.E.; Kwan, L.; Castellon, S.A.; Silverman, D.H.; Geist, C.; Breen, E.C.; Irwin, M.R.; Cole, S.W. Does tumor necrosis factor-alpha (TNF-a) play a role in post-chemotherapy cerebral dysfunction? *Brain Behav. Immun.* **2013**, *30*. [CrossRef] [PubMed]
51. Johnson, E.J.; Vishwanathan, R.; Johnson, M.A.; Hausman, D.B.; Davey, A.; Scott, T.M.; Green, R.C.; Miller, L.S.; Gearing, M.; Woodard, J.; et al. Relationship between serum and brain carotenoids, α-tocopherol, and retinol concentrations and cognitive performance in the oldest old from the georgia centenarian study. *J. Aging Res.* **2013**, *2013*, 951786. [CrossRef] [PubMed]
52. Snodderly, D.M. Evidence for protection against age-related macular degeneration by carotenoids and antioxidant vitamins. *Am. J. Clin. Nutr.* **1995**, *62*, 1448S–1461S. [CrossRef] [PubMed]

53. Chen, Y.; Jungsuwadee, P.; Vore, M.; Butterfield, D.A.; St Clair, D.K. Collateral damage in cancer chemotherapy: Oxidative stress in nontargeted tissues. *Mol. Interv.* **2007**, *7*, 147–156. [CrossRef] [PubMed]
54. Vera-Ramirez, L.; Ramirez-Tortosa, Mc.; Perez-Lopez, P.; Granados-Principal, S.; Battino, M.; Quiles, J.L. Long-term effects of systemic cancer treatment on DNA oxidative damage: The potential for targeted therapies. *Cancer Lett.* **2012**, *327*, 134–141. [CrossRef] [PubMed]
55. Yuan, T.F.; Gu, S.; Shan, C.; Marchado, S.; Arias-Carrión, O. Oxidative Stress and Adult Neurogenesis. *Stem Cell Rev. Rep.* **2015**, *11*, 706–709. [CrossRef] [PubMed]
56. Lam, V.; Hackett, M.; Takechi, R. Antioxidants and Dementia Risk: Consideration through a Cerebrovascular Perspective. *Nutrients* **2016**, *8*. [CrossRef] [PubMed]
57. Aderka, D. The potential biological and clinical significance of the soluble tumor necrosis factor receptors. *Cytokine Growth Factor Rev.* **1996**, *7*, 231–240. [CrossRef]
58. Patel, S.K.; Wong, A.L.; Wong, F.L.; Breen, E.C.; Hurria, A.; Smith, M.; Kinjo, C.; Paz, I.B.; Kruper, L.; Somlo, G.; et al. Inflammatory biomarkers, comorbidity, and neurocognition in women With newly diagnosed breast cancer. *J. Natl. Cancer Inst.* **2015**, *107*, djv131. [CrossRef] [PubMed]
59. Jenkins, V.; Thwaites, R.; Cercignani, M.; Sacre, S.; Harrison, N.; Whiteley-Jones, H.; Mullen, L.; Chamberlain, G.; Davies, K.; Zammit, C.; et al. A feasibility study exploring the role of pre-operative assessment when examining the mechanism of "chemo-brain" in breast cancer patients. *Springerplus* **2016**, *5*, 390. [CrossRef] [PubMed]
60. Kesler, S.; Janelsins, M.; Koovakkattu, D.; Palesh, O.; Mustian, K.; Morrow, G.; Dhabhar, F.S. Reduced hippocampal volume and verbal memory performance associated with interleukin-6 and tumor necrosis factor-alpha levels in chemotherapy-treated breast cancer survivors. *Brain Behav. Immun.* **2013**, *30*, S109–S116. [CrossRef] [PubMed]
61. Shibayama, O.; Yoshiuchi, K.; Inagaki, M.; Matsuoka, Y.; Yoshikawa, E.; Sugawara, Y.; Akechi, T.; Wada, N.; Imoto, S.; Murakami, K.; et al. Association between adjuvant regional radiotherapy and cognitive function in breast cancer patients treated with conservation therapy. *Cancer Med.* **2014**, *3*, 702–709. [CrossRef] [PubMed]
62. Kaulmann, A.; Bohn, T. Carotenoids, inflammation, and oxidative stress—implications of cellular signaling pathways and relation to chronic disease prevention. *Nutr. Res.* **2014**, *34*, 907–929. [CrossRef] [PubMed]
63. Thomson, C.A.; Stendell-Hollis, N.R.; Rock, C.L.; Cussler, E.C.; Flatt, S.W.; Pierce, J.P. Plasma and dietary carotenoids are associated with reduced oxidative stress in women previously treated for breast cancer. *Cancer Epidemiol. Biomarkers Prev.* **2007**, *16*, 2008–2015. [CrossRef] [PubMed]
64. Butalla, A.C.; Crane, T.E.; Patil, B.; Wertheim, B.C.; Thompson, P.; Thomson, C.A. Effects of a carrot juice intervention on plasma carotenoids, oxidative stress, and inflammation in overweight breast cancer survivors. *Nutr. Cancer* **2012**, *64*, 331–341. [CrossRef] [PubMed]
65. Institute of Medicine, Panel on Micrnutrients. *DRI: Dietary Reference Intakes for Vitamin A, Vitamin K, Arsenic, Boron, Chromium, Copper, Iodine, Iron, Manganese, Molybdenum, Nickel, Silicon, Vanadium, and Zinc*; National Academies Press: Washington, DC, USA, 2002.
66. Polidori, M.C.; Praticó, D.; Mangialasche, F.; Mariani, E.; Aust, O.; Anlasik, T.; Mang, N.; Pientka, L.; Stahl, W.; Sies, H.; et al. High fruit and vegetable intake is positively correlated with antioxidant status and cognitive performance in healthy subjects. *J. Alzheimers Dis.* **2009**, *17*, 921–927. [CrossRef] [PubMed]
67. Liu, R.H. Health-promoting components of fruits and vegetables in the diet. *Adv. Nutr.* **2013**, *4*, 384S–392S. [CrossRef] [PubMed]
68. Lamport, D.J.; Saunders, C.; Butler, L.T.; Spencer, J.P. Fruits, vegetables, 100% juices, and cognitive function. *Nutr. Rev.* **2014**, *72*, 774–789. [CrossRef] [PubMed]
69. Miller, M.G.; Thangthaeng, N.; Poulose, S.M.; Shukitt-Hale, B. Role of fruits, nuts, and vegetables in maintaining cognitive health. *Exp. Gerontol.* **2017**, *94*, 24–28. [CrossRef] [PubMed]
70. Pomykala, K.L.; Ganz, P.A.; Bower, J.E.; Kwan, L.; Castellon, S.A.; Mallam, S.; Cheng, I.; Ahn, R.; Breen, E.C.; Irwin, M.R.; et al. The association between pro-inflammatory cytokines, regional cerebral metabolism, and cognitive complaints following adjuvant chemotherapy for breast cancer. *Brain Imaging Behav.* **2013**, *7*, 511–523. [CrossRef] [PubMed]
71. Simen, A.A.; Bordner, K.A.; Martin, M.P.; Moy, L.A.; Barry, L.C. Cognitive dysfunction with aging and the role of inflammation. *Ther. Adv. Chronic Dis.* **2011**, *2*, 175–195. [CrossRef] [PubMed]
72. Sartori, A.; Vance, D. The impact of inflammation on cognitive function in older adults: Implications for health care practice and research. *J. Neurosci. Nurs.* **2012**, *44*, 206–217. [CrossRef] [PubMed]

73. Fardell, J.E.; Vardy, J.; Johnston, I.N.; Winocur, G. Chemotherapy and cognitive impairment: Treatment options. *Clin. Pharmacol. Ther.* **2011**, *90*, 366–376. [CrossRef] [PubMed]
74. Wefel, J.S.; Kesler, S.R.; Noll, K.R.; Schagen, S.B. Clinical characteristics, pathophysiology, and management of noncentral nervous system cancer-related cognitive impairment in adults. *CA Cancer J. Clin.* **2015**, *65*, 123–138. [CrossRef] [PubMed]
75. Oh, P.J.; Kim, J. The effects of nonpharmacologic interventions on cognitive function in patients with cancer: A meta-analysis. *Oncol. Nurs. Forum* **2016**, *43*, E205–E217. [CrossRef] [PubMed]
76. Treanor, C.J.; McMenamin, U.C.; O'Neill, R.F.; Cardwell, C.R.; Clarke, M.J.; Cantwell, M.; Donnelly, M. Non-pharmacological interventions for cognitive impairment due to systemic cancer treatment. *Cochrane Database Syst. Rev.* **2016**, CD011325. [CrossRef] [PubMed]
77. Demark-Wahnefried, W.; Aziz, N.M.; Rowland, J.H.; Pinto, B.M. Riding the crest of the teachable moment: Promoting long-term health after the diagnosis of cancer. *J. Clin. Oncol.* **2005**, *23*, 5814–5830. [CrossRef] [PubMed]

13

Biological Active Ecuadorian Mango 'Tommy Atkins' Ingredients—An Opportunity to Reduce Agrowaste

Jenny Ruales [1], Nieves Baenas [2], Diego A. Moreno [2], Carla M. Stinco [3], Antonio J. Meléndez-Martínez [3] and Almudena García-Ruiz [1,4,*]

1 Department of Food Science and Biotechnology, Escuela Politécnica National, Quito 17-01-2759, Ecuador; jenny.ruales@epn.edu.ec
2 Phytochemistry and Healthy Foods Lab., Department of Food Science and Technology, CEBAS-CSIC, Campus de Espinardo-Edificio 25, E-30100 Murcia, Spain; nbaenas@cebas.csic.es (N.B.); dmoreno@cebas.csic.es (D.A.M.)
3 Food Colour & Quality Lab., Department of Nutrition & Food Science, Universidad de Sevilla, Facultad de Farmacia, 41012 Sevilla, Spain; cstinco@us.es (C.M.S.); ajmelendez@us.es (A.J.M.-M.)
4 Laboratory of Epigenetics of Lipid Metabolism, Madrid Institute for Advanced Studies (IMDEA)-Food, CEI UAM + CSIC, 28049 Madrid, Spain
* Correspondence: almudena.garcia@epn.edu.ec or almudena.garcia@imdea.org;

Abstract: Mango is a commercially important tropical fruit. During its processing, peel and seed kernel are discarded as waste but they could be recovered as an excellent and cost-effective source of health-promoting ingredients. This study aimed to characterize some of them, including carotenoids like the provitamin A β-carotene and lutein, with an interest beyond its role in eye health. Other health-promoting compounds like tocopherols and polyphenols were also evaluated, as well as the in vitro antioxidant capacity of mango by-products. Regarding isoprenoids, α-tocopherol was mainly found in the peels and carotenoids concentration was higher in the pulps. β-carotene was the most abundant carotene in pulp and seed kernel, whereas peel was the only source of lutein, with violaxanthin the most abundant xanthophyll in the different mango organs tested. With regard to polyphenols, peels exhibited greater variability in its phenolic composition, being the total content up to 85 and 10 times higher than the pulp and seed kernels, respectively. On the other hand, peels also stood out for being a very rich source of mangiferin. Seed kernels and peels showed higher antioxidant capacity values than the pulps. These results contribute to the valorization of mango by-products as new natural ingredients for the pharma and food industries.

Keywords: mango by-products; lutein; β-carotene; α-tocopherol; mangiferin; food ingredients

---

1. Introduction

Mango (*Mangifera indica*) is considered one of the most consumed fresh fruits in the world, with extensive marketing and production taking place in 115 countries [1]. The global area of mangoes harvested is approximately 5.41 million hectares and its global production is 42.66 million metric tons (MMT) [2]. India, with a production of 18 MMT, is the world's largest mango producer, whereas Mexico and the United States are the main mango exporter and importer, respectively [2]. There are several hundreds of cultivars of mango; but by its long shelf life, excellent ratings in handling and transport tolerance the cultivar Tommy Atkins is the most commercialized [1,3]. Ecuador, with a global area of mangoes harvested of 13,300 hectares and a production of 61,300 metric tons, is the second and sixth mango exporter to USA and to worldwide, respectively, being an important fruit in the Ecuadorian economy [2].

Apart of being consumed fresh, about 20% of mango are processed for products such as juices, desserts, mango jam, among others [4]. During processing, 33% of the fruit is removed in the form of waste, generating, as a result, several million tons per year of mango waste from factories [4,5]. The mango fractions discarded, peel and seed kernel (35–60% total weight of the fruit) are a source of pollution, among other reasons because they are prone to microbial spoilage causing objectionable odors and environmental problems [1,3]. However, the mango peel and seed kernel may be interesting because their high levels of health-enhancing substances, such as carotenoids, polyphenols, vitamins C and E and dietary fiber, among others [6]. The benefit effect of these phytochemicals may be associated with their antioxidant capacity, since in the pathogenesis of many chronic disease is involved the overproduction of oxidants [7]. On the other hand, various studies have described that efficient, inexpensive and environmentally friendly use of agri-food industry waste is highly cost-effective and minimizes environmental impact [8,9]. In this line, the characterization, recovery and utilization of valuable compounds from mango by-products is an important challenge, whose result would have a significant positive impact both at the environmental level (reduction of pollution of mango industry) and economically (contribution to more sustainable production in the food and pharmaceutical industries). In addition, the revaluation of mango peels and seed kernels as a natural bioactive ingredient for the industry, would have a positive socio-economical effect on Ecuadorian mango and tree fruit producing areas, contributing to a reduction of nutritional deficiencies and promoting health benefits, as well as reducing the environmental implications associated with the mango processing.

In this context, the main goal of the present work was to characterize and evaluate Ecuadorian mango by-products in their phytochemical composition: two types of isoprenoids, specifically carotenoids and α-tocopherol and polyphenols by RRLC (Rapid Resolución Liquid Chromatographic) and HPLC–DAD–ESI/MS^n (High-performance Liquid Chromatographic Diode-array detector Electrospray ionization Mass Spectometry), respectively and their total antioxidant capacity by ORAC (Oxygen Radical Absorbance Capacity) and DPPH (2,2,-diphenyl-2-picrylhydrazyl) methods, as well as by Folin–Ciocalteu assay. These evaluations were carried out to establish the potential applications of these mango discards or non-commercial products (peels and seed kernels) compared with the pulp (the main fraction consumed of the mango fruits) as a valuable source of natural ingredients and/or additives for the pharmaceutical and food industry.

2. Materials and Methods

2.1. Fruit Samples

Mangoes (*Mangifera indica* L. cv. Tommy Atkins), were obtained in local markets in Quito (Ecuador). The fruits were selected free of damage. Two kilograms of samples were separated into peels, pulps and seed kernels and stored at −20 °C until freeze drying in an Alpha 2–4 LD drying manifold (Martin Christ Gefriertrocknungsanlagen GmbH, Osterode am Harz, Germany). Then, samples were ground as a fine powder and stored at −20 °C until analyses.

2.2. Standards, Chemicals and Solvents

The commercially available standards (+)-catechin and rutin (Quercetin-3-rutinoside) were acquired from Phytoplan GmbH (Heidelberg, Germany). Cyanidin 3-O-glucoside was purchased from Polyphenols (Sandnes, Norway). The β-carotene and β-cryptoxanthin were obtained from Sigma-Aldrich Chemie GmbH (Steinheim, Germany) and α-tocopherol was purchased from Calbiochem (Merck, Darmstadt, Germany). Violaxanthin and phytoene were isolated from natural sources by classical chromatographic techniques [10]. Luteoxanthin, neoxanthin and lutein were obtained as described by Meléndez-Martínez et al. [11].

Trolox (6-hydroxy-2,5,7,8-tetramethylchroman-2-carboxylic acid) was obtained from Fluka Chemika (Neu-Ulm, Switzerland). The reagents 2,2-diphenyl-1-picrylhidracyl radical (DPPH$^{\cdot}$), monobasic and dibasic sodium phosphate, Folin Ciocalteu's reagent and fluorescein (free acid) were purchased from Sigma–Aldrich (Steinheim, Germany). Finally, formic acid and solvents (ethanol, methanol, hexane, acetone, diclhoromethane and acetonitrile) were all of analytical grade and were obtained from Merck (Darmstadt, Germany).

2.3. Identification and Quantification of Isoprenoids (Carotenoids and α-Tocopherol) by Rapid Resolution Liquid Chromatography (RRLC)

The extraction and analyses of carotenoids were carried out according to the method described by Stinco et al. [12]. Mango samples (200 mg) were extracted with 1mL of hexane/acetone (1:1 *v*/*v*) using a vortex and an ultrasonic bath for 2 min. Then, samples were centrifuged at 18,000× *g* for 5 min and the colored fractions were recovered. The extraction was performed twice more until color extinction. Finally, the carotenoid extracts were concentrated to dryness in a rotary evaporator at temperature below 30 °C. To obtain saponified carotenoids, the extracts were treated with 1000 μL of dichloromethane and 1000 μL of methanolic KOH (30% *w*/*v*) for 1 h under dim light and at room temperature, after which they were washed with water to remove any trace of base. The extracts obtained were concentrated to dryness in a rotary evaporator and redissolved in ethyl acetate prior to their injection in the RRLC system. Samples were extracted and analyzed in triplicate.

The RRLC acquisitions were made by using an Agilent 1260 system equipped with a diode-array detector, which was set to scan from 200 to 770 nm and a Poroshell 120 C18 column (2.7 μm, 5 cm × 4.6 mm) (Agilent, Palo Alto, CA, USA) kept at 28 °C, according to Stinco et al. [12]. The injection volume was set at 10–20 μL. The mobile phase was pumped at 1 mL/min and consisted of three solvents: solvent A, acetonitrile, solvent B, methanol and solvent C, ethyl acetate. The linear gradient elution was 0 min, 85% A + 15% B; 5 min, 60% A + 20% B + 20% C; 7 min, 60% A + 20% B + 20% C; 9 min, 85% A + 15% B; 12 min, 85% A + 15% B. Chromatograms were monitored at 450 nm. The identification and quantification of isoprenoids were performed by comparison of their chromatographic UV–vis spectroscopic characteristics with the standards, as well as by comparison with the external calibration line calculated. Results were expressed as μg/g dry weight (D.W.).

2.4. Folin-Ciocalteu Assay

Folin assay was performed following the method described by Slinkard and Singleton [13]. Briefly, 500 μL of the extracts, blank or standards were placed in a 15 mL tube, where 2.5 mL of the Folin–Ciocalteu reagent was added, allowing to react for 2 min while shaking. Then, 2 mL of a solution of sodium carbonate (75 g/L) was added and properly mixed. The solution was thus incubated 15 min at 50 °C. After that, the absorbance was measured at 750 nm in a spectrophotometer (Shimadzu UV-160A, Kyoto, Japan). Gallic acid was used as a standard (10–90 mg/L) and the results were expressed as mg of gallic acid equivalents (GAE) per gram.

2.5. Identification and Quantification of Phenolic Compounds by HPLC–DAD–ESI-MS^n

Phenolic compounds were extracted and analyzed following the protocol and method of Gironés-Vilaplana et al. [14]. Briefly, samples were extracted with MeOH 70% using the ultrasound technology and kept at 4 °C overnight. Then, samples were filtered and the identification of phenolic compounds was carried out following their MS2 fragmentations by an HPLC–DAD–ESI-MS^n, constituted by an Agilent series model HPLC (High-performance Liquid Chromatographic) 1100 with a photodiode array detector and a mass spectrometer detector in series (model G2445A) equipped with an electrospray ionization interface (Agilent Technologies, Waldbronn, Germany). The ionization conditions were selected according to those described in the method, covering an m/z range from 100 to 1200. The acquisition of the mass spectrometry data (MS^n) was performed in the negative ionization mode for flavonoids, except for anthocyanins, where the positive ionization mode was used. The quantification equipped with a Luna C18 column (25 cm × 0.46 cm, 5 μm particle size) (Phenomenex, Macclesfield, UK) using the acquisition conditions described before. Flavan-3-ols were quantified using the external standard (+)-catechin at 280 nm, flavonols at 360 nm using the standard rutin (quercetin-3-rutinoside) and the anthocyanins by using cyanidin 3-O-glucoside at 520 nm. Samples were extracted and analyzed in triplicate. Results were expressed as μg/g D.W.

2.6. Antioxidant Capacity

The antioxidant capacity was evaluated using the methods DPPH˙ and ORAC, both adapted to a microscale and performed using 96-well micro plates (Nunc, Roskilde, Denmark), which were measured using an Infinite® M200 microplate reader (Tecan, Grödig, Austria). The power of scavenge DPPH radicals were determined according to Mena et al. [15], briefly, 2 μL of the corresponding diluted sample was added to the wells containing 250 μL of DPPH˙ dissolved in methanol up to absorbance ~1. Then, the plate was shaken and left for 50 min at 37 °C, thus, the variation in absorbance was measured at 515 nm. Regarding the ORAC method and according to Ou et al. [16], 25 μL of the properly diluted sample was added to 150 μL of fluorescein (1 μM) and, after 30 min of incubation, 25 μL of the radical AAPH (2,2′-azobis(2-methyl-propionamidine)-dihydrochloride) (250 mM) was added to the wells. Results were studied by measuring the variation in fluorescence each 2 min during 120 min of reaction with the radical. Trolox was used as a standard in both methods, following the same procedure as with the samples. Results were expressed as mmol Trolox/100 g D.W.

2.7. Statistical Analysis

All assays were conducted in triplicate. The data were processed using the software Statgraphics Centurion version 16.1.18 (Statgraphics.Net, Madrid, Spain). All values were subjected to analysis of variance (ANOVA) with a 95% confidence level. Pearson's correlation coefficients were also calculated to corroborate relationships among the selected parameters.

3. Results and Discussion

The first step to establish the potential applications of the mango by-products, peels and seed kernels, as a valuable source of natural ingredients and/or additives for the pharmaceutical and food industry is crucial to characterize the phytochemical composition with efficient techniques for the identification and quantitation of the nutrients and compounds of interest. Bearing this in mind, different chromatographic methods were used to characterize the isoprenoids, especially carotenoids and α-tocopherol and the phenolic composition of mango by-products.

3.1. Isoprenoids: Carotenoids and α-Tocopherol

Many studies have evaluated the carotenoid fraction of mango pulps but not peels and seed kernels. In this sense, this study provides information on the characterization of carotenoid in non-edible parts of the mango. In particular, six carotenoids (4 xanthophylls and 2 carotenes) were identified and quantified in the different mango organs tested (peels, pulps and seed kernels) (Table 1). The carotenoid composition, both qualitative and quantitative, showed differences between the different mango organs tested, which is in line with data previously described in the literature [17]. Violaxanthin and β-carotene stood out as the only two carotenoids present in the different mango fractions tested (Table 1). Regarding pulps and seed kernels, the most abundant carotene was β-carotene, whereas the most important xanthophyll was violaxanthin (Table 1). This is comparable with the results reported by Ornelas-Paz et al. [18] in seven Mexican mango cultivars. Moreover, several authors have described β-carotene as the most predominant carotenoid in Australian and Taiwanese mango pulps [19,20]. In terms of biological effects, β-carotene is considered, theoretically, the carotenoid with the highest provitamin A activity [21] while the health benefits of violaxanthin have yet to be established [17]. With regard to mango peels, lutein highlighted as major carotenoid (Table 1). This agrees with the result reported by Ajila et al. [22] in peels Bandami mango variety. Lutein is an essential nutrient with health promoting effects, especially for eye health. In this line, the use of lutein in the formulation of nutritional supplements have gained increasing popularity for the prevention of age-related macular degeneration, as well as for its antioxidant properties, after the public awareness of its potential to prevent the disease [23]. Thus, the particular interest of the industry, especially pharmaceutical, in the search for new cost-effective sources of lutein as could be mango peels. In addition to its effects on the retina, it has recently been reported the accumulation of lutein in brain, being its content in neural tissue positively correlated with cognitive function, which has intensified interest in identifying functions of lutein in this organ [24]. Furthermore, lutein is a natural colorant, so the mango peels could be employed as additive in the industry such as food, cosmetic and nutraceutical.

Table 1. Isoprenoid, carotenoids and α-tocopherol, composition in mango organs (peels, pulps and seed kernels).

	Concentration (μg/g D.W.)		
	Peel	**Pulp**	**Seed Kernel**
Carotenoids			
Violaxanthin *	$1.58^{b} \pm 0.13$	$3.97^{a} \pm 0.19$	$0.18^{c} \pm 0.02$
Lutein	3.26 ± 0.19	-	-
Luteoxanthin	-	$1.69^{a} \pm 0.08$	$0.16^{b} \pm 0.04$
β-cryptoxanthin	-	2.72 ± 0.04	-
β-carotene	$2.78^{b} \pm 0.05$	$4.86^{a} \pm 0.01$	$0.50^{c} \pm 0.01$
Phytoene	-	$1.23^{a} \pm 0.01$	$0.23^{b} \pm 0.03$
∑*carotenoids*	$7.62^{b} \pm 0.37$	$14.47^{a} \pm 0.33$	$1.07^{c} \pm 0.10$
α-tocopherol	$10.20^{a} \pm 1.13$	$0.39^{b} \pm 0.21$	-

* In peel, the concentration of violoxanthin corresponds to violaxanthin + neoxanthin; [a–c] Mean values with different letter on the right in the same row indicate statistically significant differences among the three treatments ($p < 0.05$).

On the other hand, the results obtained on the qualitative and quantitative characterization of carotenoid showed differences with the results reported in other mango cultivars (Keitt, Ataulfo, Haden and Kent) from Mexico, Brazil, Taiwan [18,20,25]. These differences could be due to factors such as genetics, agricultural and industrial practices, temperature, harvest, maturity, among others, which can modify the composition of carotenoids [3,17].

The total content of carotenoids (TCC), evaluated as the sum of the content of individual pigments, showed significant differences between the different fractions of mango. The mango pulps showed the highest content (Table 1). TCC obtained in the pulps (14.47 μg/g) is within the range described in other several mango cultivars (9.0 to 92 μg/g) [26]. Although the pulps showed the highest TCC, the result also reflected that mango by-products could be a valuable source of carotenoid, especially mango peels. TCC obtained in mango peels (7.62 μg/g) is higher or comparable than TCC values reported in tropical fruits (Table 2), which reflects that mango peels are not only a disposable waste but an extraordinary source natural of carotenoids. The use of mango peels offers a window of opportunity for configuring alternative food supply chains. The raw material is valuable in terms of nutritional and functional properties and besides, the use of this side stream is of great interest from the point of view of environmental concerns and for food and nutrition purposes.

Table 2. Carotenoid concentration in tropical fruits.

	Carotenoid Concentration (μg/g D.W.)
Eugenia stipitata	8.06 [27]
Solanum quitoense	7.94 [28]
Ananas comosus	4.97 [29]
Psidium guajava	6.04 [29]
Carica papaya	7.93−51.34 [30]

In relation to α-tocopherol, it is an antioxidant with an effective chemoprotectant agent against lipid oxidation. In the present study, the α-tocopherol was detected and quantified in peels and pulps but not in seed kernels. Concretely, its content was 26 times greater in peels than pulps (Table 1). Abbasi et al. [31] also detected higher content of α-tocopherol in peels than pulps in nine mango cultivars from China. α-tocopherol amount in mango pulps was higher than that described by Burns et al. [32] (0.05 μg/g) in mango from Costa Rica, in agreement with Ornelas-Paz et al. [18] (0.2–0.5 μg/g) in seven Mexican mango cultivars but lower than the content described by Vilela et al. [33] (12–94 μg/g) and Gong et al. [34] (2.0 μg/g) in twelve Portuguese mango cultivars and in mango from China, respectively. As polyphenols and carotenoids, the α-tocopherol amount depends on the genotype, the environmental factors and analytical methods, among other factors [35], which explains the differences observed among the results obtained in this study and others. On the other hand, α-tocopherol concentration obtained in peels was greater than observed in some exotic fruits such as dragon fruit (4.5 μg/g), durian (3.6 μg/g) and papaya (2.6 μg/g) [35]. This result reflects that mango peels could be exploited as natural antioxidant in cosmetic (i.e., anti-aging products), pharmaceutical and agro-industry.

3.2. Characterization of the Phenolic Composition

3.2.1. Identification of Phenolic Compounds

Seventeen phenolic compounds were separated and tentatively identified as procyanidins (1–3), anthocyanins (4, 6), xanthones (5, 7, 9, 16, 17) and flavonols (8, 10–15) by HPLC–DAD–ESI/MS^n, which are shown in Table 3. In addition, the separation of polyphenolics in mango peel is shown in Figure 1.

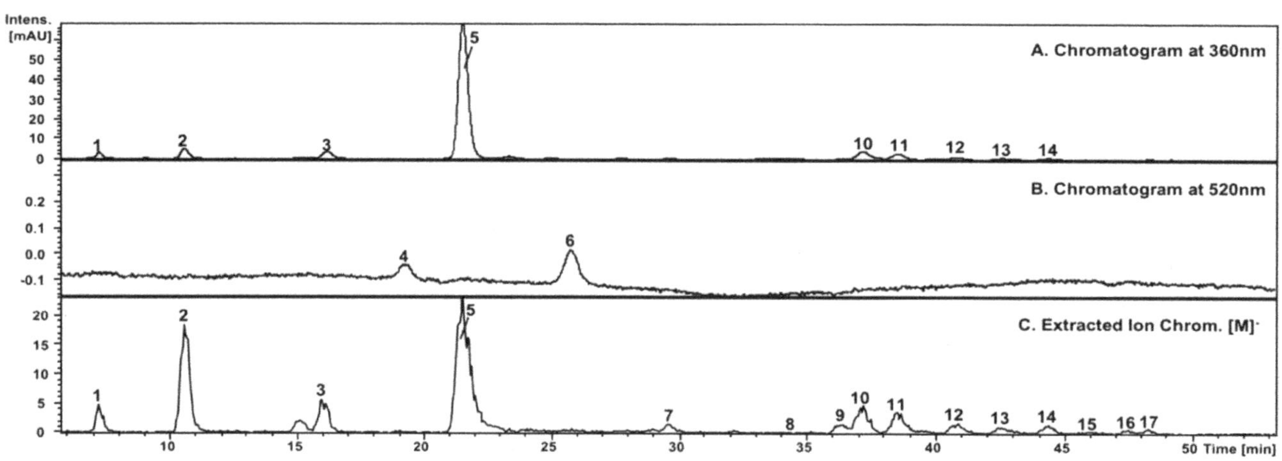

Figure 1. Typical chromatogram of mango organs (e.g., peels), registered at 360 nm (**A**) and 520 nm (**B**) for the identification; Extracted Ion Chromatogram of $(M)^-$ of parental ions (**C**) of the phenolic compounds in the mango samples is also included. For the compound assignment numbers, please see Table 3.

Table 3. Tentative identification of phenolic compounds in mango organs (peels, pulps and seed kernels) by HPLC–DAD–ESI-MS^n.

Peak Number	Rt (min)	DAD (Max. Abs.) λnm	$(M)^-$	Fragment Ions (MS^n)	Phenolic Compounds (Tentative Identification)	Peels	Pulp	Seed Kernels
1	7.2	280	423	303, 289	Procyanidin (catechin derivative)	√	-	-
2	10.5	280	575	423, 289	Procyanidin dimer	√		
3	15.9	280	559	407,289	(Epi)afzelechin-(epi)catechin dimer	√	-	-
4	19.2	280, 520	-	-	Unidentified anthocyanin	√	-	-
5	21.5	330,360	421	403, 331, 301, 258–259	Mangiferin	√	√	√
6	25.7	280, 520	-	-	Unidentified anthocyanin	√	-	-
7	29.5	360	573	421, 403, 331, 301	Mangiferin gallate	√	-	-
8	34.4	360	599	285	Kaempferol derivative	√	-	-
9	36.3	360	573	421, 403, 331, 301	Mangiferin gallate	√	-	-
10	37.1	360	463	301	Quercetin galactoside	√	-	-
11	38.5	360	463	301	Quercetin glucoside	√	-	-
12	40.8	360	433	301	Quercetin xyloside	√	-	-
13	42.5	360	433	301	Quercetin arabinopyranoside	√	-	-
14	44.4	360	433	301	Quercetin arabinofuranoside	√	-	-
15	45.8	360	447	301	Quercetin rhamnoside	√	-	-
16	47.4	330,360	421	403, 373, 331, 301	Mangiferin (isomer)	√	-	-
17	48.2	360	573	421, 403, 331, 301	Mangiferin gallate (isomer)	√	-	-

Rt: retention time; DAD: dyode-array detector.

Procyanidins

Peaks 1 and 2 showed the MS spectra of procyanidin dimers with molecular intact ions at *m/z* of 423 and 575, respectively and a characteristic deprotonated molecular ion in MS2 of *m/z* 289 that corresponds to a (epi)catechin. It is important to highlight that both phenolic compounds had never been determined in mango peels before. On the other hand, peak 3 was identified as a propelargonidin dimer due to its molecular ion (M–H) at *m/z* at 559–560 and its MS2/MS3 fragment ions *m/z* 407 and 289, corresponding probably to (epi)afzelechin-(epi)catechin. These procyanidins were only characterized in mango peels.

The compounds 4 and 6 exhibited peak absorption maximum at ~280 nm and ~520 nm wavelengths, characteristic of anthocyanins but in extremely low concentration that did not allow the tentative identification of the compounds or the isolation of their aglycones in the $(M)^-$ and its corresponding MS/MS fragmentation experiments. These compounds were detected in mango peels but not in pulps and seed kernels.

Xanthones

Peak 5 showed a molecular anion at *m/z* 421, being therefore tentatively assigned as mangiferin. Peaks 7 and 9, with a corresponding *m/z* ion of 573 $(M)^-$ and characteristic MS/MS fragmentation, were tentatively identified as mangiferin gallates [36]. In the last part of the chromatogram, tiny peaks of possible isomers of mangiferin (peak 16) and mangiferin gallate (peak 17) were also detected in the MS/MS experiments. These compounds, with exception of mangiferin, were only detected in peels. Mangiferin was also the unique xanthone detected in the pulps of the cultivar Haden, and in the seed kernels of the cultivar Ubá, but the pulps of the cultivar Ubá were constituted by a greater number of xanthones [37]. This result reflects the variability of the phenolic composition in the mango.

Flavonols

Peak 8 was identified as kaempferol derivative according to their UV spectra and MS fragmentation leading to the kaempferol aglycone at *m/z* 285 in negative mode [38]. With regard to compounds 10–14, they were identified as quercetin glycosides based on their UV-Vis data and characteristic mass spectra and elution order [39] (Table 3). In the quercetin glycosides, the most abundant fragment ion in MS2/MS3 was *m/z* 301 that corresponds with the radical anion of the aglycone quercetin. Peaks 10 and 11 displayed identical $(M)^-$ ion, *m/z* 463 and could be assigned as quercetin-galactoside and quercetin glucoside, respectively. The formation of the ion at *m/z* 433 [M]- as the main fragment ions in the peaks 12, 13 and 14 revealed the presence of three different quercetin pentosides and recognized as quercetin xyloside (12), arabinopyranoside (13) and arabinofuranoside (14), respectively. Finally, the occurrence of an ion $(M{-}H)^-$ at *m/z* 447 in the compound 15 indicated the existence of a quercetin rhamnoside. These flavonoids were observed in mango peels but not in pulps and seed kernels. This agrees with previously reported data by Berardini et al. [40] in cultivar Tommy Atkins and Gómez-Caravaca et al. [41] in Keitt mango.

These results reflected that the phenolic profile of peels was different to the profiles obtained in pulps and seed kernels (Table 3). This agrees with information previously reported in the literature, where it is indicated that of different mango phenolics differ in the different plant parts [42]. In particular, in this study the peels showed a higher number of phenolic compounds than pulps and seed kernels. This is in accordance with results previously described in mango [37,43].

3.2.2. Quantification of Phenolic Compounds

The results of the quantification of phenolic compounds in mango are shown in Table 4. Mangiferin was the predominant phenolic compound in the three mango fractions but its quantity was different in each organ. In particular, mango peels presented the highest concentration (2500 μg/g D.W.) followed by seed kernels and pulp (Table 4). This result reflected that non-edible parts of the mango fruit are good sources of mangiferin. Similar results were obtained by Luo et al. [43], Gómez-Caravaca et al. [41] and Ribeiro et al. [37] in 11 Chinese cultivars, cultivar Keitt and cultivar Ubá of mango, respectively. However, the mangiferin concentrations obtained were different to the described by other authors in cultivar Tommy Atkins (peels: 1190.9–1690.4 μg/g; pulps: 2.2 μg/g) [36,43] and cultivars Ataulfo, Keitt, Van Dyke and Ubá, among others (peels: 62.3–21530 μg/g; pulps: not detected-200 μg/g; seed kernels: traces-2340 μg/g) [37,41,43–45]. This agrees with data previously reported in the literature, where it has been reported that factors such as cultivar, environment, harvest stage, maturity as well as the method extraction, among other factors, have an effect on the phenolic composition [3,19,44,45]. Regarding the mangiferin biological effects, this phenol possesses an antioxidant capacity higher than other natural antioxidants like vitamin C and E. In this line, this phenolic compound could be used as a food preservative. In addition, mangiferin has a special particular interest for the pharmacological industry by its cancer chemopreventive potential [41].

Table 4. Concentration of phenolic composition in mango peel, pulp and seed kernel.

Peak	*Phenolic Compounds*	Concentration (μg/g D.W.)		
		Peel	Pulp	Seed Kernel
1	Procyanidin (catechin derivative)	560 ± 60	-	-
2	Procyanidin dimer	<LOQ	-	-
3	Epiafzelechin-epicatechin dimer	600 ± 60	-	-
4	Unidentified anthocyanin	<LOQ	-	-
5	Mangiferin	2500 ^{a} ± 320	50 ^{c} ± 20	430 ^{b} ± 90
6	Unidentified anthocyanin	30 ± 0	-	-
7	Mangiferin gallate	<LOQ	-	-
8	Kaempferol derivative	<LOQ	-	-
9	Mangiferin gallate	<LOQ	-	-
10	Quercetin-galactoside	220 ± 20	-	-
11	Quercetin glucoside	180 ± 10	-	-
12	Quercetin xyloside	<LOQ	-	-
13	Quercetin arabinopyranoside	80 ± 10	-	-
14	Quercetin arabinofuranoside	50 ± 0	-	-
15	Quercetin rhamnoside	50 ± 0	-	-
16	Mangiferin (isomer)	<LOQ	-	-
17	Mangiferin gallate (isomer)	<LOQ	-	-
	∑phenolic compounds	4270 ^{a} ± 480	50 ^{c} ± 20	430 ^{b} ± 90

LOQ: limit of quantification; $^{a–c}$ Mean values with different letter on the right in the same row indicate statistically significant differences among the three treatments ($p < 0.05$).

Regarding the presence of procyanidins, these compounds were found only in the peel and two of them, a catechin derivative (560 μg/g D.W.) and epiafzelechin-epicatechin (600 μg/g D.W.) dimers, constituted the most abundant phenolic compounds after mangiferin (Table 4). These compounds, accounting for the 25% of total phenolic compounds, have been described in mango peels for the first time. According to other authors, these low-molecular weight procyanidins have been described as interesting because of their potent antioxidant capacity and possible protective effects on human health [42,46], especially because dimers can be absorbed intact in the intestinal tract [47] and have recently shown to promote the growth of *Bifidobacterium* in vitro [48]. As natural antioxidants and antimicrobials, proanthocyanidins can be also used in the industry as a preservative, to stabilize food colors, to prevent rancidity due to oxidation of unsaturated fats and to avoid the growth of bacteria and molds [49].

On the other hand, flavonol glycosides obtained in mango peel were identified as quercetin glycosides, being quercetin galactoside and quercetin glucoside the most abundant (Table 4), according to the literature [36,41,50]. Quercetin glycosides biological effects are mainly associated to their antioxidant capacity which could be exploited as a food preservative and stabilizer in the agro-industry, as well as in the development of new drugs in the pharmaceutical industry, among others [51].

The total phenolic content (TPC), evaluated as the sum of the content of individual phenolic, showed significant differences between the different fractions of mango. The order observed was peels > seed kernels > pulps (Table 4). This is in line as described the literature, where it has been reported that phenolic compounds are preferentially located in non-edible parts (peels and seed kernels) and in a lesser extent in the edible part (pulps) [3,42,52].

3.3. Antioxidant Capacity and Folin Assay

The health-promoting effects of both bioactive compounds characterized, polyphenols and isoprenoids, have been strongly associated with their antioxidant capacity. Thus, in this present study has been also evaluated the antioxidant capacity of the mango by-products. As shown Table 5, antioxidant capacity of different mango organs (pulp, peel and seed kernel) was evaluated by DPPH radical and ORAC method. Mango by-products highlighted by showing a higher antioxidant capacity than pulps, being seed kernels the mango fraction that exhibited the highest values of antioxidant capacity. The order described is comparable with that obtained by Abbasi et al. [30], Guo et al. [53] and Sogi et al. [54] in nine Chinese mango cultivars, in Chinese mango cultivar and in Tommy Atkins mango from USA, respectively. However, the values obtained in mango peels and seed kernels were lower than that described by Sogi et al. [54] (seed kernels = 154.7–181.9 mmol Trolox/100 g; peels = 41.8–77.6 mmol Trolox/100 g), while mango pulp was higher than that reported by Noratto et al. [55] in five Mexican mango cultivars (15.0–32.7 mmol Trolox/100 g). In this line, it has been described that mango antioxidant capacity can be affected by different factors such as variety, maturity, agricultural and industrial practices [36]. Moreover, it is important to indicate that ORAC value of seed kernels was greater than the ORAC values reported in other tropical fruits with demonstrated high polyphenol content such as banana passion fruit and Andean blackberry [56,57]. These results suggested that mango by-products, especially seed kernels, could represent a valuable ingredient with high antioxidant capacity in the agro-industry. In spite of this, it is important to note that the results were obtained by in vitro methods, which do not take into account the (among others) the metabolic transformations and interactions that clearly affect the bioavailability and biological action of phytochemicals [58,59]. In particular, the predominant forms of polyphenols in plasma are conjugates (glucuronates or sulfates, with or without methylation), which are chemically distinct from their parent compounds and therefore their properties are also different [59]. Thus, prior to the use of mango by-product as a new ingredient in the industry is necessary to go deeper into the analysis of their antioxidant activity and carry out assays of antioxidant capacity in vivo that corroborate the results obtained in vitro; as well as analyze the synergism or antagonism between the bioactive compounds present in the mango by-product matrix both at the level of bioavailability and biological action.

Table 5. Antioxidant capacity in mango organs (peels, pulps and seed kernels).

	Antioxidant Capacity (mmol Trolox/100 g D.W.)		
	Peel	**Pulp**	**Seed Kernel**
DPPH	11.06 ^{b} ± 0.42	2.11 ^{c} ± 0.12	44.34 ^{a} ± 0.89
ORAC	29.87 ^{b} ± 2.69	1.83 ^{c} ± 0.45	126.08 ^{a} ± 2.44

$^{a-c}$ Mean values with different letter on the right in the same row indicate statistically significant differences among the three treatments ($p < 0.05$).

On the other hand, the order observed in Folin-Ciocalteu assay by mango organs, seed kernels (23,759.13 mg/100 g GAE) > peels (2,874.97 mg/100 g GAE) > pulps (563.01 mg/100 g GAE), coincided with that described in the antioxidant activity. This result makes sense, because Folin-Ciocalteu assay determines the content of polyphenols and other reducing bioactive compounds (sugars, amino acids, etc.) that have antioxidant properties.

Finally, the correlation phytochemical composition (polyphenol, carotenoid and α-tocopherol) versus antioxidant capacity (DPPH and ORAC) was positive and direct (Table 6).

Table 6. Pearson's correlation coefficients (r) between bioactive compounds (isoprenoids polyphenols and) in mango organs (peels, pulps and seed kernels) and its antioxidant capacity (DPPH and ORAC).

	Bioactive Compounds Mango		
Assay	**Peel**	**Pulp**	**Seed Kernel**
DPPH	0.97	0.89	0.92
ORAC	1.00	0.90	0.97

4. Conclusions

In summary, the results obtained demonstrate that the non-edible parts of mango, the peels and seed kernels commonly managed as a waste in the industry, are a good source of bioactive compounds like isoprenoids, especially carotenoids and α-tocopherol and polyphenols with high nutritional value and health benefit effects. In particular, mango peels constituted the great part of the fruit in terms of bioactive compounds contents, following by the seed kernels and both compared to the pulp, being some of these components essential nutrients in the human diet, such as lutein and α-tocopherol. In addition, mango by-products, especially seed kernels, exhibited higher antioxidant activity than pulps. Therefore, mango by-products could be exploited as a natural preservative by the pharmaceutical and agro-food industry, as well as being used as a natural ingredient contributing to different health benefits to consumers. Besides, the amount of waste generated during the processing of the mango could be reduced. Finally, future studies will be carried out deeply to elucidate the bioavailability and safety of bioactive compounds of mango by-products.

Author Contributions: Author N.B. carried out the assays, collecting data and helped to draft the article. Author C.M.S. carried out the assays, collecting data and helped to draft the manuscript. Authors J.R., D.A.M. and A.J.M.-M. participated in the experimental design and helped to draft the manuscript. Author A.G.-R. carried out the studies participated in collecting data, experimental design and drafted the manuscript. All authors read and approved the final manuscript.

Acknowledgments: Quality technical work from Ms. Ana Benítez González (Universidad de Sevilla) is acknowledged. AGR also thanks the Ecuadorian SENECYT for the Prometeo Postdoctoral Grants (Ref. PROMETEO-CEB-018-2015).

References

1. Torres-León, C.; Rojas, R.; Contreras-Esquivel, J.C.; Serna-Cock, L.; Belmares-Cerda, R.E.; Aguilar, C.N. Mango seed: Functional and nutritional properties. *Trends Food Sci. Technol.* **2016**, *55*, 109–117. [CrossRef]
2. Evans, E.A.; Ballen, F.H.; Siddiq, M. Mango production, global trade, consumption trends and postharvest processing and nutrition. In *Handbook of Mango Fruit*; John Wiley & Sons: Chichester, UK, 2017; pp. 1–16.
3. Burton-Freeman, B.M.; Sandhu, A.K.; Edirisinghe, I.; Trevisan, M.T.; Viana, D.d.A.; Rao, V.S.; Santos, F.A.; Gali-Muhtasib, H.; Chae, S.; Saido, T.C.; et al. Mangos and their bioactive components: Adding variety to the fruit plate for health. *Food Funct.* **2017**, *8*, 3010–3032. [CrossRef] [PubMed]
4. Ravani, A.; Joshi, D.C. Mango and it's by product utilization—A review. *Energy* **2013**, *1*, 55–67.
5. Purnachandra, M.R.; Saritha, K.V. Bio-catalysis of mango industrial waste by newly isolated *Fusarium* sp. (PSTF1) for pectinase production. *Biotech* **2015**, *5*, 893–900. [CrossRef] [PubMed]

6. Jahurul, M.H.A.; Zaidul, I.S.M.; Ghafoor, K.; Al-Juhaimi, F.Y.; Nyam, K.-L.; Norulaini, N.A.N.; Sahena, F.; Mohd Omar, A.K. Mango (*Mangifera indica* L.) by-products and their valuable components: A Review. *Food Chem.* **2015**, *183*, 173–180. [CrossRef] [PubMed]
7. Zhang, Y.J.; Gan, R.Y.; Li, S.; Zhou, Y.; Li, A.N.; Xu, D.P.; Li, H.B. Antioxidant Phytochemicals for the Prevention and Treatment of Chronic Diseases. *Molecules* **2015**, *20*, 21138–21156. [CrossRef] [PubMed]
8. De Oliveira, A.C.; Valentim, I.B.; Silva, C.A.; Bechara, E.J.H.; de Barros, M.P.; Mano, C.M.; Goulart, M.O.F. Total phenolic content and free radical scavenging activities of methanolic extract powders of tropical fruit residues. *Food Chem.* **2009**, *115*, 469–475. [CrossRef]
9. Salas, S.; Anton, A.; McLaren, S.J.; Notarnicola, B.; Saouter, E.; Sonesson, U. In quest of reducing the environmental impacts of food production and consumption. *J. Clean Prod.* **2017**, *140*, 387–398. [CrossRef]
10. Meléndez-Martínez, A.J.; Vicario, I.M.; Heredia, F.J. Carotenoids, color and ascorbic acid content of a novel frozen-marketed orange juice. *J. Agric. Food Chem.* **2007**, *55*, 1347–1355. [CrossRef] [PubMed]
11. Meléndez-Martínez, A.J.; Britton, G.; Vicario, I.M.; Heredia, F.J. The complex carotenoid pattern of orange juices from concentrate. *Food Chem.* **2008**, *109*, 546–553. [CrossRef]
12. Stinco, C.M.; Benítez-González, A.M.; Hernanz, D.; Vicario, I.M.; Meléndez-Martínez, A.J. Development and validation of a rapid resolution liquid Chromatography method for the screening of dietary plant isoprenoids: Carotenoids, tocopherols and chlorophylls. *J. Chromatogr. A* **2014**, *1370*, 162–170. [CrossRef] [PubMed]
13. Slinkard, K.; Singleton, V.L. Total Phenol Analysis: Automation and comparison with Manual Methods. *Am. J. Enol. Vitic.* **1977**, *28*, 49–55.
14. Gironés-Vilaplana, A.; Baenas, N.; Villaño, D.; Speisky, H.; García-Viguera, C.; Moreno, D.A. Evaluation of Latin-American fruits rich in phytochemicals with biological effects. *J. Funct. Foods* **2014**, *7*, 599–608. [CrossRef]
15. Mena, P.; García-Viguera, C.; Navarro-Rico, J.; Moreno, D.A.; Bartual, J.; Saura, D.; Martí, N. Phytochemical characterisation for industrial use of pomegranate (*Punica granatum* L.) cultivars grown in Spain. *J. Sci. Food Agric.* **2011**, *91*, 1893–1906. [CrossRef] [PubMed]
16. Ou, B.; Hampsch-Woodill, M.; Prior, R.L. Development and validation of an improved oxygen radical absorbance capacity assay using fluorescein as the fluorescent probe. *J. Agric. Food Chem.* **2001**, *49*, 4619–4626. [CrossRef] [PubMed]
17. Rodriguez-Amaya, D.B.; Kimura, M.; Godoy, H.T.; Amaya-Farfan, J. Updated Brazilian database on food carotenoids: Factors affecting carotenoid composition. *J. Food Compos. Anal.* **2008**, *21*, 445–463. [CrossRef]
18. Ornelas-Paz, J.D.J.; Yahia, E.M.; Gardea-Bejar, A. Identification and quantification of xanthophyll esters, carotenes and tocopherols in the fruit of seven mexican mango cultivars by liquid chromatography-atmospheric pressure chemical ionization-time-of-flight mass spectrometry [LC-(APcI+)-MS]. *J. Agric. Food Chem.* **2007**, *55*, 6628–6635. [CrossRef] [PubMed]
19. Hewavitharana, A.K.; Tan, Z.W.; Shimada, R.; Shaw, P.N.; Flanagan, B.M. Between fruit variability of the bioactive compounds, β-carotene and mangiferin, in mango (*Mangifera indica*). *Nutr. Diet.* **2013**, *70*, 158–163. [CrossRef]
20. Chen, J.P.; Tai, C.Y.; Chen, B.H. Improved liquid chromatographic method for determination of carotenoids in Taiwanese mango (*Mangifera indica* L.). *J. Chromatogr. A* **2004**, *1054*, 261–268. [CrossRef]
21. Watson, R.R.; Preedy, V.R. *Bioactive Foods in Promoting Health: Fruits and Vegetables*; Academic Press: London, UK, 2010.
22. Ajila, C.M.; Jaganmohan Rao, L.; Prasada Rao, U.J.S. Characterization of bioactive compounds from raw and ripe *Mangifera indica* L. peel extracts. *Food Chem. Toxicol.* **2010**, *48*, 3406–3411. [CrossRef] [PubMed]
23. Fernández-Sevilla, J.M.; Acién Fernández, F.G.; Molina Grima, E. Biotechnological production of lutein and its applications. *Appl. Microbiol. Biotechnol.* **2010**, *86*, 27–40. [CrossRef] [PubMed]
24. Erdman, J.W.; Smith, J.W.; Kuchan, M.J.; Mohn, E.S.; Johnson, E.J.; Rubakhin, S.S.; Wang, L.; Sweedler, J.V.; Neuringer, M.; Neuringer, M. Lutein and brain function. *Foods* **2015**, *4*, 547–564. [CrossRef] [PubMed]
25. Mercadante, A.Z.; Rodriguez-Amaya, D.B.; Britton, G. HPLC and Mass Spectrometric analysis of carotenoids from mango. *J. Agric. Food Chem.* **1997**, *45*, 120–123. [CrossRef]
26. Litz, R.E. *The Mango: Botany, Production and Uses*; CABI: Wallingford, UK, 2009.
27. Garzón, G.A.; Narváez-Cuenca, C.-E.; Kopec, R.E.; Barry, A.M.; Riedl, K.M.; Schwartz, S.J. Determination of carotenoids, total phenolic content and antioxidant activity of arazá (*Eugenia stipitata* McVaugh), an Amazonian fruit. *J. Agric. Food Chem.* **2012**, *60*, 4709–4717. [CrossRef] [PubMed]

28. Gancel, A.-L.; Alter, P.; Dhuique-Mayer, C.; Ruales, J.; Vaillant, F. Identifying Carotenoids and phenolic compounds in naranjilla (*Solanum quitoense* Lam. Var. puyo hybrid), an Andean fruit. *J. Agric. Food Chem.* **2008**, *56*, 11890–11899. [CrossRef] [PubMed]
29. Ellong, E.N.; Billard, C.; Adenet, S.; Rochefort, K. Polyphenols, carotenoids, vitamin C content in tropical fruits and vegetables and impact of processing methods. *Food Nutr. Sci.* **2015**, *6*, 299–313. [CrossRef]
30. Wall, M.M. Ascorbic acid, vitamin A and mineral composition of banana (*Musa* sp.) and papaya (*Carica papaya*) cultivars grown in Hawaii. *J. Food Compos. Anal.* **2006**, *19*, 434–445. [CrossRef]
31. Abbasi, A.M.; Liu, F.; Guo, X.; Fu, X.; Li, T.; Liu, R.H. Phytochemical composition, cellular antioxidant capacity and antiproliferative activity in mango (*Mangifera indica* L.) pulp and peel. *Int. J. Food Sci. Technol.* **2017**, *52*, 817–826. [CrossRef]
32. Burns, J.; Fraser, P.D.; Bramley, P.M. Identification and quantification of carotenoids, tocopherols and chlorophylls in commonly consumed fruits and vegetables. *Phytochemistry* **2003**, *62*, 939–947. [CrossRef]
33. Vilela, C.; Santos, S.A.O.; Oliveira, L.; Camacho, J.F.; Cordeiro, N.; Freire, C.S.R.; Silvestre, A.J.D. The ripe pulp of *Mangifera indica* L.: A rich source of phytosterols and other lipophilic phytochemicals. *Food Res. Int.* **2013**, *54*, 1535–1540. [CrossRef]
34. Gong, X.; Qi, N.; Wang, X.; Li, J.; Lin, L. A new method for determination of α-tocopherol in tropical fruits by Ultra Performance Convergence Chromatography with Diode Array Detector. *Food Anal. Methods* **2014**, *7*, 1572–1576. [CrossRef]
35. Kodad, O.; Company, R.S.i.; Alonso, J.M. Genotypic and environmental effects on tocopherol content in almond. *Antioxidants* **2018**, *7*, 6. [CrossRef] [PubMed]
36. Schieber, A.; Berardini, N.; Carle, R. Identification of flavonol and xanthone glycosides from mango (*Mangifera indica* L. cv. "Tommy Atkins") peels by High-Performance Liquid Chromatography-Electrospray Ionization Mass Spectrometry. *J. Agric. Food Chem.* **2003**, *51*, 5006–5011. [CrossRef] [PubMed]
37. Ribeiro, S.M.R.; Barbosa, L.C.A.; Queiroz, J.H.; Knödler, M.; Schieber, A. phenolic compounds and antioxidant capacity of Brazilian mango (*Mangifera indica* L.) Varieties. *Food Chem.* **2008**, *110*, 620–626. [CrossRef]
38. KajdŽanoska, M.; Gjamovski, V.; Stefova, M. HPLC-DAD-ESI-MSn Identification of phenolic compounds in cultivated strawberries from Macedonia. *Maced. J. Chem. Chem. Eng.* **2010**, *29*, 181–194.
39. Schieber, A.; Hilt, P.; Conrad, J.; Beifuss, U.; Carle, R. Elution order of quercetin glycosides from apple pomace extracts on a new HPLC stationary phase with hydrophilic endcapping. *J. Sep. Sci.* **2002**, *25*, 361–364. [CrossRef]
40. Berardini, N.; Carle, R.; Schieber, A. Characterization of gallotannins and benzophenone derivatives from mango (*Mangifera indica* L. cv. 'Tommy Atkins') peels, pulp and kernels by High-Performance Liquid Chromatography/Electrospray Ionization Mass Spectrometry. *Rapid Commun. Mass Spectrom.* **2004**, *18*, 2208–2213. [CrossRef] [PubMed]
41. Gómez-Caravaca, A.M.; López-Cobo, A.; Verardo, V.; Segura-Carretero, A.; Fernández-Gutiérrez, A. HPLC-DAD-q-TOF-MS as a powerful platform for the determination of phenolic and other polar compounds in the edible part of mango and its by-products (peel, seed and seed husk). *Electrophoresis* **2016**, *37*, 1072–1084. [CrossRef] [PubMed]
42. Masibo, M.; Qian, H. Major mango polyphenols and their potential significance to human health. *Compr. Rev. Food Sci. Food Saf.* **2008**, *7*, 309–319. [CrossRef]
43. Luo, F.; Lv, Q.; Zhao, Y.; Hu, G.; Huang, G.; Zhang, J.; Sun, C.; Li, X.; Chen, K. Quantification and purification of mangiferin from Chinese mango (*Mangifera indica* L.) cultivars and its protective effect on human umbilical vein endothelial cells under H_2O_2-induced stress. *Int. J. Mol. Sci.* **2012**, *13*, 11260–11274. [CrossRef] [PubMed]
44. Berardini, N.; Fezer, R.; Conrad, J.; Beifuss, U.; Carle, R.; Schieber, A. Screening of mango (*Mangifera indica* L.) cultivars for their contents of flavonol *O*- and xanthone *C*-glycosides, anthocyanins and pectin. *J. Agric. Food Chem.* **2005**, *53*, 1563–1570. [CrossRef] [PubMed]
45. Barreto, J.C.; Trevisan, M.T.S.; Hull, W.E.; Erben, G.; De Brito, E.S.; Pfundstein, B.; Würtele, G.; Spiegelhalder, B.; Owen, R.W. Characterization and quantitation of polyphenolic compounds in bark, kernel, leaves and peel of mango (*Mangifera indica* L.). *J. Agric. Food Chem.* **2008**, *56*, 5599–5610. [CrossRef] [PubMed]
46. Ramirez, J.E.; Zambrano, R.; Sepúlveda, B.; Simirgiotis, M.J. Antioxidant properties and hyphenated HPLC-PDA-MS Profiling of Chilean Pica mango fruits (*Mangifera indica* L. cv. Piqueño). *Molecules* **2014**, *19*, 438–458. [CrossRef] [PubMed]

47. Gu, L.; Kelm, M.A.; Hammerstone, J.F.; Beecher, G.; Holden, J.; Haytowitz, D.; Gebhardt, S.; Prior, R.L. Concentrations of proanthocyanidins in common foods and estimations of normal consumption. *J. Nutr.* **2004**, *134*, 613–617. [CrossRef] [PubMed]
48. Sáyago-Ayerdi, S.G.; Zamora-Gasga, V.M.; Venema, K. Prebiotic Effect of predigested mango peel on gut microbiota assessed in a dynamic in vitro model of the human colon (TIM-2). *Food Res. Int.* **2017**. [CrossRef]
49. Vélez-Rivera, N.; Cárdenas Perez, S.; Chanona-Pérez, J.J.; Perea-Flores, M.J.; Claderón-Domínguez, G.; Blasco Ivars, J.; Farrera-Rebollo, R.R. Industrial applications and potential pharmaceutical uses of mango (Mangifera indica) kernel. In *Seeds as Functional Foods & Nutraceuticals: New Frontiers in Food Science*; Nova Science Publishers Inc.: New York, NY, USA, 2014.
50. Ribeiro, S.M.R.; Schieber, A. Bioactive compounds in mango (*Mangifera indica* L.). In *Bioactive Foods in Promoting Health*; Elsevier: New York, NY, USA, 2010; pp. 507–523.
51. Baenas, N.; Abellán, Á.; Rivera, S.; Moreno, D.A.; García-Viguera, C.; Domínguez-Perles, R. Foods and supplements. In *Polyphenols: Properties, Recovery and Applications*; Elsevier: New York, NY, USA, 2018; pp. 327–362.
52. Ayala-Zavala, J.F.; Vega-Vega, V.; Rosas-Domínguez, C.; Palafox-Carlos, H.; Villa-Rodriguez, J.A.; Siddiqui, M.W.; Dávila-Aviña, J.E.; González-Aguilar, G.A. Agro-industrial potential of exotic fruit byproducts as a source of food additives. *Food Res. Int.* **2011**, *44*, 1866–1874. [CrossRef]
53. Guo, C.; Yang, J.; Wei, J.; Li, Y.; Xu, J.; Jiang, Y. Antioxidant activities of peel, pulp and seed fractions of common fruits as determined by FRAP assay. *Nutr. Res.* **2003**, *23*, 1719–1726. [CrossRef]
54. Sogi, D.S.; Siddiq, M.; Greiby, I.; Dolan, K.D. Total phenolics, antioxidant activity and functional properties of "Tommy Atkins" mango peel and kernel as affected by drying methods. *Food Chem.* **2013**, *141*, 2649–2655. [CrossRef] [PubMed]
55. Noratto, G.D.; Bertoldi, M.C.; Krenek, K.; Talcott, S.T.; Stringheta, P.C.; Mertens-Talcott, S.U. Anticarcinogenic effects of polyphenolics from mango (*Mangifera indica*) varieties. *J. Agric. Food Chem.* **2010**, *58*, 4104–4112. [CrossRef] [PubMed]
56. García-Ruiz, A.; Girones-Vilaplana, A.; León, P.; Moreno, D.A.; Stinco, C.M.; Meléndez-Martínez, A.J.; Ruales, J. Banana passion fruit (*Passiflora mollissima* (Kunth) L.H. Bailey): Microencapsulation, phytochemical composition and antioxidant capacity. *Molecules* **2017**, *22*, 85. [CrossRef] [PubMed]
57. Zapata, S.; Piedrahita, A.M.; Rojano, B. Capacidad Atrapadora de Radicales Oxígeno (ORAC) y fenoles totales de frutas y hortalizas de Colombia. *Perspect. Nutr. Humana* **2014**, *16*, 25–36.
58. Halliwell, B.; Rafter, J.; Jenner, A. Health promotion by flavonoids, tocopherols, tocotrienols and other phenols: Direct or indirect effects? Antioxidant or not? *Am. J. Clin. Nutr.* **2005**, *81*. [CrossRef] [PubMed]
59. Kroon, P.A.; Clifford, M.N.; Crozier, A.; Day, A.J.; Donovan, J.L.; Manach, C.; Williamson, G. How should we assess the effects of exposure to dietary polyphenols in vitro? *Am. J. Clin. Nutr.* **2005**, *80*, 15–21. [CrossRef] [PubMed]

14

Dietary Antioxidants, Macular Pigment, and Glaucomatous Neurodegeneration

Thomas Lawler [1], Yao Liu [2], Krista Christensen [3], Thasarat S. Vajaranant [4] and Julie Mares [3,*]

1 Department of Nutritional Sciences, University of Wisconsin, 1415 Linden Drive, Madison, WI 53706, USA; tlawler2@wisc.edu
2 Department of Ophthalmology and Visual Sciences, University of Wisconsin, 2870 University Avenue, Madison, WI 53705, USA; yao.liu2@wisc.edu
3 Department of Ophthalmology and Visual Sciences, University of Wisconsin, 610 N. Walnut Street, 1069 WARF Building, Madison, WI 53726, USA; krista.christensen@wisc.edu
4 Department of Ophthalmology and Visual Sciences, University of Illinois – Chicago, 1855 W. Taylor Street, Chicago, IL 60612, USA; thasarat@uic.edu
* Correspondence: jmarespe@wisc.edu;

Abstract: Primary open-angle glaucoma (POAG) is a leading cause of irreversible blindness worldwide, and the prevalence is projected to increase to 112 million worldwide by 2040. Intraocular pressure is currently the only proven modifiable risk factor to treat POAG, but recent evidence suggests a link between antioxidant levels and risk for prevalent glaucoma. Studies have found that antioxidant levels are lower in the serum and aqueous humor of glaucoma patients. In this review, we provide a brief overview of the evidence linking oxidative stress to glaucomatous pathology, followed by an in-depth discussion of epidemiological studies and clinical trials of antioxidant consumption and glaucomatous visual field loss. Lastly, we highlight a possible role for antioxidant carotenoids lutein and zeaxanthin, which accumulate in the retina to form macular pigment, as evidence has emerged supporting an association between macular pigment levels and age-related eye disease, including glaucoma. We conclude that the evidence base is inconsistent in showing causal links between dietary antioxidants and glaucoma risk, and that prospective studies are needed to further investigate the possible relationship between macular pigment levels and glaucoma risk specifically.

Keywords: glaucoma; antioxidants; oxidative stress; macular pigment; lutein

1. Introduction

Glaucoma is a progressive neurodegenerative disease in which the death of retinal ganglion cells (RGCs) in the inner retina results in characteristic visual field defects that can progress to blindness [1]. It is a leading cause of irreversible blindness worldwide and the incidence of glaucoma is expected to increase as the population ages, with a projected prevalence of 112 million worldwide by 2040 [2]. Healthcare spending related to glaucoma is estimated at roughly $5.8 billion per year in the U.S. alone [3]. Moreover, vision loss from glaucoma may make it difficult to perform activities of daily living, limit independence, and increase the risk of falls [4], depression [5], and cognitive decline [6]. Due to the lack of symptoms in the early stages, detection and treatment may be delayed until advanced stages of disease [7]. It is estimated that half of patients with glaucoma are unaware of their diagnosis [8].

Nonmodifiable glaucoma risk factors include older age, race/ethnicity (e.g., African, Asian, or Hispanic heritage), family history of glaucoma, and central corneal thickness [9]. Current treatments for glaucoma are limited to lowering of intraocular pressure (IOP) using medications, laser treatment, or surgery [7], but these interventions are not always sufficient. Some patients continue to experience disease progression and severe vision loss can occur despite achieving therapeutic IOP lowering. The identification of novel modifiable risk factors has significant implications for glaucoma prevention and may lead to new treatment modalities. In recent years, new evidence has emerged of an association between markers of oxidative stress and risk for primary open-angle glaucoma (POAG) [10,11], suggesting that consumption of dietary antioxidants may be a factor capable of modifying disease risk.

We review the growing body of evidence linking oxidative stress to the pathophysiology of POAG and review human studies linking dietary intake of antioxidants to risk for POAG. In later sections, we focus specifically on dietary carotenoids lutein and zeaxanthin (L/Z), given their well-established antioxidant activities in the retina and the ability to noninvasively estimate the density of these carotenoids within the macular region of the retina (termed macular pigment (MP)), where they accumulate at the highest density. More recent cross-sectional studies have linked MP to a reduced risk for prevalent POAG, suggesting that dietary modifications to increase MP may be one approach to lower glaucoma risk in individuals with elevated IOP [12,13].

2. Pathophysiology of Glaucoma

POAG is the most common form of glaucoma in the U.S. and worldwide [1]. In POAG, the iridocorneal angle where drainage of the aqueous humor occurs remains visibly open, yet IOP may be elevated due to either excess production of aqueous humor by the ciliary body or an impediment of aqueous humor outflow through the trabecular meshwork into the canal of Schlemm [1]. The optic nerve head, where RGC axons pass through the porous connective tissue plates of the lamina cribrosa and leave the eye to form the optic nerve in the brain, is likely the initial site of IOP-related RGC injury [14]. Elevated IOP may interfere with retrograde transport of neurotropic factors, such as brain derived neurotrophic factor [15,16]; alter cytoskeletal structure [16]; and/or induce mitochondrial dysfunction [17]. These consequences of elevated IOP can induce a bioenergetic crisis, disturb normal axonal transport, and activate RGC cell death pathways.

Although IOP reduction through the use of topical medications and/or surgery is effective, many individuals continue to develop glaucoma despite having normal eye pressures and incur progressive glaucomatous vision loss despite treatment, suggesting that there are other mechanisms contributing to RGC death. These other biological insults may include chronic inflammation, hypoxia, excitotoxicity, loss of neurotrophic factors, and oxidative stress [18] that may be independent of pressure related injury. Consequently, there may be opportunities to develop novel treatment approaches to use in conjunction with pharmaceutical or surgical approaches to reduce IOP. A large body of evidence implicates oxidative stress, as there is evidence for oxidative damage (and depletion of antioxidants) in the aqueous humor [19,20] and trabecular meshwork [21,22] of glaucoma cases compared with age and sex-matched controls.

3. Oxidative Stress in Primary Open-Angle Glaucoma Pathogenesis

Current evidence suggests that oxidative stress is relevant to the pathophysiology of POAG and may contribute to damage in the retina and the anterior chamber of the eye (the space between the iris and the corneal endothelium containing aqueous humor). An imbalance between reactive oxygen species (ROS) and antioxidants in these tissues can result in excessive generation of ROS, including hydrogen peroxide, superoxide, and peroxynitrate, tipping the balance in favor of oxidative stress. These insults may damage cellular macromolecules (nucleic acids, structural proteins, and lipids [23]) and organelles, including mitochondria, and may promote cell death via apoptosis [24]. Prior studies have observed diminished total antioxidant capacity in plasma or serum of glaucoma cases compared to matched controls [10,11,25,26], as well as increased levels of oxidation products in the serum (e.g., malonyldialdehyde, a lipid peroxidation product) [25–27]. The total antioxidant capacity in aqueous humor has been observed to be lower in POAG patients compared to age- and sex-matched controls [20,25,26], along with levels of some specific antioxidants including vitamins C and E [28]. There is evidence for greater activity of antioxidant enzymes (glutathione peroxidase and superoxide dismutase) in the aqueous humor of glaucoma cases compared to control individuals [19,20,28], which may signal the body's attempt to combat oxidative stress [20]. In a recent meta-analysis containing pooled data from 22 case–control studies, there was consistent evidence for a significant increase in oxidative stress markers (e.g., malonyldialdehyde) and a decrease in antioxidant level in both serum and aqueous humor in cases from several glaucoma subtypes (including but not limited to POAG) compared to age- and sex-matched controls [29].

Mechanisms by which oxidative stress may contribute to glaucomatous neurodegeneration are complex and multifactorial. One mechanism by which oxidative stress may contribute to glaucoma is by damaging cells in the trabecular meshwork [30], leading to interference with normal drainage of aqueous humor [31] and an increase in IOP [21]. Consistent with oxidative stress in the aqueous humor, there is evidence that cells within the trabecular meshwork of glaucoma cases have higher levels of 8-hydroxy-2′-deoxyguanosine (8-OHdG) [21,22], a marker of oxidative damage to the DNA. Oxidative damage to trabecular meshwork cells may cause remodeling of the cytoskeleton [30] and decrease outflow facility [31] and it has been observed that presence of 8-OHdG in trabecular meshwork cells correlates with several measures of glaucoma disease severity, including degree of visual field loss and IOP [21,22].

Oxidative stress may also contribute directly to the apoptotic death of RGCs of the inner retina [32] and activation of the immune system [33–35]. Animal models of glaucoma suggest that elevated IOP causes oxidative stress in RGCs [32,36,37]. In a rat model of elevated IOP, induced by injection of hyaluronic acid in the anterior chamber, retinal levels of antioxidant enzymes SOD and catalase were decreased over 10 weeks, as were levels of glutathione, while markers of lipid peroxidation were markedly increased [36]. Another group reported that elevated IOP (induced in rats by episcleral vein cauterization) can increase levels of malonyldialdehyde and the free radical superoxide [32], while others have reported that acute elevation of IOP or hydrostatic pressure can induce markers of oxidative stress in both mouse retina and RGC-5 cell culture in a matter of hours [38].

Unstable perfusion of the optic nerve head and retina, characterized by large fluctuations in the ocular perfusion pressure, has emerged as another source of oxidative stress that may cause glaucomatous damage, evidenced by new imaging technologies that allow measurement of retinal vessel caliper, ocular blood flow, and ocular perfusion pressure [39]. Vascular diseases, including stroke, cardiovascular disease, migraine, and hypertension, are associated with increased risk for glaucoma, strongly suggesting that vascular abnormalities and impaired blood flow to the retina play a role in development of the disease [39]. Decreased ocular blood flow is a risk factor for prevalent glaucoma in large epidemiological studies [40,41], as well as progression of glaucoma over time [42]. Similar associations are seen for vessel narrowing [43]. It has also been noted that glaucoma is associated with primary vascular dysregulation [44,45], leading to speculation that unstable perfusion of the retina may be an important mechanism in damage to the optic nerve head. Unstable retinal blood flow may lead to oxidative stress-related injury, as periods of relative ischemia may be succeeded by periods of reperfusion in which blood supply to the retina exceeds the need for oxygen, contributing to the formation of ROS [46].

Mitochondrial dysfunction in RGCs may also contribute to the generation of ROS [47], as mitochondria are abundant in RGC axons to provide ATP for sodium/potassium ATPase activity needed to maintain electrical conductivity, and to support axonal transport of organelles and other materials [48]. Mitochondria are the cell's primary consumers of oxygen, and hence contribute significantly to generation of reactive oxygen species. Glaucoma patients have significantly lower rates of complex-1 driven ATP synthesis, which is inversely associated with disease severity [49]. Further, glaucoma cases may have higher rates of mitochondrial DNA (mtDNA) mutations and lower mean mitochondrial respiratory activity than controls [50], consistent with mitochondrial dysfunction and oxidative stress.

Oxidative stress may promote RGC death directly by activating apoptotic cell signaling pathways [51], or indirectly by interacting with the retinal immune system [33–35,52]. Oxidative stress arising from glaucomatous stimuli can cause retinal glial cells (including Mueller cells and astrocytes) to adapt an 'immune-activated' phenotype, characterized by greater expression of major histocompatibility complex (MHC) II [52] and toll-like receptors [33]. In cell culture experiments, oxidative stress increases the expression of MHCII by glial cells, consequently improving their ability to stimulate T cell proliferation and secretion of cytokines (including TNF-α) that can induce ganglion cell apoptosis [52]. Activation of the innate and adaptive immune systems under conditions of cell stress may help to promote homeostasis and the removal of dead or dying cells. However, it has also been suggested that chronic immune activation under pathologic conditions may also exacerbate the disease state in glaucoma [34].

4. Dietary Antioxidants and Risk for POAG

Given the body of evidence linking oxidative stress to the etiology of POAG, several researchers have proposed the potential utility of antioxidant treatments [53,54]. However, there is limited evidence that long-term antioxidant intake lowers risk for glaucoma incidence or severity. Four large-scale epidemiological studies have examined this relationship using estimated dietary intake and a handful of intervention trials have been conducted (see Table 1).

Table 1. Summary of human studies of dietary antioxidants (and antioxidant food sources) and primary open-angle glaucoma.

Author, Year	Study Design	Participants (age)	Exposure/Treatment	Outcome	Follow-Up Period	Significant Findings ($p < 0.05$)
Kang, 2003 [55]	Cohort	116,505 health professionals free from glaucoma (≥40 years)	Dietary antioxidant vitamins and carotenoids: Vitamins A, C, E, α and β carotene, lutein/zeaxanthin, lycopene, and β-cryptoxanthin (Total and from foods only)	Incident self-reported primary open-angle glaucoma confirmed by medical record review ($n = 474$)	9.3 years (average)	Vitamin E (foods only) (p-trend = 0.02) OR: 0.67 (quintile 5 vs. 1)
Wang, 2013 [56]	Cross-sectional	2912 NHANES participants (≥40 years)	Vitamins A, C, E (from supplements) Vitamins A, C, E (in serum)	Self-reported glaucoma ($n = 203$)	N/A	Vitamin C from supplements ($p = 0.13$) OR: 0.34 (quartile 1 vs. no consumption)
Garcia-Medina, 2015 [57]	RCT	117 POAG cases	Placebo ($n = 63$) Supplement containing vitamins, A, C, E, and B-complex, lutein and zeaxanthin, zinc, copper, selenium, and omega 3 fatty acids ($n = 54$)	-Visual fields: Mean deviation, pattern standard deviation -Retinal nerve fiber layer thickness -Ganglion cell complex thickness	2 years	No effect of treatment was observed for any of the three outcomes.
Kang, 2016 [58]	Cohort	104,987 health professionals (≥40 years)	Total green leafy vegetables	Incident self-reported open-angle glaucoma confirmed by medical record review ($n = 1483$)	16.0 years (average)	Green leafy vegetables inversely associated with glaucoma risk (p-trend = 0.02) OR 0.82, (quintile 5 vs. 1)
Ramdas, 2012 [59]	Cohort	3502 adults without POAG (≥55 years)	Dietary antioxidant vitamins and carotenoids: α and β carotene, lutein/zeaxanthin, β-cryptoxanthin, retinol, vitamins B1, B6, B12, C, and E.	Incident POAG, detected by visual field testing ($n = 91$)	9.7 years (average)	Vitamin B1 ($p = 0.03$) HR: 0.31 (tertile 3 vs. 1) Retinol equivalents ($p = 0.01$) HR: 0.33 (tertile 3 vs. 1)

Table 1. *Cont.*

Author, Year	Study Design	Participants (age)	Exposure/Treatment	Outcome	Follow-Up Period	Significant Findings ($p < 0.05$)
Coleman, 2008 [60]	Cross-sectional	1155 women (67–97 years)	Dietary fruits and vegetables Dietary vitamins and carotenoids (vitamins A, C, E, B-complex, α and β carotene, lutein/zeaxanthin, cryptoxanthin, and lycopene	Prevalent POAG, detected by visual field testing and optic disc examination ($n = 95$)	N/A	Canned/dried peaches ($p = 0.04$) OR: 0.53 (≥1 serving/week, vs. <1/month) Fresh carrots ($p = 0.009$) OR: 0.36, (>2 servings/week vs. <1/month) -Collard greens/kale ($p = 0.34$) OR: 0.31 (≥1 serving/month vs. <1/month) -Vitamin B2 ($p = 0.02$) OR: 0.19 (≥2 mg/day vs. <1 mg/day)
Giaconi, 2012 [61]	Cross-sectional	584 African American women	Dietary fruits and vegetables Dietary vitamins and carotenoids (vitamins A, C, E, B-complex, α and β carotene, lutein/zeaxanthin, cryptoxanthin, and lycopene	Prevalent POAG, detected by visual field testing and optic disc examination ($n = 77$)	N/A	Retinol (p-trend 0.11) Vitamin C (p-trend = 0.018) α-carotene (p-trend = 0.21) All fruits and fruit juices (p-trend = 0.023) Oranges (p-trend = 0.002) Peaches (p-trend = 0.002) Collard greens/kale (p-trend = 0.014)

4.1. Epidemiological Studies

A cross-sectional analysis of data from the National Health and Nutrition Examination Survey showed a statistically significant decrease in the odds of self-reported glaucoma among those currently using vitamin C supplements, with no association seen for use of vitamin A or E supplements, and no association for levels of vitamins A, C, or E in serum; carotenoid use in supplements or serum levels of carotenoids were not assessed in this study [56]. These analyses were limited by reliance on self-reported glaucoma as the main outcome measure, which is known to be of limited accuracy and many individuals with glaucoma are unaware of the disease, limiting the ability to detect an association if it exists [8]. Also, given that glaucoma may take decades to develop, it is unlikely that the use of antioxidant containing supplements at any single point in time would be an etiologically relevant exposure.

In the Nurses' Health Study (NHS) and Health Professionals Follow-up Study (HPFS), which included 116,484 participants ≥40 years of age, there was no strong evidence that dietary intake of carotenoids (α-carotene, β-carotene, β-cryptoxanthin, lycopene, and L/Z) or antioxidant vitamins (A, C, and E) was associated with risk for incident glaucoma over an average follow-up period of 9.1 years, except for vitamin E from foods (odds ratio (OR) of 0.67 comparing highest to lowest quintile of intake) [55]. The study authors made a considerable effort to prevent misclassification, by excluding individuals who did not attend regular eye checkups, and by confirming cases of self-reported glaucoma by reviewing medical records (including visual fields). Although this should be considered a strength of this study, it is still possible that misclassification of participants (especially those unaware that they had glaucoma) may have biased the results towards the null. It is also not clear that results from a cohort of healthcare professionals generalize to other populations due to differences in diet and other health-related behaviors; perhaps most importantly, dietary intake of antioxidants may not reflect the quantity available to the eye due to differences in absorption and transport of antioxidants related to genetic heterogeneity [62,63], bioavailability [64,65], and reliance on circulating lipoproteins for transport of lipid soluble molecules (e.g., carotenoids) [66–68]. In this study, it was not determined whether serum antioxidant levels were predictive of incident glaucoma.

In the Rotterdam Study, glaucoma was assessed by visual field testing and 91 of 3502 eligible participants, age 55 years and older, developed glaucoma over an average of 9.7 years of follow-up [59]. There was no association between the intake of the majority of antioxidant carotenoids and vitamins evaluated (including carotenoids α-carotene, β-carotene, lutein, zeaxanthin, and β cryptoxanthin, and vitamins C and E) and risk for glaucoma, although protective associations were observed for thiamine and retinol equivalents. This study is limited by lack of serum antioxidant measures, and may have been underpowered given the relatively small number of glaucoma cases.

A cross-sectional analysis of African American women greater than 65 years old participating in the Study of Osteoporotic Fractures found that specific antioxidant-rich fruits and vegetables (including oranges, peaches, and collard greens/kale) were associated with reduced risk for prevalent glaucoma ($p < 0.05$), ascertained via visual field testing and the appearance of the optic nerve head [61]. Specific dietary antioxidant vitamins and carotenoids (vitamins A and C and α-carotene) were also associated with significantly reduced risk after adjustment for potential confounders. Trends were also observed for β-carotene and L/Z, although the trends did not reach significance ($p = 0.05$–0.08). In an earlier report from the Study of Osteoporotic Fractures, including 1155 participants of Caucasian or African American background, there was a significant protective association for collard greens/kale (OR: 0.31 for ≥1 serving per month) [60]. α-carotene and β-carotene were also inversely associated with glaucoma risk in this sample, although the association between L/Z consumption and risk for glaucoma did not approach significance in this sample.

In summary, there is limited evidence from epidemiological studies that consumption of dietary antioxidants is associated with reduced risk for incident or prevalent glaucoma. Inconsistencies may arise from differences in diagnostic criteria to ascertain glaucoma cases (i.e., visual field testing vs. self-report) and heterogeneity in the racial/genetic background of participants, which may influence genetic disease risks and dietary habits. Measuring diet during the lengthy, etiologically relevant time frame for glaucoma remains a persistent challenge in nutritional epidemiology, and this may be considered a limitation in cross-sectional studies of glaucoma prevalence [56,60,61].

4.2. Clinical Trials

There have been few randomized controlled trials (RCTs) to determine whether the administration of high dose antioxidant supplements can prevent new cases of glaucoma or slow the progression of visual field loss in glaucoma patients. In one trial, a supplement containing B-vitamins; vitamins A, C, and E; carotenoids; and antioxidant minerals with or without omega 3 fatty acids consumed over 2 years, did not prevent visual field loss or thinning of the retinal nerve fiber layer or ganglion cell complex (GCC) in a study of older adults with glaucoma [57]. There is more evidence from trials of Ginkgo Biloba extract (GBE) indicating that this substance may be a useful therapeutic tool for those with glaucoma, possibly slowing the rate of visual field loss and thinning of the neuronal retina [69–74]. Results from animal studies are also supportive, as the administration of GBE can prevent RGC death related to chronic elevation of IOP and destruction of the optic nerve [70,72]. GBE has approximately 60 bioactive substances, including antioxidants, and may possibly influence glaucoma progression through several unique mechanisms, including effects on ocular blood flow [73].

5. Antioxidant Effects of Lutein and Zeaxanthin in the Retina

Although research consistently demonstrates increased oxidative stress and depletion of antioxidants in the serum and aqueous humor of adults with glaucoma [29], there is not consistent evidence from epidemiological or clinical studies to implicate specific antioxidants. However, a growing body of evidence from animal models and cell culture indicates that antioxidant carotenoids L/Z, which uniquely accumulate in the retina in humans, may prevent RGC death related to glaucomatous stimuli [75–79].

L/Z are polar dietary carotenoids and potent antioxidants that may hold special relevance for retinal health, integrity, and long-term risk for age-related eye disease [80]. L/Z are unique among other major carotenoids found in serum in that they cross the blood–retinal barrier and bind to specific binding proteins in the retina [81,82]. Their highest concentration in human body is located in the macular region located centrally in the retina where they contribute to the pigmentation level (hence the term macular pigment), but macular concentrations of these carotenoids are also correlated with levels in peripheral retinal areas [83]. MP peaks in the center fovea and rapidly declines toward the periphery, and is generally undetectable at 7 degrees from the foveal center [84]. Although the majority of MP is concentrated in the outer retina, in the photoreceptor outer segments and outer plexiform layer, considerable amounts of MP are detectable in the inner plexiform layer [85], adjacent to the ganglion cell layer that is damaged in glaucoma. Due to a backbone of conjugated carbon–carbon double bonds, L/Z act as potent retinal antioxidants [86], able to scavenge ROS including superoxide, hydroxyl radical, and hydrogen peroxide without being 'used up' in the process [80]. L/Z also have the unique capacity to filter short-wavelength blue light before it reaches the outer retina [87], thought to protect the retinal pigment epithelium and photoreceptors from the effects of photooxidative stress [88,89]. MP is modifiable with diet and supplement interventions [90,91], and has become an attractive target to treat or prevent age-related eye diseases that have high levels of oxidative stress.

6. Lutein and Zeaxanthin and POAG

6.1. Protective Mechanisms of L/Z in the Retina

Evidence, which links these carotenoids to diseases of the inner retina, like glaucoma, is now emerging. A recent study of Chinese adults demonstrated that serum concentrations of L/Z, but not other carotenoids, were positively associated with measures of retinal blood flow [92]. This provides preliminary evidence that L/Z may help to stabilize retinal perfusion, which has been linked to glaucoma risk [45]. Additional evidence has emerged that L/Z may also have protective effects on the inner retina in response to glaucomatous stimuli in animal models [75,76,79], with additional evidence that the mechanism of protection involves suppression of apoptotic signaling pathways. Lutein reduced the number of TUNEL-positive RGCs (a marker of apoptotic cell death) in mouse retina after ischemia/reperfusion injury (2 h of retinal ischemia followed by 22 h of reperfusion) and increased the number of viable cells to approximately control levels [75]. These results corroborate those of an earlier study in rats, in which intravitreous or intraperitoneal lutein almost completely prevented RGC loss after 1 h of ischemia and 24 h of reperfusion [93]. Likewise, lutein significantly increased the number of viable RGCs after intravitreal injection of an NMDA receptor agonist, meant to stimulate excitotoxic cell death in the inner retina, although cell viability did not approach control levels [79]. Reduced expression of the proapoptotic Bax protein and increased expression of antiapoptotic Bcl2 in the inner retina mirrored this finding, as well as reduced release of proapoptotic cytochrome C from the mitochondria, a key player in the activation of caspases, the primary effectors of apoptotic cell death. Similar effects on Bax and Bcl2 expression were seen in a cell culture model of rat Mueller cells (a prominent glial cell type in the retina whose activity is linked to onset of glaucomatous pathology), where it was also observed that lutein could reduce levels of cleaved caspase 3 after simulated hypoxia [94]. Antiapoptotic effects of lutein were also apparent in a model of retinal detachment, as lutein treatment reduced levels of cleaved caspase 3 and 8 [95].

While the results from animal models indicate that administration of L/Z may protect the inner retina from glaucomatous insults, the relevance for humans is unclear. Unlike humans, rodents do not accumulate MP in appreciable quantities (although mouse models of MP have recently been developed) [96], and animal models of RGC death based on short-term elevations in IOP or ischemia do not perfectly mimic the complex mechanisms that underlie human glaucoma. Cell culture models of physiologically relevant L/Z concentrations show that L/Z can maintain murine RGC-5 cell viability after cell stress, including simulated hypoxia and serum deprivation [77,97], helping to corroborate results from animal studies. However, cell culture does not perfectly mimic disease pathophysiology, and RGC-5 cells lack several key characteristics of human RGCs, including excitability [98].

6.2. L/Z and POAG—Epidemiological Studies

Several groups have evaluated the association between L/Z consumption and risk for POAG in epidemiological studies, with mixed results. In data pooled from the NHS and HPFS, individuals in the highest quintile of dietary L/Z had lower risk than individuals in the lowest quintile OR = 0.68. CI: 0.49–0.93), after excluding the four most recent years of dietary data (to account for a lag in disease diagnosis) [55]. Although there was no significant linear trend, these results are consistent with a possible threshold effect. In contrast, there was no association between for L/Z and glaucoma in the Rotterdam Study [59]. More recently, greater consumption of green leafy vegetables, the predominant source of L/Z in the diet, was linearly associated with reduced risk for incident POAG (p-trend = 0.01) in the NHS and HPFS [58]. However, the authors attribute this beneficial association to the presence of nitrates in leafy green vegetables, hypothesized to influence ocular blood flow and regulation of IOP, rather than L/Z content. There was a significant negative association between dietary nitrate consumption (OR: 0.67 for Q5 vs. Q1) and risk of POAG that maintained statistical significance after adjustment for dietary L/Z and other antioxidants. However, it may be difficult to identify independent effects among highly correlated nutrient intakes, and differences in the degree of measurement error between nutrients exacerbate this difficulty. Other groups have also observed a negative association for leafy green vegetables, and it is not clear whether this is attributable to the L/Z content, nitrates, and/or another bioactive component [60,61].

Accumulation of L/Z in the retina as MP may be a more relevant exposure metric than L/Z in the diet, as the quantity of L/Z that reaches the retina is highly dependent on genetic heterogeneity [99,100] and other factors, including body composition and metabolic health [101,102]. Several low-cost, noninvasive approaches to reliably measure MP have been developed in recent years [103], making it feasible to investigate MP level as a potential modifiable risk factor for POAG. Currently, the literature contains only four studies directly addressing the association between MP and the presence of POAG and glaucomatous optic neuropathy (see Table 2). In the first, a study of 40 glaucoma cases and 54 normal controls, it was determined that MP optical density (MPOD), assessed using customized heterochromatic flicker photometry (cHFP), was approximately 36% lower in cases, although there was no association with disease severity [12]. However, in a follow-up study of 88 glaucoma cases, they discovered that MPOD at multiple eccentricities was significantly lower ($p < 0.0001$) in cases with foveal GCC loss (an indicator of greater disease severity) compared to cases without foveal involvement [13]. Although the associations with disease severity differ in these studies, the authors suggest that the differences in sample size and methodology may explain the different results, as the first study did not include optical coherence tomography scans to assess foveal GCC loss. In the second study, MPOD was also significantly and positively associated with glaucoma-related structural parameters including optic disc rim area, GCC thickness, and thickness of the inner retina, although the results were only marginally significant (p = 0.02–0.05). MPOD was negatively associated with cup to disc ratio, suggesting maintenance of RGC number. The results obtained by this group were later corroborated by another group utilizing the one-wavelength reflectometry approach for measuring MP, as both maximum and mean MPOD were reduced in 30 POAG patients relative to 52 controls, by 19% and 14%, respectively [104]. However, in the recent San Diego Macular Pigment Study, MP volume did not differ between 85 glaucoma patients and 22 controls when measured utilizing the two-wavelength autofluorescence technique [105]. There was also no association between MP volume and retinal nerve fiber layer thickness, as assessed by optical coherence tomography imaging of the retina.

Table 2. Summary of cross-sectional studies of macular pigment optical density (MPOD) and primary open-angle glaucoma.

Author, Year	Participants	MPOD Measurement Technique	Exposure Variable	Mean ± SD (Controls)	Mean ± SD (Cases)	p-Value
Igras, 2013 [12]	40 POAG cases 54 healthy controls	HFP	MPOD at 0.5°	0.36 (median)	0.23 (median)	0.03
Siah, 2015 [13]	52 foveal-involved POAG cases 33 controls without foveal involvement	HFP	MPOD at 0.5° [1]	0.24 ± 0.12	0.15 ± 0.10	<0.001
Ji, 2016 [104]	30 POAG cases 52 healthy controls	Reflectometry	MPOD mean over 7° [2]	0.14 ± 0.03	0.12 ± 0.03	<0.001
Daga, 2018 [105]	85 POAG cases 22 healthy controls	2-wavelength autofluorescence	MP volume over 7°	7661 ± 3750	8717 ± 3903	0.44

[1] Significant results also observed for MPOD at 0.25° and 1° targets ($p < 0.001$); [2] Significant results also obtained for maximum MPOD ($p < 0.001$).

It is not clear why there have been inconsistent results, but it is possible that reliance on different testing approaches for MPOD may have led to different conclusions [103]. Some approaches are biased by the health of the lens and retina [103]. While cHFP is reliable in older adults [106] and controls for differences in lens density and retinal health [103], it is time-consuming, possibly leading to participant fatigue, and otherwise relies on the skill of the examiner and patient to produce valid measurements. It is not known whether the peculiar changes to retinal health and vision function that occur in glaucoma could also bias results of MPOD testing, or whether bias would be limited to cases of late-stage, foveal-involved glaucoma, as MP accumulates almost exclusively in the fovea [107]. Given the inconsistent results of MP levels in relation to glaucoma and the small samples used to evaluate this association, this is an interesting area for further investigation.

As all of these are studies cross-sectional, it is not possible to determine whether high MPOD is associated with risk for incident glaucoma over time. To help clarify this issue, long-term prospective studies of MP and glaucomatous visual field loss and changes to the retina are required. In addition, reverse causality cannot be ruled out, as glaucomatous changes to the retina, including thinning of the GCC and impaired blood flow to the retina, may make it difficult to accrue MP. Although MP attenuates oxidative stress by filtering short wavelength light and by directly neutralizing ROS [80], the biological rationale for a protective effect is not entirely clear, as the primary site of RGC injury is believed to be located at the optic nerve head [14], rather, not within the retina. Further, although L/Z accumulate throughout the macula, concentrations are highest in the photoreceptors of the outer retina and in the fovea [107], which usually remains unaffected until later stages of glaucoma [108]. Despite this, multiple studies showing an inverse association between MPOD and risk for glaucoma provide a strong rationale for prospective studies, as interventions to increase MPOD would be a low cost and low risk approach to prevent disease.

7. Conclusions and Future Directions

Given the increasing prevalence of glaucoma among older adults and lack of known modifiable risk factors other than lowering of IOP, interventions, such as increasing consumption of antioxidants targeted to those who are at high risk for disease development or progression, may have a considerable population health impact. Despite the evidence supporting oxidative stress in glaucoma, there is still inconsistent evidence as to whether dietary antioxidant intake predicts the incidence or prevalence of POAG, and no prospective evidence that interventions to increase antioxidant consumption can prevent or slow glaucomatous visual field loss or thinning of the neural retina. This may reflect persistent challenges in accurately measuring dietary intake, as well as high levels of interindividual variability in the absorption of antioxidants. Future prospective studies of serum antioxidants and incident visual field loss, or thinning of the inner retina, may help to clarify the effect of antioxidants on the health of the neural retina. Older adults at increased risk for glaucoma are currently advised to consume an overall healthy diet rich in fruits and vegetables, as this diet pattern is linked to reduced risk [61,109], and because maintaining a healthy body weight and good metabolic health through diet and exercise may help to prevent disease.

Despite the limitations of the current evidence, there is a strong rationale for continuing to investigate MP as risk factor for POAG, given its unique antioxidant/protective activities in the retina [80], and ease of modification with diet [91,110] and supplements [90]. The majority of recent cross-sectional research, made possible by low-cost, noninvasive approaches to MPOD testing, suggests an association between higher MPOD and reduced risk for POAG [12,13,104,105]. A protective association is also supported by observations that L/Z may protect the neural retina from glaucomatous stressors, at least in animal models [75,79]. There is currently a need for prospective studies of MPOD and glaucomatous visual field loss to further elucidate whether the relationship is likely to be causal in humans. There is a strong precedent for this type of research, given longstanding interest in MPOD as a modifiable risk factor for AMD (a disease characterized by oxidative stress), and evidence from large-scale clinical trials that high doses of L/Z (12 mg/day) may reduce risk for progression of AMD in some individuals [111] without increased risk for side effects [112]. Prospective studies showing reduced risk for visual field loss with higher MPOD may support the development of low-cost interventions to increase MPOD in individuals at high risk for POAG, administered alongside treatment to lower IOP, and monitoring of MPOD in a clinical setting.

Author Contributions: T.L.; Writing—Original Draft Preparation, K.C., J.M., Y.L., and T.S.V.; Writing—Review & Editing, J.M. and Y.L.; Supervision and funding acquisition.

References

1. Quigley, H.A. Glaucoma. *Lancet* **2011**, *377*, 1367–1377. [CrossRef]
2. Tham, Y.C.; Li, X.; Wong, T.Y.; Quigley, H.A.; Aung, T.; Cheng, C.Y. Global prevalence of glaucoma and projections of glaucoma burden through 2040: A systematic review and meta-analysis. *Ophthalmology* **2014**, *121*, 2081–2090. [CrossRef] [PubMed]
3. John Wittenborn, D.R. *Cost of Vision Problems: The Economic Burden of Vision Loss and Eye Disorders in the United States*; University of Chicago: Chicago, IL, USA, 2013; p. 8.
4. Kannus, P.; Sievanen, H.; Palvanen, M.; Jarvinen, T.; Parkkari, J. Prevention of falls and consequent injuries in elderly people. *Lancet* **2005**, *366*, 1885–1893. [CrossRef]
5. Zhang, X.; Bullard, K.M.; Cotch, M.F.; Wilson, M.R.; Rovner, B.W.; McGwin, G., Jr.; Owsley, C.; Barker, L.; Crews, J.E.; Saaddine, J.B. Association between depression and functional vision loss in persons 20 years of age or older in the United States, NHANES 2005–2008. *JAMA Ophthalmol.* **2013**, *131*, 573–581. [CrossRef] [PubMed]
6. Rogers, M.A.; Langa, K.M. Untreated poor vision: A contributing factor to late-life dementia. *Am. J. Epidemiol.* **2010**, *171*, 728–735. [CrossRef]
7. Cohen, L.P.; Pasquale, L.R. Clinical characteristics and current treatment of glaucoma. *Cold Spring Harb. Perspect. Med.* **2014**, *4*. [CrossRef]
8. Vajaranant, T.; Maki, P.; Pasquale, L.; Khan, F.; Mares, J.; Meyer, K.; Haan, M. The accuracy of self-reported glaucoma in the Women's Health Initiative. In Proceedings of the American Glaucoma Society Annual Meeting, Fort Lauderdale, FL, USA, 3–6 March 2016.
9. Cook, C.; Foster, P. Epidemiology of glaucoma: What's new? *Can. J. Ophthalmol. J. Can. Ophtalmol.* **2012**, *47*, 223–226. [CrossRef]
10. Abu-Amero, K.K.; Kondkar, A.A.; Mousa, A.; Osman, E.A.; Al-Obeidan, S.A. Decreased total antioxidants in patients with primary open angle glaucoma. *Curr. Eye Res.* **2013**, *38*, 959–964. [CrossRef] [PubMed]

11. Mousa, A.; Kondkar, A.A.; Al-Obeidan, S.A.; Azad, T.A.; Sultan, T.; Osman, E.; Abu-Amero, K.K. Association of total antioxidants level with glaucoma type and severity. *Saudi Med. J.* **2015**, *36*, 671–677. [CrossRef] [PubMed]
12. Igras, E.; Loughman, J.; Ratzlaff, M.; O'Caoimh, R.; O'Brien, C. Evidence of lower macular pigment optical density in chronic open angle glaucoma. *Br. J. Ophthalmol.* **2013**, *97*, 994–998. [CrossRef] [PubMed]
13. Siah, W.F.; Loughman, J.; O'Brien, C. Lower Macular Pigment Optical Density in Foveal-Involved Glaucoma. *Ophthalmology* **2015**, *122*, 2029–2037. [CrossRef]
14. Nickells, R.W.; Howell, G.R.; Soto, I.; John, S.W. Under pressure: Cellular and molecular responses during glaucoma, a common neurodegeneration with axonopathy. *Annu. Rev. Neurosci.* **2012**, *35*, 153–179. [CrossRef]
15. Morrison, J.C.; Johnson, E.C.; Cepurna, W.; Jia, L. Understanding mechanisms of pressure-induced optic nerve damage. *Prog. Retin. Eye Res.* **2005**, *24*, 217–240. [CrossRef]
16. Chidlow, G.; Ebneter, A.; Wood, J.P.; Casson, R.J. The optic nerve head is the site of axonal transport disruption, axonal cytoskeleton damage and putative axonal regeneration failure in a rat model of glaucoma. *Acta Neuropathol.* **2011**, *121*, 737–751. [CrossRef]
17. Wu, J.H.; Zhang, S.H.; Nickerson, J.M.; Gao, F.J.; Sun, Z.; Chen, X.Y.; Zhang, S.J.; Gao, F.; Chen, J.Y.; Luo, Y.; et al. Cumulative mtDNA damage and mutations contribute to the progressive loss of RGCs in a rat model of glaucoma. *Neurobiol. Dis.* **2015**, *74*, 167–179. [CrossRef]
18. Almasieh, M.; Wilson, A.M.; Morquette, B.; Cueva Vargas, J.L.; Di Polo, A. The molecular basis of retinal ganglion cell death in glaucoma. *Prog. Retin. Eye Res.* **2012**, *31*, 152–181. [CrossRef]
19. Ghanem, A.A.; Arafa, L.F.; El-Baz, A. Oxidative stress markers in patients with primary open-angle glaucoma. *Curr. Eye Res.* **2010**, *35*, 295–301. [CrossRef]
20. Ferreira, S.M.; Lerner, S.F.; Brunzini, R.; Evelson, P.A.; Llesuy, S.F. Oxidative stress markers in aqueous humor of glaucoma patients. *Am. J. Ophthalmol.* **2004**, *137*, 62–69. [CrossRef]
21. Sacca, S.C.; Pascotto, A.; Camicione, P.; Capris, P.; Izzotti, A. Oxidative DNA damage in the human trabecular meshwork: Clinical correlation in patients with primary open-angle glaucoma. *Arch. Ophthalmol.* **2005**, *123*, 458–463. [CrossRef]
22. Izzotti, A.; Sacca, S.C.; Cartiglia, C.; De Flora, S. Oxidative deoxyribonucleic acid damage in the eyes of glaucoma patients. *Am. J. Med.* **2003**, *114*, 638–646. [CrossRef]
23. Aslan, M.; Cort, A.; Yucel, I. Oxidative and nitrative stress markers in glaucoma. *Free Radic. Biol. Med.* **2008**, *45*, 367–376. [CrossRef]
24. Pinazo-Duran, M.D.; Zanon-Moreno, V.; Gallego-Pinazo, R.; Garcia-Medina, J.J. Oxidative stress and mitochondrial failure in the pathogenesis of glaucoma neurodegeneration. *Prog. Brain Res.* **2015**, *220*, 127–153. [CrossRef] [PubMed]
25. Nucci, C.; Di Pierro, D.; Varesi, C.; Ciuffoletti, E.; Russo, R.; Gentile, R.; Cedrone, C.; Pinazo Duran, M.D.; Coletta, M.; Mancino, R. Increased malondialdehyde concentration and reduced total antioxidant capacity in aqueous humor and blood samples from patients with glaucoma. *Mol. Vis.* **2013**, *19*, 1841–1846.
26. Sorkhabi, R.; Ghorbanihaghjo, A.; Javadzadeh, A.; Rashtchizadeh, N.; Moharrery, M. Oxidative DNA damage and total antioxidant status in glaucoma patients. *Mol. Vis.* **2011**, *17*, 41–46.
27. Yildirim, O.; Ates, N.A.; Ercan, B.; Muslu, N.; Unlu, A.; Tamer, L.; Atik, U.; Kanik, A. Role of oxidative stress enzymes in open-angle glaucoma. *Eye* **2005**, *19*, 580–583. [CrossRef]
28. Goyal, A.; Srivastava, A.; Sihota, R.; Kaur, J. Evaluation of oxidative stress markers in aqueous humor of primary open angle glaucoma and primary angle closure glaucoma patients. *Curr. Eye Res.* **2014**, *39*, 823–829. [CrossRef]
29. Benoist d'Azy, C.; Pereira, B.; Chiambaretta, F.; Dutheil, F. Oxidative and Anti-Oxidative Stress Markers in Chronic Glaucoma: A Systematic Review and Meta-Analysis. *PLoS ONE* **2016**, *11*, e0166915. [CrossRef]
30. Zhou, L.; Li, Y.; Yue, B.Y. Oxidative stress affects cytoskeletal structure and cell-matrix interactions in cells from an ocular tissue: The trabecular meshwork. *J. Cell. Physiol.* **1999**, *180*, 182–189. [CrossRef]
31. Kahn, M.G.; Giblin, F.J.; Epstein, D.L. Glutathione in calf trabecular meshwork and its relation to aqueous humor outflow facility. *Investig. Ophthalmol. Vis. Sci.* **1983**, *24*, 1283–1287.
32. Ko, M.L.; Peng, P.H.; Ma, M.C.; Ritch, R.; Chen, C.F. Dynamic changes in reactive oxygen species and antioxidant levels in retinas in experimental glaucoma. *Free Radic. Biol. Med.* **2005**, *39*, 365–373. [CrossRef]

33. Luo, C.; Yang, X.; Kain, A.D.; Powell, D.W.; Kuehn, M.H.; Tezel, G. Glaucomatous tissue stress and the regulation of immune response through glial Toll-like receptor signaling. *Investig. Ophthalmol. Vis. Sci.* **2010**, *51*, 5697–5707. [CrossRef]
34. Tezel, G. The immune response in glaucoma: A perspective on the roles of oxidative stress. *Exp. Eye Res.* **2011**, *93*, 178–186. [CrossRef]
35. Tezel, G.; Yang, X.; Luo, C.; Kain, A.D.; Powell, D.W.; Kuehn, M.H.; Kaplan, H.J. Oxidative stress and the regulation of complement activation in human glaucoma. *Investig. Ophthalmol. Vis. Sci.* **2010**, *51*, 5071–5082. [CrossRef]
36. Moreno, M.C.; Campanelli, J.; Sande, P.; Sanez, D.A.; Keller Sarmiento, M.I.; Rosenstein, R.E. Retinal oxidative stress induced by high intraocular pressure. *Free Radic. Biol. Med.* **2004**, *37*, 803–812. [CrossRef]
37. Muller, A.; Pietri, S.; Villain, M.; Frejaville, C.; Bonne, C.; Culcas, M. Free radicals in rabbit retina under ocular hyperpressure and functional consequences. *Exp. Eye Res.* **1997**, *64*, 637–643. [CrossRef]
38. Liu, Q.; Ju, W.K.; Crowston, J.G.; Xie, F.; Perry, G.; Smith, M.A.; Lindsey, J.D.; Weinreb, R.N. Oxidative stress is an early event in hydrostatic pressure induced retinal ganglion cell damage. *Investig. Ophthalmol. Vis. Sci.* **2007**, *48*, 4580–4589. [CrossRef]
39. Nakazawa, T. Ocular Blood Flow and Influencing Factors for Glaucoma. *Asia-Pac. J. Ophthalmol.* **2016**, *5*, 38–44. [CrossRef]
40. Tielsch, J.M.; Katz, J.; Sommer, A.; Quigley, H.A.; Javitt, J.C. Hypertension, perfusion pressure, and primary open-angle glaucoma. A population-based assessment. *Arch. Ophthalmol.* **1995**, *113*, 216–221. [CrossRef]
41. Leske, M.C.; Connell, A.M.; Wu, S.Y.; Hyman, L.G.; Schachat, A.P. Risk factors for open-angle glaucoma. The Barbados Eye Study. *Arch. Ophthalmol.* **1995**, *113*, 918–924. [CrossRef]
42. Zeitz, O.; Galambos, P.; Wagenfeld, L.; Wiermann, A.; Wlodarsch, P.; Praga, R.; Matthiessen, E.T.; Richard, G.; Klemm, M. Glaucoma progression is associated with decreased blood flow velocities in the short posterior ciliary artery. *Br. J. Ophthalmol.* **2006**, *90*, 1245–1248. [CrossRef]
43. Wang, S.; Xu, L.; Wang, Y.; Wang, Y.; Jonas, J.B. Retinal vessel diameter in normal and glaucomatous eyes: The Beijing eye study. *Clin. Exp. Ophthalmol.* **2007**, *35*, 800–807. [CrossRef]
44. Grieshaber, M.C.; Mozaffarieh, M.; Flammer, J. What is the link between vascular dysregulation and glaucoma? *Surv. Ophthalmol.* **2007**, *52* (Suppl. 2), S144–S154. [CrossRef]
45. Leske, M.C. Ocular perfusion pressure and glaucoma: Clinical trial and epidemiologic findings. *Curr. Opin. Ophthalmol.* **2009**, *20*, 73–78. [CrossRef]
46. Mozaffarieh, M.; Grieshaber, M.C.; Flammer, J. Oxygen and blood flow: Players in the pathogenesis of glaucoma. *Mol. Vis.* **2008**, *14*, 224–233.
47. Osborne, N.N.; Nunez-Alvarez, C.; Joglar, B.; Del Olmo-Aguado, S. Glaucoma: Focus on mitochondria in relation to pathogenesis and neuroprotection. *Eur. J. Pharmacol.* **2016**, *787*, 127–133. [CrossRef]
48. Osborne, N.N. Mitochondria: Their role in ganglion cell death and survival in primary open angle glaucoma. *Exp. Eye Res.* **2010**, *90*, 750–757. [CrossRef]
49. Lee, S.; Sheck, L.; Crowston, J.G.; Van Bergen, N.J.; O'Neill, E.C.; O'Hare, F.; Kong, Y.X.; Chrysostomou, V.; Vincent, A.L.; Trounce, I.A. Impaired complex-I-linked respiration and ATP synthesis in primary open-angle glaucoma patient lymphoblasts. *Investig. Ophthalmol. Vis. Sci.* **2012**, *53*, 2431–2437. [CrossRef]
50. Abu-Amero, K.K.; Morales, J.; Bosley, T.M. Mitochondrial abnormalities in patients with primary open-angle glaucoma. *Investig. Ophthalmol. Vis. Sci.* **2006**, *47*, 2533–2541. [CrossRef]
51. Martindale, J.L.; Holbrook, N.J. Cellular response to oxidative stress: Signaling for suicide and survival. *J. Cell. Physiol.* **2002**, *192*, 1–15. [CrossRef]
52. Tezel, G.; Yang, X.; Luo, C.; Peng, Y.; Sun, S.L.; Sun, D. Mechanisms of immune system activation in glaucoma: Oxidative stress-stimulated antigen presentation by the retina and optic nerve head glia. *Investig. Ophthalmol. Vis. Sci.* **2007**, *48*, 705–714. [CrossRef]
53. Grover, A.K.; Samson, S.E. Antioxidants and vision health: Facts and fiction. *Mol. Cell. Biochem.* **2014**, *388*, 173–183. [CrossRef]
54. Mozaffarieh, M.; Grieshaber, M.C.; Orgul, S.; Flammer, J. The potential value of natural antioxidative treatment in glaucoma. *Surv. Ophthalmol.* **2008**, *53*, 479–505. [CrossRef]
55. Kang, J.H.; Pasquale, L.R.; Willett, W.; Rosner, B.; Egan, K.M.; Faberowski, N.; Hankinson, S.E. Antioxidant intake and primary open-angle glaucoma: A prospective study. *Am. J. Epidemiol.* **2003**, *158*, 337–346. [CrossRef]

56. Wang, S.Y.; Singh, K.; Lin, S.C. Glaucoma and vitamins A, C, and E supplement intake and serum levels in a population-based sample of the United States. *Eye* **2013**, *27*, 487–494. [CrossRef]
57. Garcia-Medina, J.J.; Garcia-Medina, M.; Garrido-Fernandez, P.; Galvan-Espinosa, J.; Garcia-Maturana, C.; Zanon-Moreno, V.; Pinazo-Duran, M.D. A two-year follow-up of oral antioxidant supplementation in primary open-angle glaucoma: An open-label, randomized, controlled trial. *Acta Ophthalmol.* **2015**, *93*, 546–554. [CrossRef]
58. Kang, J.H.; Willett, W.C.; Rosner, B.A.; Buys, E.; Wiggs, J.L.; Pasquale, L.R. Association of Dietary Nitrate Intake with Primary Open-Angle Glaucoma: A Prospective Analysis from the Nurses' Health Study and Health Professionals Follow-up Study. *JAMA Ophthalmol.* **2016**, *134*, 294–303. [CrossRef]
59. Ramdas, W.D.; Wolfs, R.C.; Kiefte-de Jong, J.C.; Hofman, A.; de Jong, P.T.; Vingerling, J.R.; Jansonius, N.M. Nutrient intake and risk of open-angle glaucoma: The Rotterdam Study. *Eur. J. Epidemiol.* **2012**, *27*, 385–393. [CrossRef]
60. Coleman, A.L.; Stone, K.L.; Kodjebacheva, G.; Yu, F.; Pedula, K.L.; Ensrud, K.E.; Cauley, J.A.; Hochberg, M.C.; Topouzis, F.; Badala, F.; et al. Glaucoma risk and the consumption of fruits and vegetables among older women in the study of osteoporotic fractures. *Am. J. Ophthalmol.* **2008**, *145*, 1081–1089. [CrossRef]
61. Giaconi, J.A.; Yu, F.; Stone, K.L.; Pedula, K.L.; Ensrud, K.E.; Cauley, J.A.; Hochberg, M.C.; Coleman, A.L. The association of consumption of fruits/vegetables with decreased risk of glaucoma among older African-American women in the study of osteoporotic fractures. *Am. J. Ophthalmol.* **2012**, *154*, 635–644. [CrossRef]
62. Borel, P.; Desmarchelier, C.; Nowicki, M.; Bott, R.; Morange, S.; Lesavre, N. Interindividual variability of lutein bioavailability in healthy men: Characterization, genetic variants involved, and relation with fasting plasma lutein concentration. *Am. J. Clin. Nutr.* **2014**, *100*, 168–175. [CrossRef]
63. Borel, P. Genetic variations involved in interindividual variability in carotenoid status. *Mol. Nutr. Food Res.* **2012**, *56*, 228–240. [CrossRef]
64. Failla, M.L.; Chitchumronchokchai, C.; Ferruzzi, M.G.; Goltz, S.R.; Campbell, W.W. Unsaturated fatty acids promote bioaccessibility and basolateral secretion of carotenoids and alpha-tocopherol by Caco-2 cells. *Food Funct.* **2014**, *5*, 1101–1112. [CrossRef]
65. Chung, H.Y.; Rasmussen, H.M.; Johnson, E.J. Lutein bioavailability is higher from lutein-enriched eggs than from supplements and spinach in men. *J. Nutr.* **2004**, *134*, 1887–1893. [CrossRef]
66. Clevidence, B.A.; Bieri, J.G. Association of carotenoids with human plasma lipoproteins. *Methods Enzymol.* **1993**, *214*, 33–46.
67. Connor, W.E.; Duell, P.B.; Kean, R.; Wang, Y. The prime role of HDL to transport lutein into the retina: Evidence from HDL-deficient WHAM chicks having a mutant ABCA1 transporter. *Investig. Ophthalmol. Vis. Sci.* **2007**, *48*, 4226–4231. [CrossRef] [PubMed]
68. Loane, E.; Nolan, J.M.; Beatty, S. The respective relationships between lipoprotein profile, macular pigment optical density, and serum concentrations of lutein and zeaxanthin. *Investig. Ophthalmol. Vis. Sci.* **2010**, *51*, 5897–5905. [CrossRef] [PubMed]
69. Cybulska-Heinrich, A.K.; Mozaffarieh, M.; Flammer, J. Ginkgo biloba: An adjuvant therapy for progressive normal and high tension glaucoma. *Mol. Vis.* **2012**, *18*, 390–402.
70. Hirooka, K.; Tokuda, M.; Miyamoto, O.; Itano, T.; Baba, T.; Shiraga, F. The Ginkgo biloba extract (EGb 761) provides a neuroprotective effect on retinal ganglion cells in a rat model of chronic glaucoma. *Curr. Eye Res.* **2004**, *28*, 153–157. [CrossRef]
71. Lee, J.; Sohn, S.W.; Kee, C. Effect of Ginkgo biloba extract on visual field progression in normal tension glaucoma. *J. Glaucoma* **2013**, *22*, 780–784. [CrossRef] [PubMed]
72. Ma, K.; Xu, L.; Zhang, H.; Zhang, S.; Pu, M.; Jonas, J.B. The effect of ginkgo biloba on the rat retinal ganglion cell survival in the optic nerve crush model. *Acta Ophthalmol.* **2010**, *88*, 553–557. [CrossRef] [PubMed]
73. Ritch, R. Potential role for Ginkgo biloba extract in the treatment of glaucoma. *Med. Hypotheses* **2000**, *54*, 221–235. [CrossRef] [PubMed]
74. Shim, S.H.; Kim, J.M.; Choi, C.Y.; Kim, C.Y.; Park, K.H. Ginkgo biloba extract and bilberry anthocyanins improve visual function in patients with normal tension glaucoma. *J. Med. Food* **2012**, *15*, 818–823. [CrossRef] [PubMed]

75. Li, S.Y.; Fu, Z.J.; Ma, H.; Jang, W.C.; So, K.F.; Wong, D.; Lo, A.C. Effect of lutein on retinal neurons and oxidative stress in a model of acute retinal ischemia/reperfusion. *Investig. Ophthalmol. Vis. Sci.* **2009**, *50*, 836–843. [CrossRef] [PubMed]
76. Li, S.Y.; Fung, F.K.; Fu, Z.J.; Wong, D.; Chan, H.H.; Lo, A.C. Anti-inflammatory effects of lutein in retinal ischemic/hypoxic injury: In vivo and in vitro studies. *Investig. Ophthalmol. Vis. Sci.* **2012**, *53*, 5976–5984. [CrossRef] [PubMed]
77. Li, S.Y.; Lo, A.C. Lutein protects RGC-5 cells against hypoxia and oxidative stress. *Int. J. Mol. Sci.* **2010**, *11*, 2109–2117. [CrossRef] [PubMed]
78. Ozawa, Y.; Sasaki, M.; Takahashi, N.; Kamoshita, M.; Miyake, S.; Tsubota, K. Neuroprotective effects of lutein in the retina. *Curr. Pharm. Des.* **2012**, *18*, 51–56. [CrossRef] [PubMed]
79. Zhang, C.; Wang, Z.; Zhao, J.; Li, Q.; Huang, C.; Zhu, L.; Lu, D. Neuroprotective Effect of Lutein on NMDA-Induced Retinal Ganglion Cell Injury in Rat Retina. *Cell. Mol. Neurobiol.* **2016**, *36*, 531–540. [CrossRef] [PubMed]
80. Bernstein, P.S.; Li, B.; Vachali, P.P.; Gorusupudi, A.; Shyam, R.; Henriksen, B.S.; Nolan, J.M. Lutein, zeaxanthin, and meso-zeaxanthin: The basic and clinical science underlying carotenoid-based nutritional interventions against ocular disease. *Prog. Retin. Eye Res.* **2016**, *50*, 34–66. [CrossRef]
81. Li, B.; Vachali, P.; Frederick, J.M.; Bernstein, P.S. Identification of StARD3 as a lutein-binding protein in the macula of the primate retina. *Biochemistry* **2011**, *50*, 2541–2549. [CrossRef]
82. Bhosale, P.; Larson, A.J.; Frederick, J.M.; Southwick, K.; Thulin, C.D.; Bernstein, P.S. Identification and characterization of a Pi isoform of glutathione S-transferase (GSTP1) as a zeaxanthin-binding protein in the macula of the human eye. *J. Biol. Chem.* **2004**, *279*, 49447–49454. [CrossRef]
83. Bone, R.A.; Landrum, J.T.; Dixon, Z.; Chen, Y.; Llerena, C.M. Lutein and zeaxanthin in the eyes, serum and diet of human subjects. *Exp. Eye Res.* **2000**, *71*, 239–245. [CrossRef]
84. Chen, S.F.; Chang, Y.; Wu, J.C. The spatial distribution of macular pigment in humans. *Curr. Eye Res.* **2001**, *23*, 422–434. [CrossRef] [PubMed]
85. SanGiovanni, J.P.; Neuringer, M. The putative role of lutein and zeaxanthin as protective agents against age-related macular degeneration: Promise of molecular genetics for guiding mechanistic and translational research in the field. *Am. J. Clin. Nutr.* **2012**, *96*, 1223s–1233s. [CrossRef] [PubMed]
86. Khachik, F.; Bernstein, P.S.; Garland, D.L. Identification of lutein and zeaxanthin oxidation products in human and monkey retinas. *Investig. Ophthalmol. Vis. Sci.* **1997**, *38*, 1802–1811.
87. Ahmed, S.S.; Lott, M.N.; Marcus, D.M. The macular xanthophylls. *Surv. Ophthalmol.* **2005**, *50*, 183–193. [CrossRef]
88. Sparrow, J.R.; Nakanishi, K.; Parish, C.A. The lipofuscin fluorophore A2E mediates blue light-induced damage to retinal pigmented epithelial cells. *Investig. Ophthalmol. Vis. Sci.* **2000**, *41*, 1981–1989.
89. Leung, I.Y.; Sandstrom, M.M.; Zucker, C.L.; Neuringer, M.; Snodderly, D.M. Nutritional manipulation of primate retinas, II: Effects of age, n-3 fatty acids, lutein, and zeaxanthin on retinal pigment epithelium. *Investig. Ophthalmol. Vis. Sci.* **2004**, *45*, 3244–3256. [CrossRef] [PubMed]
90. Ma, L.; Liu, R.; Du, J.H.; Liu, T.; Wu, S.S.; Liu, X.H. Lutein, Zeaxanthin and Meso-zeaxanthin Supplementation Associated with Macular Pigment Optical Density. *Nutrients* **2016**, *8*, 426. [CrossRef] [PubMed]
91. Hammond, B.R., Jr.; Johnson, E.J.; Russell, R.M.; Krinsky, N.I.; Yeum, K.J.; Edwards, R.B.; Snodderly, D.M. Dietary modification of human macular pigment density. *Investig. Ophthalmol. Vis. Sci.* **1997**, *38*, 1795–1801.
92. Kumari, N.; Cher, J.; Chua, E.; Hamzah, H.; Wong, T.Y.; Cheung, C.Y. Association of serum lutein and zeaxanthin with quantitative measures of retinal vascular parameters. *PLoS ONE* **2018**, *13*, e0203868. [CrossRef]
93. Choi, J.S.; Kim, D.; Hong, Y.M.; Mizuno, S.; Joo, C.K. Inhibition of nNOS and COX-2 expression by lutein in acute retinal ischemia. *Nutrition* **2006**, *22*, 668–671. [CrossRef]
94. Fung, F.K.; Law, B.Y.; Lo, A.C. Lutein Attenuates Both Apoptosis and Autophagy upon Cobalt (II) Chloride-Induced Hypoxia in Rat Muller Cells. *PLoS ONE* **2016**, *11*, e0167828. [CrossRef]
95. Woo, T.T.; Li, S.Y.; Lai, W.W.; Wong, D.; Lo, A.C. Neuroprotective effects of lutein in a rat model of retinal detachment. *Graefe's Arch. Clin. Exp. Ophthalmol.* **2013**, *251*, 41–51. [CrossRef]
96. Li, B.; Rognon, G.T.; Mattinson, T.; Vachali, P.P.; Gorusupudi, A.; Chang, F.Y.; Ranganathan, A.; Nelson, K.; George, E.W.; Frederick, J.M.; et al. Supplementation with macular carotenoids improves visual performance of transgenic mice. *Arch. Biochem. Biophys.* **2018**. [CrossRef]

97. Nakajima, Y.; Shimazawa, M.; Otsubo, K.; Ishibashi, T.; Hara, H. Zeaxanthin, a retinal carotenoid, protects retinal cells against oxidative stress. *Curr. Eye Res.* **2009**, *34*, 311–318. [CrossRef] [PubMed]
98. Moorhouse, A.J.; Li, S.; Vickery, R.M.; Hill, M.A.; Morley, J.W. A patch-clamp investigation of membrane currents in a novel mammalian retinal ganglion cell line. *Brain Res.* **2004**, *1003*, 205–208. [CrossRef]
99. Meyers, K.J.; Johnson, E.J.; Bernstein, P.S.; Iyengar, S.K.; Engelman, C.D.; Karki, C.K.; Liu, Z.; Igo, R.P., Jr.; Truitt, B.; Klein, M.L.; et al. Genetic determinants of macular pigments in women of the Carotenoids in Age-Related Eye Disease Study. *Investig. Ophthalmol. Vis. Sci.* **2013**, *54*, 2333–2345. [CrossRef] [PubMed]
100. Liew, S.H.; Gilbert, C.E.; Spector, T.D.; Mellerio, J.; Marshall, J.; van Kuijk, F.J.; Beatty, S.; Fitzke, F.; Hammond, C.J. Heritability of macular pigment: A twin study. *Investig. Ophthalmol. Vis. Sci.* **2005**, *46*, 4430–4436. [CrossRef]
101. Mares, J.A.; LaRowe, T.L.; Snodderly, D.M.; Moeller, S.M.; Gruber, M.J.; Klein, M.L.; Wooten, B.R.; Johnson, E.J.; Chappell, R.J.; Group, C.M.P.S.; et al. Predictors of optical density of lutein and zeaxanthin in retinas of older women in the Carotenoids in Age-Related Eye Disease Study, an ancillary study of the Women's Health Initiative. *Am. J. Clin. Nutr.* **2006**, *84*, 1107–1122.
102. Bovier, E.R.; Lewis, R.D.; Hammond, B.R., Jr. The relationship between lutein and zeaxanthin status and body fat. *Nutrients* **2013**, *5*, 750–757. [CrossRef] [PubMed]
103. Hammond, B.R., Jr.; Wooten, B.R.; Smollon, B. Assessment of the validity of in vivo methods of measuring human macular pigment optical density. *Optom. Vis. Sci. Off. Publ. Am. Acad. Optom.* **2005**, *82*, 387–404. [CrossRef]
104. Ji, Y.; Zuo, C.; Lin, M.; Zhang, X.; Li, M.; Mi, L.; Liu, B.; Wen, F. Macular Pigment Optical Density in Chinese Primary Open Angle Glaucoma Using the One-Wavelength Reflectometry Method. *J. Ophthalmol.* **2016**, *2016*, 2792103. [CrossRef] [PubMed]
105. Daga, F.B.; Ogata, N.G.; Medeiros, F.A.; Moran, R.; Morris, J.; Zangwill, L.M.; Weinreb, R.N.; Nolan, J.M. Macular Pigment and Visual Function in Patients With Glaucoma: The San Diego Macular Pigment Study. *Investig. Ophthalmol. Vis. Sci.* **2018**, *59*, 4471–4476. [CrossRef]
106. Snodderly, D.M.; Mares, J.A.; Wooten, B.R.; Oxton, L.; Gruber, M.; Ficek, T. Macular pigment measurement by heterochromatic flicker photometry in older subjects: The carotenoids and age-related eye disease study. *Investig. Ophthalmol. Vis. Sci.* **2004**, *45*, 531–538. [CrossRef]
107. Bone, R.A.; Landrum, J.T.; Fernandez, L.; Tarsis, S.L. Analysis of the macular pigment by HPLC: Retinal distribution and age study. *Investig. Ophthalmol. Vis. Sci.* **1988**, *29*, 843–849.
108. Rapp, L.M.; Maple, S.S.; Choi, J.H. Lutein and zeaxanthin concentrations in rod outer segment membranes from perifoveal and peripheral human retina. *Investig. Ophthalmol. Vis. Sci.* **2000**, *41*, 1200–1209.
109. Moise, M.M.; Benjamin, L.M.; Doris, T.M.; Dalida, K.N.; Augustin, N.O. Role of Mediterranean diet, tropical vegetables rich in antioxidants, and sunlight exposure in blindness, cataract and glaucoma among African type 2 diabetics. *Int. J. Ophthalmol.* **2012**, *5*, 231–237. [CrossRef]
110. Wenzel, A.J.; Gerweck, C.; Barbato, D.; Nicolosi, R.J.; Handelman, G.J.; Curran-Celentano, J. A 12-wk egg intervention increases serum zeaxanthin and macular pigment optical density in women. *J. Nutr.* **2006**, *136*, 2568–2573. [CrossRef] [PubMed]
111. Chew, E.Y.; Clemons, T.E.; Sangiovanni, J.P.; Danis, R.P.; Ferris, F.L., 3rd; Elman, M.J.; Antoszyk, A.N.; Ruby, A.J.; Orth, D.; Bressler, S.B.; et al. Secondary analyses of the effects of lutein/zeaxanthin on age-related macular degeneration progression: AREDS2 report No. 3. *JAMA Ophthalmol.* **2014**, *132*, 142–149. [CrossRef] [PubMed]
112. Chew, E.Y.; Clemons, T.E.; SanGiovanni, J.P.; Danis, R.; Ferris, F.L.; Elman, M.; Antoszyk, A.; Ruby, A.; Orth, D.; Bressler, S.; et al. Lutein + zeaxanthin and omega-3 fatty acids for age-related macular degeneration: The Age-Related Eye Disease Study 2 (AREDS2) randomized clinical trial. *JAMA* **2013**, *309*, 2005–2015. [CrossRef]

Permissions

All chapters in this book were first published by MDPI; hereby published with permission under the Creative Commons Attribution License or equivalent. Every chapter published in this book has been scrutinized by our experts. Their significance has been extensively debated. The topics covered herein carry significant findings which will fuel the growth of the discipline. They may even be implemented as practical applications or may be referred to as a beginning point for another development.

The contributors of this book come from diverse backgrounds, making this book a truly international effort. This book will bring forth new frontiers with its revolutionizing research information and detailed analysis of the nascent developments around the world.

We would like to thank all the contributing authors for lending their expertise to make the book truly unique. They have played a crucial role in the development of this book. Without their invaluable contributions this book wouldn't have been possible. They have made vital efforts to compile up to date information on the varied aspects of this subject to make this book a valuable addition to the collection of many professionals and students.

This book was conceptualized with the vision of imparting up-to-date information and advanced data in this field. To ensure the same, a matchless editorial board was set up. Every individual on the board went through rigorous rounds of assessment to prove their worth. After which they invested a large part of their time researching and compiling the most relevant data for our readers.

The editorial board has been involved in producing this book since its inception. They have spent rigorous hours researching and exploring the diverse topics which have resulted in the successful publishing of this book. They have passed on their knowledge of decades through this book. To expedite this challenging task, the publisher supported the team at every step. A small team of assistant editors was also appointed to further simplify the editing procedure and attain best results for the readers.

Apart from the editorial board, the designing team has also invested a significant amount of their time in understanding the subject and creating the most relevant covers. They scrutinized every image to scout for the most suitable representation of the subject and create an appropriate cover for the book.

The publishing team has been an ardent support to the editorial, designing and production team. Their endless efforts to recruit the best for this project, has resulted in the accomplishment of this book. They are a veteran in the field of academics and their pool of knowledge is as vast as their experience in printing. Their expertise and guidance has proved useful at every step. Their uncompromising quality standards have made this book an exceptional effort. Their encouragement from time to time has been an inspiration for everyone.

The publisher and the editorial board hope that this book will prove to be a valuable piece of knowledge for researchers, students, practitioners and scholars across the globe.

List of Contributors

Homer S. Black
Department of Dermatology, Baylor College of Medicine, Houston, TX 77030, USA

Fritz Boehm
Photobiology Research, Internationales Handelszentrum (IHZ), Friedrichstraße 95, 10117 Berlin, Germany

Ruth Edge
Dalton Cumbrian Facility, Westlakes Science Park, The University of Manchester, Cumbria CA24 3HA, UK

T. George Truscott
School of Chemical and Physical Sciences, Keele University, Keele, Staffordshire ST5 5BG, UK

Shabnam Jalili-Moghaddam
Faculty of Health and Environmental Studies, Auckland University of Technology, Auckland 1142, New Zealand

Elaine Rush, Isaac Amoah and Tung Diep
Riddet Centre of Research Excellence, Palmerston North 0632, New Zealand

Catherine C. Applegate and Joe L. Rowles III
Division of Nutritional Sciences, University of Illinois at Urbana-Champaign, Urbana, IL 61801, USA

John W. Erdman Jr.
Division of Nutritional Sciences, University of Illinois at Urbana-Champaign, Urbana, IL 61801, USA
Department of Food Science and Human Nutrition, University of Illinois at Urbana-Champaign, Urbana, IL 61801, USA

Huilin Liu and Xueqi Fu
School of Life Sciences, Jilin University, Changchun 130012, China

Jingsheng Liu and Meihong Liu
College of Food Science and Engineering, Jilin Agricultural University, Changchun 130118, China
National Engineering Laboratory for Wheat and Corn Deep Processing, Changchun 130118, China

Ziqi Zhang, Lingyu Zhu and Xin Zheng
College of Animal Science and Technology, Jilin Agricultural University, Changchun 130118, China

Thomas Lawler
Department of Nutritional Sciences, University of Wisconsin, 1415 Linden Drive, Madison, WI 53706, USA

Ana A. O. Xavier, Juan Garrido-Fernández and Antonio Pérez-Gálvez
Department of Food Phytochemistry, Instituto de la Grasa (CSIC), Campus Universitario, Building 46, 41013 Sevilla, Spain

Elena Díaz-Salido, Isabel Arenilla-Vélez and Josefa Aguayo-Maldonado
Unidad de Neonatología, Hospital Virgen del Rocío, 41013 Sevilla, Spain

Javier Fontecha
Institute of Food Science Research (CSIC-UAM), 28049 Madrid, Spain

Alicia Sánchez-García
Laboratorio de Espectrometría de Masas, Instituto de la Grasa (CSIC), 41013 Sevilla, Spain

Ji Hyun Kim, Jeonghee Lee and Jeongseon Kim
Graduate School of Cancer Science and Policy, National Cancer Center, 323 Ilsan-ro, Ilsandong-gu, Goyang-si, Gyeonggi-do 10408, Korea

Ju Choi and Young-Il Kim
Center for Gastric Cancer, National Cancer Center Hospital, National Cancer Center, 323 Ilsan-ro, Ilsandong-gu, Goyang-si, Gyeonggi-do 10408, Korea

Oran Kwon and Hyesook Kim
Department of Nutritional Science and Food Management, Ewha Womans University, 52, Ewhayeodae-gil, Seodaemun-gu, Seoul 03760, Korea

Corinne N. Cannavale
Neuroscience Program, University of Illinois at Urbana-Champaign, Champaign, IL 61801, USA

Kelsey M. Hassevoort
Beckman Institute for Advanced Science and Technology, University of Illinois at Urbana-Champaign, Champaign, IL 61801, USA
Center for Brain Plasticity, University of Illinois at Urbana-Champaign, Champaign, IL 61801, USA

Caitlyn G. Edwards and Sharon V. Thompson
Division of Nutritional Sciences, University of Illinois at Urbana-Champaign, Champaign, IL 61801, USA

Nicholas A. Burd
Division of Nutritional Sciences, University of Illinois at Urbana-Champaign, Champaign, IL 61801, USA
Department of Kinesiology and Community Health, University of Illinois at Urbana-Champaign, Champaign, IL 61801, USA

Naiman A. Khan
Neuroscience Program, University of Illinois at Urbana-Champaign, Champaign, IL 61801, USA
Division of Nutritional Sciences, University of Illinois at Urbana-Champaign, Champaign, IL 61801, USA
Department of Kinesiology and Community Health, University of Illinois at Urbana-Champaign, Champaign, IL 61801, USA

Hannah D. Holscher
Division of Nutritional Sciences, University of Illinois at Urbana-Champaign, Champaign, IL 61801, USA
Department of Kinesiology and Community Health, University of Illinois at Urbana-Champaign, Champaign, IL 61801, USA
Department of Food Science and Human Nutrition, University of Illinois at Urbana-Champaign, Champaign, IL 61801, USA

Neal J. Cohen
Neuroscience Program, University of Illinois at Urbana-Champaign, Champaign, IL 61801, USA
Beckman Institute for Advanced Science and Technology, University of Illinois at Urbana-Champaign, Champaign, IL 61801, USA
Center for Brain Plasticity, University of Illinois at Urbana-Champaign, Champaign, IL 61801, USA
Department of Psychology, University of Illinois at Urbana-Champaign, Champaign, IL 61801, USA

Paula Mapelli-Brahm
Food Colour & Quality Laboratory, Area of Nutrition & Food Science, Universidad de Sevilla, 41012 Seville, Spain

Emmanuelle Reboul
Aix-Marseille University, INRA, INSERM, C2VN, 13005 Marseille, France

Talia Wolak and Esther Paran
Hypertension Unit, Soroka University Medical center and Ben-Gurion University of the Negev, Beer Sheva 84101, Israel

Yoav Sharoni, Joseph Levy and David Stepensky
Department of Clinical Biochemistry and Pharmacology, Ben-Gurion University of the Negev, Beer Sheva 84105, Israel

Karin Linnewiel-Hermoni
Lycored Ltd., Secaucus, NJ 07094, USA

Krystle E. Zuniga
Nutrition and Foods, Family and Consumer Sciences, Texas State University, 601 University Drive, San Marcos, TX 78666, USA

Nancy E. Moran
United States Department of Agriculture/Agricultural Research Service Children's Nutrition Research Center, Department of Pediatrics, Baylor College of Medicine, Houston, TX 77030, USA

Jenny Ruales
Department of Food Science and Biotechnology, Escuela Politécnica National, Quito 17-01-2759, Ecuador

Nieves Baenas and Diego A. Moreno
Phytochemistry and Healthy Foods Lab., Department of Food Science and Technology, CEBAS-CSIC, Campus de Espinardo-Edificio 25, E-30100 Murcia, Spain

Carla M. Stinco and Antonio J. Meléndez-Martínez
Food Colour & Quality Lab., Department of Nutrition & Food Science, Universidad de Sevilla, Facultad de Farmacia, 41012 Sevilla, Spain

Almudena García-Ruiz
Department of Food Science and Biotechnology, Escuela Politécnica National, Quito 17-01-2759, Ecuador
Laboratory of Epigenetics of Lipid Metabolism, Madrid Institute for Advanced Studies (IMDEA)-Food, CEI UAM + CSIC, 28049 Madrid, Spain

Yao Liu
Department of Ophthalmology and Visual Sciences, University of Wisconsin, 2870 University Avenue, Madison, WI 53705, USA

Krista Christensen and Julie Mares
Department of Ophthalmology and Visual Sciences, University of Wisconsin, 610 N. Walnut Street, 1069WARF Building, Madison, WI 53726, USA

Thasarat S. Vajaranant
Department of Ophthalmology and Visual Sciences, University of Illinois - Chicago, 1855W. Taylor Street, Chicago, IL 60612, USA

Index

www.ingramcontent.com/pod-product-compliance
Lightning Source LLC
LaVergne TN
LVHW061511220926
848485LV00017B/800

* 9 7 8 1 6 4 6 4 7 5 3 5 3 *